NUTRITION AND BONE DEVELOPMENT

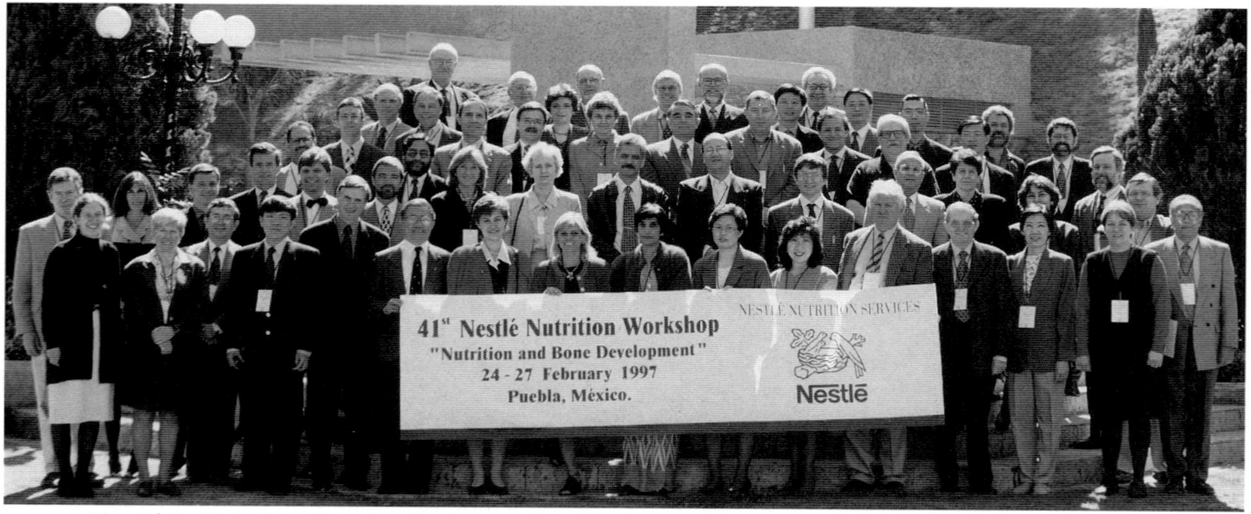

The 41st Nestlé Nutrition Workshop, Nutrition and Bone Development, *was held in Puebla, México, 24–27 February 1997.*

Workshop participants *(left to right, from front to back):* A. Prentice, M.C. Secretin, E. Vasquez Garibay, P. Mahachoklertwattana, J-Ph. Bonjour, R.C. Tsang, J. De Bruyne, M.B. Oliveri, V. Kumari Ponhampalan, R. Namgung, L. Hsieh, M. Moya, M. Casanova Bellido, S. Charoenkiatkul, B.L. Specker, P. Arroyo Acevedo, J. Caverzasio, C. Brown, F. Haschke, J.M. Pettifor, H. Jüppner, Ph. Steenhout, L.K. Bachrach, I. Rumba, R. Calva Rodríguez, M. Menchaca Marín, J. Farrugia, E. Domenech, S. Heller Rouassant, M. Garabédian, V. Gilsanz, M.Z. Mughal, Ph. Alliet, F. Pohlandt, A.A. Pollak, A. Mithal, R. Rizzoli, R.J. Schanler, C.E. Teodorescu, E. Tomberg, P. Guesry, J. Rigo, M. De Curtis, A. Marini, L. Chyi-Her Lin, J. Eisman, S.S. Potter, W. Klish, S. Frenk, W. Kachel, O. Schofer, R. Sandrini, X. Shen, E.P. Ciofu, P. Jianping, Y.H. Chen, E. Seeman.

Nestlé Nutrition Workshop Series
Volume 41

NUTRITION AND BONE DEVELOPMENT

Editors

Jean-Philippe Bonjour
WHO Collaborating Center
for Osteoporosis and Bone Diseases
Department of Internal Medicine
Division of Bone Diseases
University Hospital
1211 Geneva 14
Switzerland

Reginald C. Tsang
Pediatric Bone Research Center
University of Cincinnati
Cincinnati, Ohio, USA

NESTLÉ NUTRITION SERVICES

Nestlé

LIPPINCOTT-RAVEN ■ PHILADELPHIA

Acquisitions Editor: Beth Barry
Developmental Editor: Glenda Insua
Manufacturing Manager: Kevin Watt
Production Manager: Robert Pancotti
Production Editor: Brandy Mui
Indexer: Robert Elwood
Compositor: Maryland Composition Company
Printer: Quebecor Printing, Kingsport

Nestec, Ltd., 55 Avenue Nestlé,
CH-1800 Vevey, Switzerland
Lippincott–Raven Publishers,
227 East Washington Square,
Philadelphia, Pennsylvania 19106

Printed in the United States of America

9 8 7 6 5 4 3 2 1

Library of Congress Cataloging-in-Publication Data

Nutrition and bone development / editors, Jean-Philippe Bonjour,
Reginald C. Tsang.
p. cm.—(Nestlé Nutrition workshop series ; v. 41)
"Based on presentations given during the 41NNW in Puebla, Mexico,
February 1997"—Foreword.
Includes bibliographical references and index.
ISBN 0-7817-1753-1
1. Bones—Growth—Congresses. 2. Children—Nutrition—Congresses.
3. Bones—Metabolism—Congresses. I. Bonjour, Jean-Philippe.
II. Tsang, Reginald C. III. Nestlé Nutrition Services, IV. Nestlé
Nutrition Workshop (41st : 1997 : Puebla, Mexico) V. Series.
[DNLM: 1. Bone and Bones—metabolism congresses. 2. Bone
Development congresses. 3. Diet congresses. W1 NE228 v.41 1999 /
WE 200 N9761 1999]
QP88.2.N873 1999
612.7'5—dc21
DNLM/DLC
for Library of Congress 98-22556
CIP

The material contained in this volume was submitted as previously unpublished material, except in the instances in which credit has been given to the source from which some of the illustrative material was derived.

Great care has been taken to maintain the accuracy of the information contained in the volume. However, neither Nestec nor Lippincott–Raven Publishers can be held responsible for errors or for any consequences arising from the use of the information contained herein.

Preface

This workshop brought together scientists studying various fundamental and clinical aspects of skeletal development, and exploring the impact of nutritional factors on bone mass growth, from fetal life through postadolescence. By negatively influencing peak bone mass, inadequate skeletal development largely contributes to the risk of osteoporosis, a disease affecting a large proportion of the elderly population. Therefore, advances in understanding how environmental factors can influence the genetic program of bone development will greatly help to devise adequate strategies for achieving optimal peak bone mass and thus prevent osteoporosis.

The meeting began with a fascinating report on the developmental genetic program that controls skeletogenesis. It was followed by new information on the complex autocrine-paracrine system that governs bone elongation at the level of the growth cartilage. An updated review examined the handling and role of inorganic phosphate in osteogenic cells and skeletal matrix mineralization. The supply of the main bone mineral constituents during fetal development is insured by specific placental transport systems. The state of our current knowledge on the mechanisms and regulation of calcium translocation across the placenta was reviewed. Several important issues concerning nutritional and other environmental factors that affect skeletal mass at birth, as well as bone growth in premature and full-term infants, were discussed in detail.

Then, presentations focused on calcium and phosphate requirements for optimizing postnatal accrual of bone mineralized tissue that can now be safely and precisely assessed by non-invasive techniques even applicable to small preterm infants. In this respect, a critical review on the currently available quantitative imaging techniques for the assessment of bone mass development was a topic of great interest. The relation between maternal calcium intake, lactational performance, and bone development was an important subject of discussion, since it raised a number of questions regarding the calcium requirements of infants and women of reproductive age.

The association between changes in the noncoding regions of certain gene products that are implicated in calcium-phosphate economy and bone metabolism was also an issue critically presented and discussed. Several presentations followed on the role of vitamin D, calcium, proteins, and fluoride on bone mass acquisitions during childhood and adolescence. The molecular mechanisms whereby nutrients such as calcium, some amino acids, and fluoride can affect bone formation, resorption, and the process of matrix mineralization was also discussed. Thus, experimental and clinical evidence for the probable involvement of insulin-like growth factor I (IGF-1) in the stimulatory osteogenic effect of proteins was reviewed. The important question of whether delayed puberty in absence of any pathological condition affects bone mass acquisition was also critically documented in relation to the differential rapidity of bone mass accrual in various parts of the skeleton.

Finally, a report focused on the impact of malnutrition and conditions such as anorexia nervosa, exercise-associated amenorrhea, cystic fibrosis, and various endocrinopathies on bone mass acquisition during childhood and adolescence. It emphasized the importance of recognizing those conditions leading to osteopenia and the need to better define the appropriate therapy to normalize the skeletal growth of these pathological conditions.

All presentations were followed by lively discussions which complemented or modulated the viewpoints of the referents. This volume, which faithfully reports most of the issues that were presented and discussed at this workshop, would be a helpful source of information for pediatricians, nutritionists, endocrinologists, and scientists interested in bone development and metabolism in health and disease. Furthermore, it is hoped that the new insights presented in this book will stimulate more basic and clinical research, particularly on the molecular mechanism whereby nutrients may act, and influence the genetic program of bone development. With my co-chairman, Dr. Reginald Tsang, we are thankful to all authors and speakers for their most valuable participation at this workshop and their readiness to contribute to the production of this book.

JEAN-PHILIPPE BONJOUR, M.D.
Geneva, Switzerland

Foreword

In humans, normal growth and bone development can occur in the face of substantial differences in dietary calcium supply. It is a challenge for the future to evaluate the limits of human adaptive response to different calcium intakes. In order to do this, we need to understand cellular and hormonal regulation of bone development and metabolism.

Peak bone mass is the major determinant of bone mass in women after menopause. Factors which contribute to the development of peak bone mass by early adulthood have become more evident in recent years: 70–80% of peak bone mass is genetically determined. Calcium supplements with fortified foods can increase the bone mass of adolescent girls, but the long-term effect of this preventive measure is not yet known. Other dietary and lifestyle factors may also influence bone mass: protein intake, body mass, and the level of physical exercise—during adolescence and early adulthood—can have an effect on bone mineralization 60 years later.

This volume summarizes our current knowledge of bone mass development, based on the presentations given during the 41st Nestlé Nutrition Workshop in Puebla, Mexico, February 1997. In addition, a critical evaluation on methodology to determine bone mass is presented. We express our sincere thanks and appreciation to Prof. J-Ph. Bonjour and Prof. R.C. Tsang, whose valued contribution and efforts have made this workshop possible.

PROFESSOR F. HASCHKE, M.D.
Vice President
Nestec Ltd., Vevey, Switzerland

Contents

Contributing Authors

Speakers

Laura K. Bachrach
Department of Pediatrics
Stanford University School of Medicine
Stanford University Medical Center
Pasteur Drive
Stanford, California 94305-5208
USA

Jean-Philippe Bonjour
WHO Collaborating Center for Osteoporosis and Bone Diseases
Department of Internal Medicine
Division of Bone Diseases
University Hospital
Rue Micheli-du-Crest
1211 Geneva 14
Switzerland

Joseph Caverzasio
WHO Collaborating Center for Osteoporosis and Bone Diseases
Department of Internal Medicine
Division of Bone Diseases
University Hospital
Rue Micheli-du-Crest
1211 Geneva 14
Switzerland

John Eisman
Bone and Mineral Research Program
Garvan Institute of Medical Research
384 Victoria Street
Sydney, NSW 2010
Australia

Michèle Garabédian
CNRS UPR 1524
Hôpital Saint Vincent de Paul
82, Avenue Denfert-Rochereau
Paris 75014
France

Vicente Gilsanz
Professor of Radiology
Department of Radiology
University of Southern California
School of Medicine
Los Angeles, California 90033
USA

Harald Jüppner
Endocrine Unit
Departments of Pediatrics and Medicine
Massachusetts General Hospital and Harvard Medical School
50 Blossom Street
Boston, Massachusetts 02114
USA

Ketan C. Mehta
Department of Pediatrics
Division of Neonatology
Children's Hospital Medical Center
University of Cincinnati Medical Center
231 Bethesda Avenue
P.O. Box 670541
Cincinnati, Ohio 45267-0541
USA

Ambrish Mithal
Department of Medical Endocrinology
Sanjay Gandhi Post Graduate Institute of Medical Sciences
Rae Bareli Road
Lucknow, 226014
India

M. Zulf Mughal
Department of Paediatrics
St. Mary's Hospital for Women and Children
Hathersage Road
Manchester M13-OJH
United Kingdom

Ran Namgung
Department of Pediatrics
Yonsei University College of Medicine
134 Shinchon-Dong
Sudaemoon-Ku
Seoul 120-752
Korea

John M. Pettifor
Department of Paediatrics
University of Witwatersrand
7 York Road
Parktown, Johannesburg, 2193
South Africa

S. Steven Potter
Department of Pediatrics
The Children's Hospital Research Foundation
Room 3003
3333 Burnet Avenue
Cincinnati, Ohio 45229-3039
USA

Ann Prentice
MRC Dunn Nutrition Unit
University of Cambridge and Medical Research Council
Downhams Lane
Milton Road
Cambridge CB4 1XJ
United Kingdom

Jacques Rigo
Department of Pediatrics
University of Liège, CHR Citadelle
Boulevard du 12e de Ligne 1
4000 Liège
Belgium

René Rizzoli
WHO Collaborating Center for Osteoporosis and Bone Diseases
Department of Internal Medicine
Division of Bone Diseases
University Hospital
Rue Micheli-du-Crest
1211 Geneva 14
Switzerland

Richard J. Schanler
Department of Pediatrics
Baylor College of Medicine
1100 Bates Street
Houston, Texas 77030-3498
USA

Ego Seeman
Department of Endocrinology
Austin Hospital
Heidelberg, Melbourne
Victoria 3084
Australia

Bonny L. Specker
Ethel Austin Martin Program in Human Nutrition
Box 2275A
South Dakota State University
NFA Building
Rotunda Drive
Brookings, South Dakota 57007
USA

Session Chairmen
Jean-Philippe Bonjour, *Switzerland*
Reginald C. Tsang, *USA*

Invited Attendees
Pedro Arroyo Acevedo, *Mexico*
Steve Allen, *USA*
Philippe Alliet, *Belgium*
Yuri Antipkin, *Ukraine*
Alberto García Aranda, *Mexico*
Manuel Casanova Bellido, *Spain*
Jessie de Bruyne, *Malaysia*
Somsri Charoenkiatkul, *Thailand*
Yuan-Had Chen, *Taiwan*
Eugeniu Pascal Ciofu, *Rumania*
Mario de Curtis, *Italy*
Eduardo Domenech, *Spain*
Jimmy Farrugia, *Malta*
Silvestre Frenk, *Mexico*
Edgar Vasquez Garibay, *Mexico*
Pan Jainping, *China*
Walter Kachel, *Germany*
William Klish, *USA*
Chyi-Her Lin, *Taiwan*
Elena Lukyanova, *Ukraine*
Pat Mahachoklertwattana, *Thailand*
Mario Menchaca Marín, *Mexico*
Antonio Marini, *Italy*
Christian Moelgaard, *Denmark*
Manuel Moya, *Spain*
Maria Bealtriz Oliveri, *Argentina*
Frank Pohlandt, *Germany*
Arnold Pollak, *Austria*
Vasantha Kumari Ponhampalan, *Malaysia*
Robert Calva Rodríguez, *Mexico*
Solange Heller Rouassant, *Mexico*
Ingrida Rumba, *Latvia*
Romolo Sandrini, *Brazil*
Otto Schofer, *Germany*
Xiaoming Shen, *China*
Carmen Ecaterina Teodorescu, *Rumania*
Ene Tomberg, *Estonia*

Nestlé Representatives
Pierre Guesry/Lausanne, *Switzerland*
Cindy Brown/Vevey, *Switzerland*
Ferdinand Haschke/Vevey, *Switzerland*
Linda Hsieh/Glendale, *USA*
Nicholas Melachouris/New Milford, *USA*
Marie Christine Secretin/Vevey, *Switzerland*
Philippe Steenhout/Vevey, *Switzerland*
Ernie Strapazon/Glendale, *USA*

Nestlé Nutrition Workshop Series

Volume 41: Nutrition and Bone Development
Jean-Philippe Bonjour and Reginald C. Tsang, Editors; 304 pp., 1999.

Volume 40: Clinical Trials in Infant Nutrition
Jay A. Perman and Jean Rey, Editors; 304 pp., 1998.

Volume 39: Placental Function and Fetal Nutrition
Frederick C. Battaglia, Editor; 288 pp., 1997.

Volume 38: Diarrheal Disease
Michael Gracey and John A. Walker-Smith, Editors; 368 pp., 1997.

Volume 37: Feeding from Toddlers to Adolescence
Angel Ballabriga, Editor; 320 pp., 1996.

Volume 36: Long-Term Consequences of Early Feeding
John Boulton, Zvi Laron, and Jean Rey, Editors; 256 pp., 1996.

Volume 35: Diabetes
Richard M. Cowett, Editor; 320 pp., 1995.

Volume 34: Intestinal Immunology and Food Allergy
Alain L. de Weck and Hugh A. Sampson, Editors; 320 pp., 1995.

Volume 33: Protein Metabolism During Infancy
Niels C.R. Räihä, Editor; 264 pp., 1994.

Volume 32: Nutrition of the Low Birthweight Infant
Bernard L. Salle and Paul R. Swyer, Editors; 240 pp., 1993.

Volume 31: Birth Risks
J. David Baum, Editor; 256 pp., 1993.

Volume 30: Nutritional Anemias
Samuel J. Fomon and Stanley Zlotkin, Editors; 232 pp., 1992.

Volume 29: Nutrition of the Elderly
Hamish N. Munro and Günter Schlierf, Editors; 248 pp., 1992.

Volume 28: Polyunsaturated Fatty Acids in Human Nutrition
Umberto Bracco and Richard J. Deckelbaum, Editors; 256 pp., 1992.

Volume 27: For a Better Nutrition in the 21st Century
Peter Leathwood, Marc Horisberger, and W. Philip T. James, Editors; 272 pp., 1993.

Volume 26: Perinatology
Erich Saling, Editor; 208 pp., 1992.

Volume 25: Sugars in Nutrition
Michael Gracey, Norman Kretchmer, and Ettore Rossi, Editors; 304 pp., 1991.

Volume 24: Inborn Errors of Metabolism
Jürgen Schaub, François Van Hoof, and Henri L. Vis, Editors; 320 pp., 1991.

Volume 23: Trace Elements in Nutrition of Children—II
Ranjit Kumar Chandra, Editor; 248 pp., 1991.

Volume 22: History of Pediatrics 1850–1950
Buford L. Nichols, Jr., Angel Ballabriga, and Norman Kretchmer, Editors; 320 pp., 1991.

Volume 21: Rickets
Francis H. Glorieux, Editor; 304 pp., 1991.

NUTRITION AND BONE DEVELOPMENT

Nutrition and Bone Development, edited by
Jean-Philippe Bonjour and Reginald C. Tsang,
Nestlé Nutrition Workshop Series, Vol. 41, Nestec Ltd.,
Vevey/Lippincott–Raven Publishers,
Philadelphia © 1999.

Hox Genes Involved in Fetal Bone Development

S. Steven Potter

Division of Developmental Biology, Children's Hospital Research Foundation and Department of Pediatrics, University of Cincinnati College of Medicine, Cincinnati, Ohio 45267, USA

The skeletal system is a remarkably exact and intricate structure. During development bones must be generated in correct numbers in correct positions. Furthermore, each bone has a precise three-dimensional contour shape that must be properly recapitulated from one generation to the next. In several respects it appears that the developmental genetic program that controls skeletogenesis must be extraordinary. It seems likely that the study of this process would provide insight into the basic mechanisms of the genetic control of development as well as an understanding of how flaws in the program can yield congenital malformations.

The homeobox genes are known to be master switch genetic regulators of development in simpler organisms. Mutations in these genes were found by classical geneticists to result in striking alterations in patterning during development. A mutation in the *Antennapedia* gene, for example, could cause the cells of the antennal imaginal disks of *Drosophila* to form legs instead of antennae protruding from the head (1). And mutation of the *Bithorax* gene resulted in the formation of a second thoracic segment equipped with a second pair of wings. Such alterations of one body segment into another were termed homeotic transformations. It seemed a profound observation that mutation of a single gene could render such a dramatic effect on phenotype. Presumably hundreds or even thousands of genes would be required to program the formation of an appendage or body segment, yet mutation of but a single gene, a minute fraction of the total involved, could have profound effects on the outcome. This suggested that not all genes are equal in the process of development.

The molecular cloning of the first *Drosophila* homeotic genes quickly revealed a possible mechanism of their function in development. When the first three of these genes were sequenced, it was observed that their coding sequences carried a common block of homology (2,3). This stretch of highly conserved sequence was about 180 bp in size and was named the *homeobox*. This homeobox in turn encoded the homeodomain at the protein level. Of great interest, the amino acid sequence of the homeodomain suggested that it carried a helix–turn–helix motif. This motif had previously been observed in bacterial proteins involved in the regulation of transcription, suggesting that the homeotic genes encoded transcription factors. Such proteins regulate the expression levels of batteries of downstream genes, some of which may encode additional transcription factors. These genes can therefore initiate genetic cascades that can result in the altered expression of hundreds or even thousands of other genes. It appeared that the homeotic genes functioned as master switch regulators by serving in the upper levels of the genetic hierarchy of development, controlling entry into different developmental genetic programs and thereby regulating the developmental destinies of groups of cells.

To better define the roles of homeobox genes in mammalian development, it was first necessary to clone them and analyze their genomic organization, DNA sequences, and developmental expression patterns. Much of this work was accomplished in the late 1980s and early 1990s, although it still carries on as novel homeobox genes continue to be cloned and these and previously cloned genes continue to be analyzed. A screen of a mouse genomic DNA library using a degenerate oligonucleotide with a mixture of all nucleotide sequences capable of encoding the most conserved region of the homeodomain yielded ten previously undescribed homeobox genes (4).

The early studies of the mammalian homeobox genes produced several interesting findings. First, the sequences of the encoded homeodomains are evolutionarily extremely well conserved (2). The mouse cognates of the *Drosophila Antennapedia* gene, for example, encode homeodomains that are approximately 95% identical to the *Drosophila* one. Outside of the 60 amino acid homeodomains, however, the proteins showed very little similarity. This suggests that the DNA-binding component of the protein, which defines target gene specificity, has very tight sequence restraints, whereas the other domains of the protein, such as transcription activator and repressor domains, allow a greater variety of amino acid sequences. This is consistent with observations in simpler organisms, suggesting that, for example, apparently any collection of acidic amino acids can function as a transcription activator (5).

The genomic organization of the *Hox* genes is also remarkably well conserved (6). In *Drosophila* nine homeobox genes are localized to the two *Antennapedia* and *Bithorax* clusters. There is evidence from comparisons with other organisms that these two *Drosophila* clusters result from the splitting of a single primordial cluster. In mammals, in contrast, this single primordial cluster has been quadruplicated to give four distinct clusters of homeobox genes (Fig. 1). Sequence comparisons reveal that gene order within the clusters has been conserved between *Drosophila* and mammals. In mammals the clustered homeobox genes are termed *Hox* genes, and the individual genes are named in matrix fashion, with a letter (A to D) representing the cluster and a number (1 to 13) designating the gene position within the cluster. Because of their evolutionary history, genes at equivalent positions within the *Hox* clusters are most closely related. Such genes, designated paralogs, are derived from a single gene on the primordial cluster and are more similar to each other than to other genes on the same cluster. As shown in Fig. 1, the 13 paralogous groups of

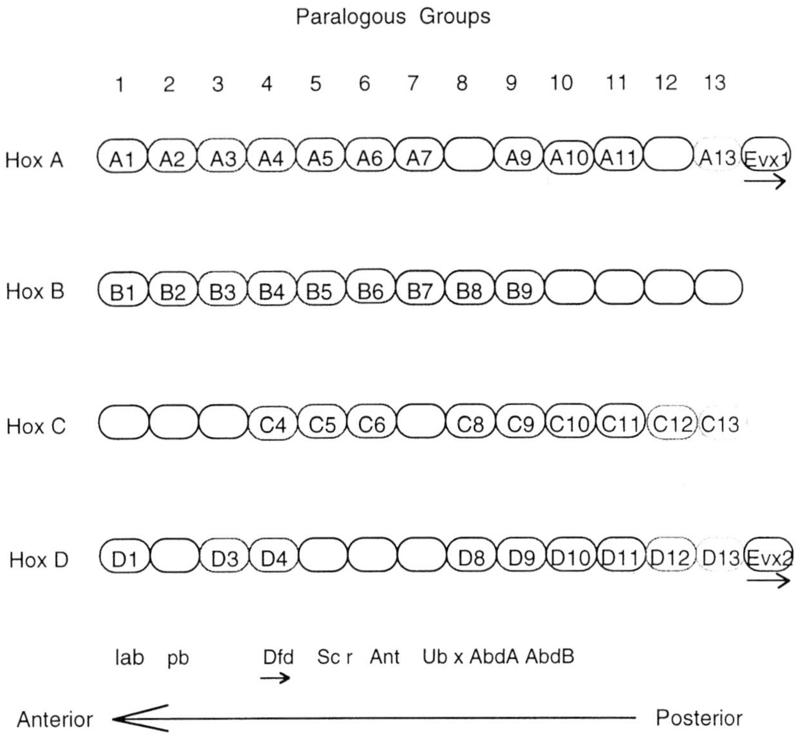

FIG. 1. The *Hox* gene clusters. The four clusters are labeled A–D, with the 13 paralogous groups of most closely related genes vertically aligned and labeled 1–13. *Evx1* and *-2* represent distinct categories of homeobox genes associated with the clustered *Hox* genes. The *arrow* at the bottom represents the direction of transcription for all genes except for the three genes with *opposite arrows*. The genes of the *Drosophila Hom-C* are listed in order just above the bottom *arrow*. For both *Drosophila* and mammals, genes at the left ends of the clusters are expressed earlier in development and in more anterior positions.

Hox genes of the four clusters can be vertically aligned. Because of unequal crossing over during evolution, not every cluster has a member of every group, and conversely, some regions, such as the *Abdominal-b (Abd-b)* genes, have been amplified in number. The preservation of the clustered arrangement during evolution is thought to reflect a required sharing of *cis*-regulatory elements by the genes of a cluster that are necessary to achieve correct developmental expression patterns.

In addition to this evolutionary conservation of gene order, there is also a remarkable conservation of collinearity (1). It has been found that the genes located at more 3′ positions within the clusters are expressed earlier in development and at more anterior positions than genes located more 5′. It has also been noted that the 3′ genes are more readily induced by retinoic acid. Furthermore, all *Hox* genes within a cluster are oriented in the same 5′-to-3′ direction.

ECTOPIC EXPRESSION STUDIES

To begin to define developmental function in the patterning of the skeletal and other systems, it was necessary to perform mutational studies in developing systems. Debra Wolgemuth and colleagues performed the first such studies, generating transgenic mice that carried additional copies of the *Deformed*-type *Hoxa 4* gene (7). The resulting overexpression of this gene resulted in a megacolon phenotype, in which the animals suffered a terminal constipation. The analysis of *Hox* function in patterning was then carried to the next level, first by Peter Gruss and colleagues, when they made transgenic mice that carried the chicken β-actin promoter, driving widespread ectopic expression of the *Hoxa 7* gene (8,9). Several interesting observations were made. Although the β-actin promoter was active almost ubiquitously, the resulting developmental defects were restricted, suggesting that most regions of the developing embryo were buffered from the effects of ectopic expression. The craniocervical transition region appeared particularly sensitive to ectopic *Hoxa 7* expression. The atlas and axis bones experienced segment identity transformations that were interpreted to support the *Hox* code hypothesis originally proposed by Lewis to explain homeotic mutants in *Drosophila* (10). This model states that segment identity is determined by the combination of *Hox* genes expressed. That is, a combinatorial code of *Hox* gene expression defines the developmental destinies of segments. According to this model, the ectopic expression of *Hox* genes would be predicted to change expressed *Hox* codes and hence segment identities, as observed.

Similar ectopic expression assays were conducted for the *Hoxb 5, Hoxb 6,* and *Hoxb 7* genes by Potter and colleagues (11,12). These studies also used the β-actin promoter to drive misexpression. This promoter offered the efficient screening of multiple tissues for developmental perturbation. This appeared an important advantage because previous experiments in both *Drosophila* and mouse suggested that only a small subset of regions experiencing ectopic expression would consequently develop abnormally (8,13). Ectopic expression of *Antennapedia* with the heat shock promoter in *Drosophila,* for example, which drives ubiquitous expression, resulted only in abnormal development of antennae. The *Hox* codes in other developing domains were apparently not sufficiently altered to disrupt normal developmental outcome. The use of the same β-actin promoter previously used in mice also offered another advantage. By comparing the developmental perturbations resulting from the substitution of different *Hox* genes, all driven by the same promoter, one gains insight into the functional similarities of the different *Hox* coding sequences. If, for example, the different *Hox* genes all resulted in identical malformations when ectopically expressed with this single β-actin promoter, then this would suggest that the coding sequences were functionally equivalent and that the different developmental functions of *Hox* genes simply result from their normally different expression patterns. This ectopic expression functional assay provided some interesting results.

Ectopic expression of *Hoxa 7, Hoxb 6,* and *Hoxb 7* (Fig. 2) each resulted in alterations of segment identity determination along the anterior–posterior axis. Ectopic expression of *Hoxb 7,* for example, resulted in the posteriorization of the

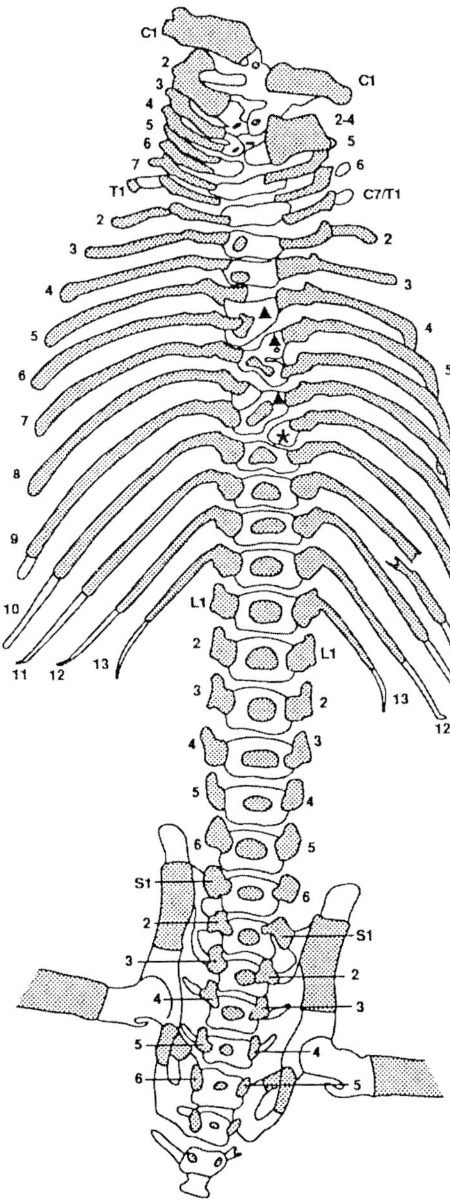

FIG. 2. Ectopic expression of the *Hoxb 7* gene during development results in anterior–posterior shifts in segment identity. In this chimeric mouse, left–right comparisons reveal homeotic transformations of segment identity. Note, for example, that the L1 segment on the left carries a rib and the identity of a T13 segment on the right. From Kaur *et al.* (11).

seventh cervical vertebra, with an additional pair of ribs now articulating with this vertebral segment. Also, in each case there were multiple ossification defects in the craniocervical transition region. For each gene there were deficient or absent supraoccipital bones, and the basioccipital and exoccipital bones were similarly malformed. Also, similar ossification defects were seen in the atlas for each of these three ectopic expression assay studies. This strong overlap in phenotypes observed suggests that these three genes have overlapping functions. One interpretation is that these transcription factor genes share overlapping sets of gene targets that they regulate. Their functions are not, however, identical, as in each case there are some unique distinguishing features to the phenotype.

HOXA 11 KNOCKOUT PHENOTYPE

The *Abd-b* type homeobox genes are located at the 5′ ends of the *Hox* gene clusters. These genes are considerably expanded in number in vertebrates compared to simpler organisms. *Drosophila* have but one, whereas mammals have a total of 16. In accord with their position within the clusters, these genes tend to be expressed in more caudal positions at later times in development. These genes show overlapping domains of expression, which suggest important roles in the development of both the axial and appendicular skeleton.

The mouse *Hoxa 11* gene, within this group, was originally described as a result of a degenerate oligonucleotide screen for novel homeobox genes (4). Whole-mount *in situ* hybridizations were used to define the expression of *Hoxa 11* in both the body and the developing limbs (14). As expected, the gene was expressed in only the most caudal regions of the body. The expression in the developing limbs was dynamic with time. At early time points (E 9.5), the entire limb bud showed *Hoxa 11* expression. Later, however, at around E 10.5, *Hoxa 11* transcripts became restricted to proximal regions of the limbs, with transcripts now absent in the more distal domains. With time this region of distal exclusion of *Hoxa 11* transcripts expanded as the expression became restricted to a more proximal zone.

Gene targeting provides a very powerful tool for the dissection of developmental function. Genes can be precisely inactivated by homologous recombination in embryonic stem cells, which can then be used to generate mice carrying the mutation. This *in vivo* developing system can then be used to determine the functions of the targeted gene. If a gene were required for proper limb development, for example, then in the mice with a targeted mutation of the gene, limb development should not proceed normally. To begin to understand the functions of the *Abd-b* type *Hox* genes we used gene targeting to generate a deletion of the *Hoxa 11* gene.

The resulting mice showed a variety of interesting developmental defects (14). First, in the axial skeletons, we observed alterations in segment identity determination. There was posteriorization of the 13th thoracic segment toward a first lumbar segment. Surprisingly, there were partial homeotic segment transformations of this segment identity even in heterozygotes, with only one copy of the *Hoxa 11* gene inactivated. In homozygotes there was a complete loss of the ribs normally associated with this segment, whereas in the heterozygotes there was a partial loss of ribs, with some individual-to-individual variation in severity. This heterozygote effect suggested that the *Hox* code hypothesis needed revision, as gene dosage was apparently also important, and not only the combinations of *Hox* genes expressed. It is interesting to note that this phenotypic effect in heterozygotes was apparently a function of the mixed genetic background of these original mutants, as in subsequent studies outlined below, following additional generations of breeding, this heterozygote effect largely disappeared.

It was also surprising to find that although there was a posteriorization at the thoracolumbar boundary, with T13 converted to L1, there was an anteriorization at the lumbosacral boundary, with a conversion of the first sacral segment into a lumbar segment. The net effect was that homozygote mutants often had eight lumbar segments instead of the normal six.

The limbs also showed developmental abnormalities, although they were milder than expected and could not readily be interpreted in terms of homeotic transformations of one body segment into another. In particular, the contour shapes of the ulna and radius of the forelimb, and the tibia and fibula of the hindlimb, were altered. In addition, two carpal bones of the wrist, the triangular and pisiform, were fused in the mutants although they are normally separate.

MALE AND FEMALE INFERTILITY IN *HOXA 11* MUTANTS

Both male and female *Hoxa 11* homozygous mutants were found to be sterile (15). Because *Hox* genes determine developmental destinies of groups of cells in a combinatorial code fashion, it is possible for a single *Hox* gene to participate in the development of multiple components of the embryo. Hence, it was observed that the *Hoxa 11* gene is important in the development of the skeletal system and also of the urogenital system.

In men, the seminiferous tubules showed a block in spermatogenesis. Leydig cells, Sertoli cells, and spermatogonia were present and, at the histologic level, appeared normal. The process of spermatogenesis, however, was disrupted, with only cell debris and few if any mature sperm found in the lumen. This disruption appeared to be the result of cryptorchidism or undescended testes. Indeed, the gubernaculum, which is the canal through which the testes normally descend, was absent in mutants. In mammals the testes generally require the reduced temperature found outside the body wall for spermatogenesis to proceed normally.

In addition, the vas deferens of the male mutants showed a striking partial homeotic transformation toward an epididymis. At the gross level this was evident in the smaller diameter of the mutant vas deferens and by its more convoluted, coiled path. It was also apparent at the histologic level, with the cells of the epithelial and stromal layers more resembling those of the epididymis. These observations reflected the first observed partial homeotic transformation of a soft tissue reported in a *Hox* mutant. The anteriorization toward an epididymis is what would be predicted by the *Hox* code hypothesis and what is known about the normal expression patterns of

Hox genes in the urogenital tract. The *11* paralogous group is normally expressed in the vas deferens but not in the epididymis, so mutation of *Hoxa 11* converts the code in the vas toward that normally found in the epididymis.

The female *Hoxa 11* mutants are also sterile, but not as a result of failed gametogenesis. Indeed, the female mutants produce normal eggs that can be fertilized and transferred to surrogate mothers, where they develop normally. The failure instead appears to be at the level of uterine support of development. This is also consistent with the expression pattern of *Hoxa 11,* which is transcribed not in the developing gonads but rather in the mesenchymal cells that give rise to the stroma of the uterus and vas deferens. The mutant uterus, like the mutant vas deferens, appears to be partially anteriorized, in this case toward an oviduct.

The role of *Hoxa 11* in female fertility was studied further. It was observed that the expression of *Hoxa 11* in the stroma of the uterus cycles as a function of the estrous cycle. This was shown by both Western blot analysis and *in situ* hybridizations. Expression was also examined in the pregnant uterus, where the highest levels were found in the secondary zone of decidualization. It was also observed that the mutant uterus has reduced numbers of uterine glands. Because a previous knockout of the leukemia inhibitory factor (LIF) gene had shown resulting female infertility, this suggested that a perturbation of LIF synthesis in the mutant uterine glands might partially explain the female infertility. Western blot analysis confirmed that the mutant uterus produced very low levels of LIF and did not generate the normal burst of LIF associated with implantation at E 4.5. This was further pursued by immunohistochemistry to determine if the deficit in LIF was just the result of the reduced numbers of uterine glands or if the glands that were present were defective and did not make LIF. It was shown that, indeed, the few mutant uterine glands that were present did not synthesize LIF.

HOXA 11 ANTISENSE RNA

During the normal characterization of the *Hoxa 11* genomic DNA and cDNA sequences a very surprising finding was made. It was observed that there is an antisense RNA made from the *Hoxa 11* locus (15) (Fig. 3). By several measures the antisense RNA actually appeared significantly more abundant than the normal *Hoxa 11* sense RNA. In screening of limb cDNA libraries with a probe that hybridized to the 5′ ends of both sense and antisense RNAs, over 90% of the resulting positive clones were found to correspond to antisense RNA. Also on Northern blots, probes specific to the antisense RNAs gave much stronger hybridization signals. And similarly, for *in situ* hybridizations the antisense RNA appeared much more abundant at several time points in limb development.

The antisense RNA was truly antisense. This was apparent from the locations of the poly-A tails on the cDNA clones and also from the splice donor and acceptor sequences of the introns of the antisense transcripts. The first exons of the sense and antisense transcripts overlapped by over 500 base pairs. The antisense RNA showed several variant forms of RNA processing that reflected alternate exon usage

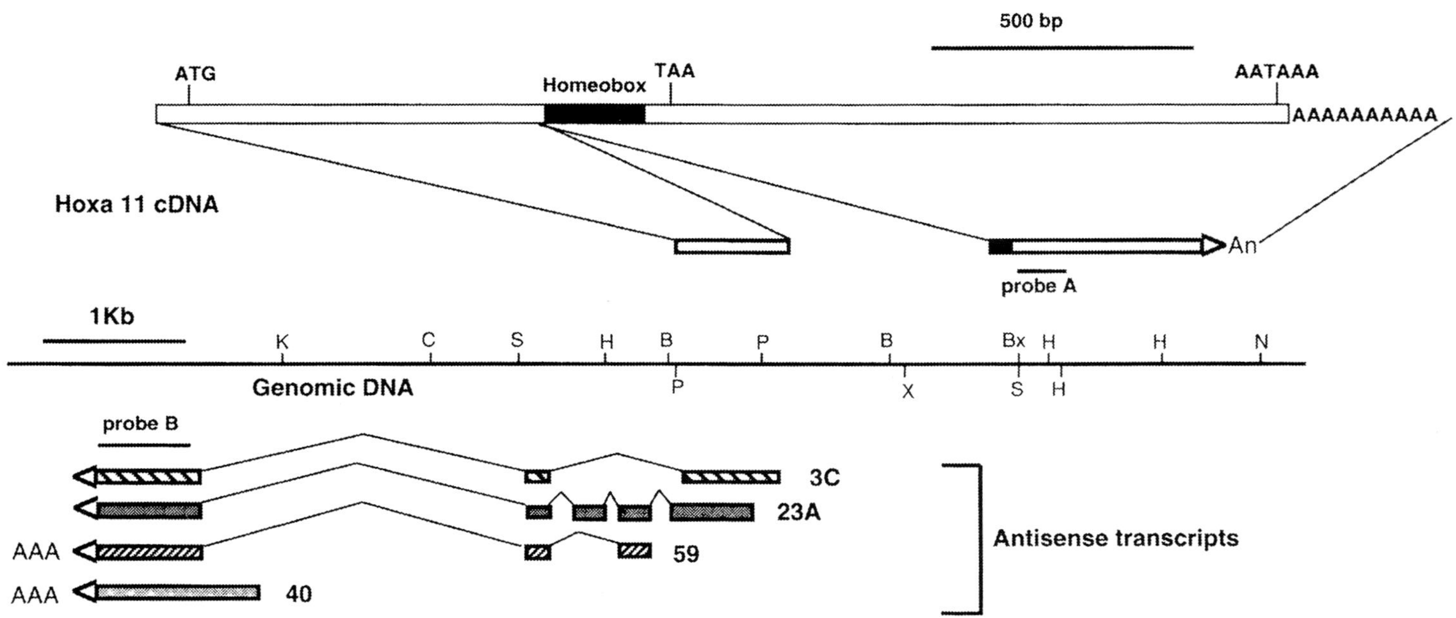

FIG. 3. *Hoxa 11* antisense transcripts. The standard *Hoxa 11* sense cDNA is shown at the top, with a restriction map of the genomic DNA shown in the center. Four different antisense cDNAs are shown at the bottom, with *thin lines* representing introns and *rectangles* representing exons. From Hsieh-Li *et al.* (15).

and variable splice sites for exons (Fig. 3). The antisense RNA carried significantly long open reading frames that suggested coding potential. Predicted amino acid sequences included proline-rich regions, often found in transcription factor proteins.

The expression pattern of the *Hoxa 11* antisense gene showed a striking complementarity to that of the *Hoxa 11* sense transcript. At early time points in development (E 9.5), the sense transcript was detected throughout the developing limb, whereas the antisense transcript was not present. At a later time point (E 10.5), however, just as the sense transcripts are disappearing at the most distal tip, the antisense transcripts were present in that same region in great abundance. And as time moves forward, the domain of expression of the antisense transcripts expands to include more proximal regions, and in a corresponding fashion, the domain where sense transcripts are found diminishes to become more proximally localized.

These observations suggest that the antisense RNA may have a functional role in the regulation of *Hoxa 11* expression. If the antisense RNA is indeed functional and not simply a spurious transcript of no significance, then one might expect it to be evolutionarily conserved, and this appears to be the case. Several possible models of regulation by the antisense genes can be envisioned. First, the antisense RNA could duplex with the sense RNA and trigger its degradation. There is certainly ample precedent for this in the world of prokaryotes and in the laboratory. Another model is that the promoters of the sense and antisense genes could, in opposing each other directionally, perhaps compete with each other. In yet a third model the products of the antisense gene could themselves function to block transcription of the sense RNA. These models are now being tested.

HOXA 11–HOXD 11 DOUBLE MUTANTS

Paralogous *Hox* genes at equivalent positions on different *Hox* clusters typically show similar sequence and expression patterns, suggesting overlapping function. To test this the Potter and Capecchi laboratories exchanged the *Hoxa 11* and *Hoxd 11* mutant mice and bred them to make double homozygous mice as well as intermediate genotypes and analyzed the resulting phenotypes (16). If the two genes were largely redundant in function, then one would predict that in the single mutant the absence of one gene was compensated by the presence of the other, whereas in the double mutants the phenotype would be much more severe than in either single mutant.

For each of these two *Hox* genes the limb mutant phenotype for the single mutant was relatively mild. In the wrists the single *Hoxa 11* or *Hoxd 11* homozygous mutants each show fusion of carpal bones. For the individual heterozygotes the carpals are normal, but in the double heterozygotes, for both *Hoxa 11* and *Hoxd 11,* there is again carpal fusion. This suggests that these two genes are functionally redundant and that it is the total dosage of wild-type allele that determines phenotype. With three of the four alleles mutant, the phenotype becomes more severe, with the triangular and pisiform bones of the wrist now severely malformed. With four mutant alleles all of the proximal carpal bones are dramatically affected, with the pisiform now missing, the triangular also missing or fused to a distal carpal, and the last proximal carpal, the navicular lunate, now deformed.

The zeugopod of the double mutants is also synergistically altered. The zeugopod of the forelimb, consisting of the ulna and radius, is relatively normal in both the *Hoxa 11* and *Hoxd 11* single homozygous mutants. For the double homozygous mutant, however, almost the entire zeugopod is missing (Fig. 4). Tiny remnants of the ulna and radius remain, with the paw now attached to the elbow at an odd angle.

These results show that the *Hox* genes are indeed very important in limb development but that they have functional overlap. It is therefore necessary to generate mice mutant for multiple genes before the function is revealed in the phenotype.

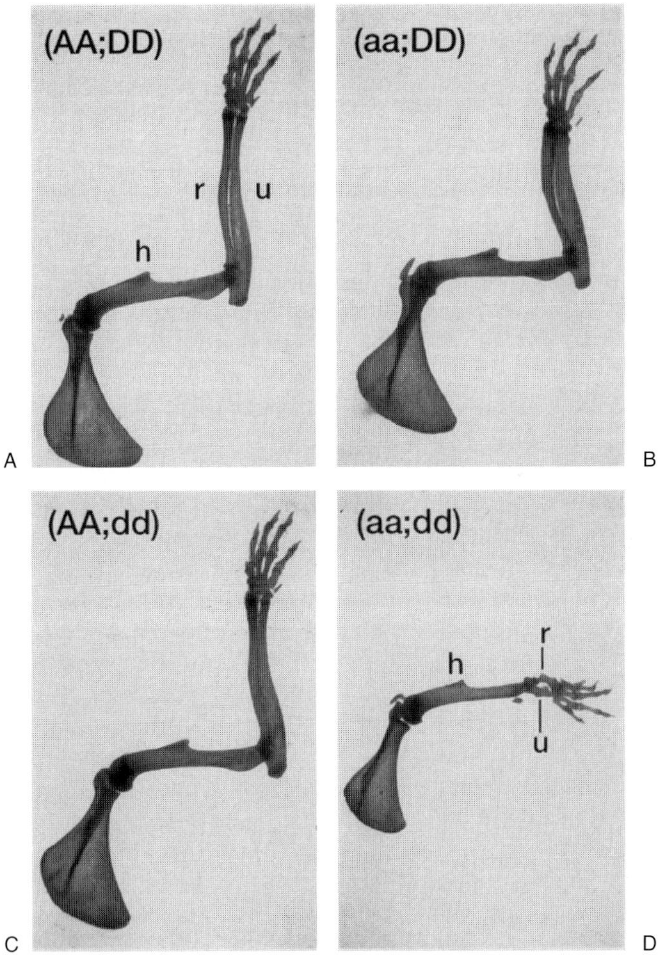

FIG. 4. Forelimb phenotype of mice with mutations in *Hoxa 11* and *Hoxd 11*. **A:** Wild type. **B:** Homozygote *Hoxa 11* mutant. **C:** Homozygote *Hoxd 11* mutant. **D:** Double homozygote mutant for both *Hoxa 11* and *Hoxd 11*. r, radius; u, ulna; h, humerus. From Davis *et al.* (16).

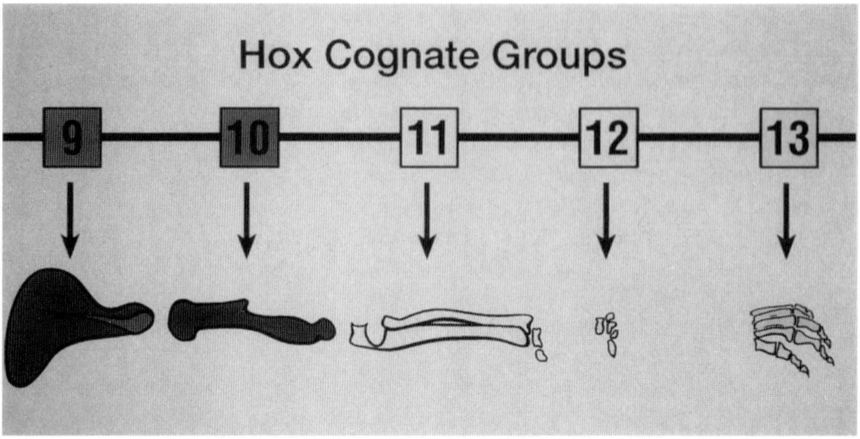

FIG. 5. Model of *Hox* function. As shown, each paralogous group is predicted to be responsible for genetic programming of a different component of the limb. From Davis *et al.* (16).

These studies directly demonstrate that the number-11 *Hox* paralogous series is essential for the production of the zeugopod. Based on known expression patterns of the other *Abd-b* type *Hox* genes, one can predict that in similar fashion the number-13 paralogs are necessary for autopod development, number 12 for the distal wrist, and number 10 for the more proximal development of the humerus and femur (Fig. 5). Recently, double *Hoxa 13–Hoxd 13* mutants have been described with severe failure of autopod development, as predicted by this model (17).

The *Hoxa 11–Hoxd 11* double mutants also revealed redundant function for these two genes in the development of the urogenital system. Each single mutant has normal kidneys, but the double mutants have kidneys very severely reduced in size, which typically results in death within 1 day of birth. In addition, both the vas deferens and uterus transformations toward epididymis and oviduct, respectively, are more complete in the double mutants.

HOX GENE FUNCTION

It has been suggested that *Hox* genes have fundamentally different functions in flies and mammals. Duboule (18) has stated that although it is clear that *Hox* genes play an important role in pattern formation in flies, in mammals it is likely that they are mere regulators of cell proliferation. This statement is indeed consistent with several observations. For example, it explains the failure to observe homeotic transformations in the limbs of single *Abd-b Hox* mutants. There are also several independent reports that now implicate a variety of homeobox genes in the control of cell proliferation (19–27).

Nevertheless, the overwhelming body of evidence indicates that homeobox genes fulfill similar roles in the development of flies and mammals. Perhaps most dramatic in illustrating this point are the early experiments of McGinnis and co-workers (28,29), who showed that mammalian homeobox genes can functionally substitute for *Drosophila* homeobox genes in transgenic flies. These results strongly suggest that upper developmental genetic hierarchies are astonishingly well conserved across enormous phylogenetic distance. It should also be noted that in *Drosophila* one of the most common results of a homeobox gene mutation is the deletion of a structure (1). If the genes that normally drive a developmental program forward are not present, then the program cannot be executed, and the structure does not form. In the double *Hoxa 11–Hoxd 11* mutants, and in increasing numbers of other multiple *Hox* mutants being described, there are reported failures of structures to form. This strongly suggests that in mammals, as in *Drosophila, Hox* genes control genetic cascades that generate components of the embryo.

REFERENCES

1. McGinnis W, Krumlauf R. Homeobox genes and axial patterning. *Cell* 1992; 68: 283–302.
2. McGinnis W, Levine MS, Hafen E, Kuroiwa A, Gehring WJ. A conserved DNA sequence in homoeotic genes of the *Drosophila melanogaster Antennapedia* and *Bithorax* complexes. *Nature* 1984; 308: 428–433.
3. McGinnis W, Garber RL, Wirz J, Kuroiwa A, Gehring WJ. A homologous protein coding sequence in *Drosophila* homoeotic genes and its conservation in other metagoans. *Cell* 1984; 38: 403–409.
4. Singh G, Kaur S, Stock JL, *et al.* Identification of 10 murine homeobox genes. *Proc Natl Acad Sci USA* 1991; 88: 10706–10710.
5. Ma J, Ptashne M. A new class of yeast transcriptional activators. *Cell* 1987; 51: 113–119.
6. Graham H, Papalopulu N, Krumlauf R. The murine and *Drosophila* homeobox gene complexes have common features of organization and expression. *Cell* 1989; 57: 367–378.
7. Wolgemuth DJ, Behringer RR, Mostoller MP, Brinster RL, Palmiter RD. Transgenic mice overexpressing the mouse homeobox-containing gene *Hox-1.4* exhibit abnormal gut development. *Nature* 1989; 337: 464–467.
8. Balling R, Mutter G, Gruss P, Kessel M. Craniofacial abnormalities induced by ectopic expression of the homeobox gene *Hox-1.1* in transgenic mice. *Cell* 1989; 58: 337–347.
9. Kessel M, Balling R, Gruss P. Variations of cervical vertebrae after expression of *Hox-1.1* in transgenic mice. *Cell* 1990; 61: 301–308.
10. Lewis EB. A gene complex controlling segmentation in *Drosophila. Nature* 1978; 276: 565–570.
11. Kaur S, Singh G, Stock J, *et al.* Dominant mutation of the murine *Hox-2.2* gene results in developmental abnormalities. *J Exp Zool* 1992; 264: 323–336.
12. McLain K, Schreiner C, Yager K, Stock J, Potter S. Ectopic expression of *Hox-2.3* induces craniofacial and skeletal malformations in transgenic mice. *Mech Dev* 1992; 39: 3–16.
13. Gibson G, Gehring WJ. Head and thoracic transformations caused by ectopic expression of *Antennapedia* during *Drosophila* development. *Development* 1988; 102: 657–675.
14. Small KM, Potter SS. Homeotic transformations and limb defects in *Hox A11* mutant mice. *Genes Dev* 1993; 7: 2318–2328.
15. Hsieh-Li HM, Witte DP, Weinstein M, *et al. Hoxa 11* structure, extensive antisense transcription, and function in male and female fertility. *Development* 1995; 121: 1373–1385.
16. Davis AP, Witte DP, Hsieh-Li HM, Potter SS, Capecchi MR. Absence of radius and ulna in mice lacking *hoxa-11* and *hoxd-11. Nature* 1995; 375: 791–795.
17. Fromental-Ramain C, Warot X, Messadecq N, LeMeur M, Dollé P, Chambon P. *Hoxa-13* and *Hoxd-13* play a crucial role in the patterning of the limb autopod. *Development* 1996; 122: 2997–3011.
18. Duboule D. Vertebrate *Hox* genes and proliferation: an alternative pathway to homeosis? *Curr Opin Genet Dev* 1995; 5: 525–528.
19. Perkins AC, Cory S. Conditional immortalization of mouse myelomonocytic, megakaryocytic and mast cell progenitors by the *Hox-2.4* homeobox gene. *EMBO J* 1993; 12: 3835–3846.
20. Blatt C, Aberdam D, Schwartz R, Sachs L. DNA rearrangement of a homeobox gene in myeloid leukaemic cells. *EMBO J* 1988; 7: 4283–4290.

21. Zhang N, Gong Z-Z, Minden M, Lu M. The *HOX-11* (TCL-3) homeobox proto-oncogene encodes a nuclear protein that undergoes cell cycle-dependent regulation. *Oncogene* 1993; 8: 3265–3270.
22. Dear TN, Sanchez-Garcia I, Rabbitts TH. The *HOX11* gene encodes a DNA-binding nuclear transcription factor belonging to a distinct family of homeobox genes. *Proc Natl Acad Sci USA* 1993; 90: 4431–4435.
23. Kongsuwan K, Allen J, Adams JM. Expression of *Hox-2.4* homeobox gene directed by proviral insertion in a myeloid leukemia. *Nucl Acids Res* 1989; 17: 1881–1891.
24. Perkins A, Kongsuwan K, Visvader J, Adams JM, Cory S. Homeobox gene expression plus autocrine growth factor production elicits myeloid leukemia. *Proc Natl Acad Sci USA* 1990; 87: 8398–8402.
25. Woloshin P, Song K, Degnin C, *et al.* MSX1 inhibits myoD expression in fibroblast × 10T 1/2 cell hybrids. *Cell* 1995; 82: 611–620.
26. Hatano M, Roberts CWM, Minden M, Crist WM, Korsmeyer SJ. Deregulation of a homeobox gene, *HOX11,* by the t(10;14) in T cell leukemia. *Science* 1991; 253: 79–82.
27. Song K, Wang Y, Sassoon D. Expression of *Hox-7.1* in myoblasts inhibits terminal differentiation and induces cell transformation. *Nature* 1992; 360: 477–481.
28. Malicki J, Schughart K, McGinnis W. Mouse *Hox-2.2* specifies thoracic segmental identity in *Drosophila* embryos and larvae. *Cell* 1990; 63: 961–967.
29. McGinnis N, Kuziora MA, McGinnis W. Human *Hox 4.2* and *Drosophila Deformed* encode similar regulatory specificities in *Drosophila* embryos and larvae. *Cell* 1990; 63: 969–976.

DISCUSSION

Dr. Guesry: The transgenic mouse that you showed us at the beginning has a neural tube defect that is quite similar to spina bifida in the newborn human infant. Have you analyzed the genetic makeup of newborn infants with spina bifida, and did you find this modification that you induced in mice? This might give us a better understanding of the role of folate deficiency, which is also important in the genesis of these neural tube defects in humans.

Dr. Potter: The homeobox genes are expressed in the developing neural tube, and mutations in these genes certainly can result in neural tube defects. We have generated mice that have delayed closure of both the anterior and posterior neuropores. There are other genes involved in this process too—for example, the *Pax* genes: the *Pax 3* mouse (the *splotch* mouse) has neural tube defects. The *Pax* genes are genes with both paired boxes and in some cases homeoboxes as well. People are certainly very interested in trying to define the genetic program of neural tube closure. How the homeobox genes relate to folate metabolism and spina bifida in humans is still to be resolved.

Dr. Tsang: Is there more than one kind of redundancy of *Hoxa* or *Hoxd* among the master genes?

Dr. Potter: It turns out that more primitive organisms typically have one of these clusters of homeobox genes, and only one. In organisms such as the fruit fly, if you mutate one gene you get a dramatic phenotype. In more complex organisms like the human, these primitive clusters have been quadruplicated so we have four of them. Thus, from a single primal cluster, this quadruplication has generated four copies of each gene that was present on the original cluster. Not all of these genes have been preserved during evolution; unequal crossing over has deleted some and duplicated others. So we can't say there are exactly four copies of each gene now in mammals, but as a general rule there are four copies of the clusters now, and as a rule there are four copies of each gene that is present in a more primitive organism. Now presumably we have four copies because they are useful to us, and not each copy is completely redundant. They have evolved to assume slightly divergent functions though they have retained a considerable overlap in function.

Dr. Klish: I was fascinated by your pictures of these abnormalities. It appeared that the malformed bones also had increased density. Do these *Hox* genes not only control morphology but also histology of these elements?

Dr. Potter: That is a very interesting question. We have not done much histology on these animals. But it is probably something we should do, especially in the *Hoxa 11* single mutant animals, where the tibia–fibula region does appear more dense after skeletal staining.

Dr. Mughal: The skeletal malformations that you showed in the mice are also seen in, for example, pups born to diabetic rats, especially the cordal regression syndrome and many of the spinal malformations. I just wonder whether the diabetic environment in the mother might modify the expression of some of these *Hox* genes.

Dr. Potter: I don't think that has ever been looked at either. We are inclined to think that many of the malformations that we see from folate deficiency or diabetes or from environmental teratogens might indeed function through alteration of *Hox* gene expression patterns.

Dr. Pettifor: Taking the model further, although the *Hox* genes fit somewhere close to the top of your pyramid, there is obviously something above it that controls its expression, particularly in the early embryonic phase. What is the controlling factor for *Hox* gene expression in the early embryo?

Dr. Potter: That is of major interest to my laboratory right now. In addition to looking at downstream targets, we are also looking at the upstream regulation of the *Hox* genes. I drew the *Hox* genes at the top of the pyramid, but of course they are not—there has to be something above them, as you point out. The answer to that question is fairly well worked out in fruit flies but not in mammals yet. In fruit flies there is a genetic hierarchy that begins with maternal genes that are expressed in nurse cells that feed the zygote and that set up maternal gradients in the egg of the fruit fly. These genes in turn then regulate the expression of gap genes and segment polarity genes, such as *hunchback,* which are zinc finger genes, and again, there are genes that regulate other genes, but they are at a different position in the hierarchy. These segmentation genes in the fruit fly are known to regulate the expression pattern of homeobox genes; thus the segmentation genes in the fruit fly set up the partitioning of the embryo and define the segments. Then the homeobox genes define segment identity, so they establish what each segment will actually become. So the hierarchy in the fruit fly is fairly well worked out, and using that as a model, we are trying to work out a similar hierarchy in mammals. There are zinc finger genes in mammals that are under investigation and that are believed to be upstream regulators of our homeobox genes, but the details remain to be defined.

Dr. Eisman: Is it not one of the problems with using that approach that the *Hox* genes themselves regulate each other and turn each other on and off? Aren't you going to identify 100 *Hox* genes before you find your wonderful upstream segmentation gene?

Dr. Potter: You are right. *Hox* genes do tend to cross-regulate both in *Drosophila* and, we think, in mammals. Many of them actually autoregulate, so both in *Drosophila* and in mammals, once you turn the gene on it turns itself on, and that is believed to play a role in maintaining the determined state. So it is a complex network without a doubt, rather like a neural network where each neuron can interconnect with a large number of others, both on the input and the output sides, and that is clearly happening in these genetic networks. They do cross-regulate each other, but there are clearly other things from above that are regulating them as well. It is going to be a lot of work to define all these interactions. I don't think it is impossible though.

Dr. Eisman: With the Brazilian family you described with the skeletal defects that look very much like your *Hoxa 11* or *Hoxd 11* double knockout, what do you think you are going to find? I mean if you are describing a fairly simple recessive trait you would imagine this is a single gene knockout. Do you think there is another gene that is already knocked out widely in that population, which allows the expression of the defect, or do you think you will be looking for something which is not a homologue of any of the homeobox genes?

Dr. Potter: I suspect that, based on the genetics of this family, there is a single gene involved. The inheritance pattern looks like a single autosomal recessive. I am not proposing that it is necessarily a homeobox gene—it could be any of a large number of interesting genes that are important in limb development. We have some interesting clues already as to what it might be, based on our experimental systems. We know for example that if you experimentally remove the apical ectodermal ridge from a chick limb you get a truncated limb: the proximal distal access is truncated so growth stops and you get just a femur, for example, like these people have. So it could well be an apical ectodermal ridge gene that is involved, and the important signaling genes in the ridge are fibroblast growth factors 2, 4, and 8. So it is quite possible that these people are suffering a mutation of FGF 2, 4 or 8. Another project in my laboratory is pursuing a transgene insertional mutation that we have made, where the mice have truncated limbs. The mice I showed you with *Hoxa 11* and *Hoxd 11* missing actually have paws stuck on at the elbow, so they don't have everything missing from there out. However, we have generated another mouse model that does have everything missing distally. This is the transgene insertional mutation mouse, and we have recently shown that mutated gene is a dynein gene. Dyneins aren't gene regulators—they encode molecular motor proteins that move things along microtubules. These mice with truncated limbs also have situs inversus, with left–right asymmetry reversal, and we believe that this dynein gene plays an important role both in limb outgrowth and in correct situs development in mammals.

Dr. Jüppner: If *Hox* genes are so important for limb development, and if there is some degree of redundancy but also of gene dosage effect, do you see any abnormalities if you look carefully in the nonaffected individuals in these families?

Dr. Potter: Heterozygotes appeared to be absolutely normal. So for that particular gene, there don't appear to be any gene dosage effects. For homeobox genes there generally are, so that might suggest this is not a homeobox gene defect.

Dr. Guesry: In your transgenic mice with the homeobox gene defect, is the defect confined to the bone so that there is still some atrophic muscle attached to the part, or have the muscle and vessels disappeared as well? In other words, does this gene control only the bone or the whole limb?

Dr. Potter: It is the whole limb. I don't know what follows what, but I am told that the muscle tends to follow the bone, and if you remove the bone you will have no formation of muscle either.

Dr. Guesry: But this a consequence of the missing bone, it is not the direct effect of the gene?

Dr. Potter: All I can say is when we look at these animals we don't see muscle or bone present. They are both missing. Which came first—which is the primal cause and which is the effect—I am not personally certain of.

Dr. Pettifor: Thalidomide produces defects similar to that you just described. How does thalidomide have its effects?

Dr. Potter: Thalidomide generates phocomelia as you know, and that is similar in many respects to what we see, with distal components of limbs sometimes being attached to more proximal components, with the portions in between missing. So the phenotype is quite similar. The molecular mechanisms of how thalidomide works remain unresolved after decades of intensive research. So how thalidomide phocomelia ties in with the phenotypes that we see at a molecular level is not known.

Dr. Gilsanz: My understanding was that many of these defects are believed to follow injury to the neural crest of the embryo, and it is from these that the abnormalities originate. Thalidomide was known to have produced peripheral neuropathy in some women.

Dr. Potter: So you believe the primal effect is actually in neural crest cells. I am surprised to hear that. I didn't think neural crest cells made a major contribution to, for example, the zeugopod development of the limb, but I could be wrong in that.

Dr. Gilsanz: Infants of diabetic mothers have similar abnormalities.

Dr. Eisman: So when you were talking about the *Hoxa 11–Hoxd 11* knockout, you said that these animals did not have any renal development. Am I right?

Dr. Potter: That's right. It was proposed many years ago by Ed Lewis that homeobox genes are expressed in a coded fashion to define developmental destinies of regions, and that if you express homeobox gene A plus C plus D you will define a portion of the limb, but if you express homeobox genes A plus C plus F you will define another structure. So in fact each homeobox gene can play an important role in the coding of multiple components of the embryo. For example, in our *Hoxa 11* mutants we don't see only limb defects; we also see kidney defects and both male and female subjects are sterile. There are homeotic transformations of reproductive parts, with the vas deferens homeotically transformed toward an epididymis and the uterus homeotically transformed toward an oviduct, because of the changing *Hox* expression patterns and the changing codes that are present in these mutant mice. So yes, the kidneys are absent in the A11–D11 mutants—absent or very rudimentary.

Dr. Eisman: In the fruit fly with A11 absence, is the equivalent of the kidney missing?

Dr. Potter: The modeling breaks down when you are comparing mammals with flies because flies don't have an equivalent to a kidney. In fact, the abdominal B gene is present in only one copy in a fly, and yet it is present in about 17 or 18 copies in a mouse because of the quadruplication and then unequal crossing over generating multiple additional copies on top of that. So it is a much more complex story in mammals compared to the fly, and the phenotypes that you get with the mutation in a fly don't always mimic very closely what you see in a mouse when you mutate a corresponding gene.

Dr. Tsang: What teratogens are known to interact with the *Hox* genes, particularly in terms of limb or bone development?

Dr. Potter: The only really good example that I am aware of is retinoic acid, which is a powerful teratogen. It turns out that homeobox genes have retinoic acid response elements that regulate their expression and can easily be up-regulated by retinoic acid.

Dr. Alliet: Are homeobox genes less prone to mutation compared to structural genes or genes lower in the pyramid?

Dr. Potter: I think that is true. The data argue strongly that the upper components of these genetic pyramids or genetic hierarchy are strongly conserved in evolution, and as you move down the pyramid towards structural component genes, there is more flexibility. It makes eminent good sense to me that if you mess up a gene at the top of the pyramid, you are going to perturb not only that gene but the expression of all the genes beneath it in the cascade, and the effects would be dramatic, whereas mutation at the bottom of the pyramid may change the structural component gene protein in some modest way, but it would not have such a far-reaching effect on so many genes.

Dr. Pollak: If these genes are of such fundamental importance and high in the cascade, as you say they are, is anything known about repair mechanisms?

Dr. Potter: I don't believe it is going to be a special repair mechanism for these genes. I believe instead that there is simply natural selection at work. When these genes are mutated, there are dramatic phenotypic consequences, and such mutations would be selected against.

Nutrition and Bone Development, edited by
Jean-Philippe Bonjour and Reginald C. Tsang,
Nestlé Nutrition Workshop Series, Vol. 41, Nestec Ltd.,
Vevey/Lippincott–Raven Publishers,
Philadelphia © 1999.

Role of Parathyroid Hormone-Related Peptide in Skeletal Development

Harald Jüppner

Endocrine Unit, Departments of Pediatrics and Medicine, Massachusetts General Hospital and Harvard Medical School, Boston, Massachusetts 02114, USA

Apart from 1,25$(OH)_2$vitamin D_3, parathyroid hormone (PTH) is the major regulator of mammalian calcium and phosphorus homeostasis (1). Until recently, PTH was thought to be produced exclusively by the parathyroid glands. However, small amounts of its mRNA were detected in the rat hypothalamus (2), suggesting that it may be produced in the central nervous system as well, where it could serve as yet unknown functions that are unrelated to its role in mineral ion homeostasis. The existence of a second hormone with biological properties largely indistinguishable from those of PTH was first proposed in the early 1940s, when Fuller Albright discussed a patient with malignancy-associated severe hypercalcemia. The clinical and biochemical characterization of similarly affected patients subsequently established the humoral hypercalcemia of malignancy syndrome (3) and led to the molecular cloning of parathyroid hormone-related peptide (PTHrP) from several different tumors (4–7). Despite this important breakthrough in understanding the pathogenesis of tumor-associated humoral hypercalcemia, only limited conclusions could be drawn about the physiological role of PTHrP in normal fetal and adult life. Recently, however, remarkable insights into its biological role were gained through the application of gene-targeting and disruption strategies and through the molecular definition of Jansen's metaphyseal chondrodysplasia, a rare genetic disorder of calcium/phosphorus homeostasis and growth. The cumulative evidence from these studies indicates that PTHrP plays a major role in normal endochondral bone formation and bone elongation.

PARATHYROID HORMONE-RELATED PEPTIDE

The search for the humoral factor that causes the hypercalcemia of malignancy syndrome led to the discovery of PTHrP (4–7). Its amino-terminal portion, but not its mid- and carboxyl-terminal regions, resembles that of PTH. Because of this limited structural homology, PTH and PTHrP can activate a common G-protein-

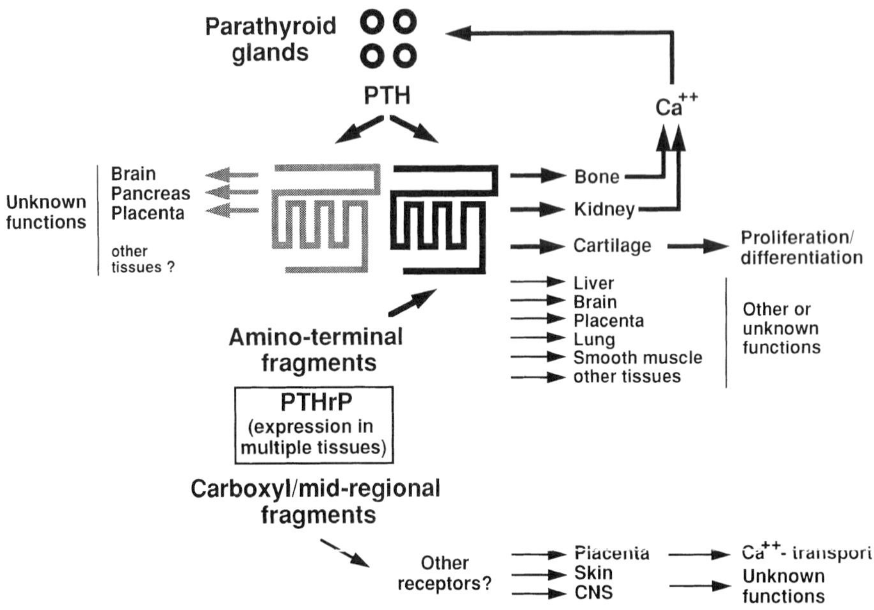

FIG. 1. Biological functions of PTH and PTHrP fragments that are mediated through the PTH/PTHrP receptor (black pathway), the PTH2 receptor (gray pathway), and possibly other receptors.

coupled receptor, the PTH/PTHrP receptor, with indistinguishable efficacy (Fig. 1) (8,9). Consequently, amino-terminal fragments of both peptides have largely indistinguishable biological properties *in vivo,* at least with respect to their roles in regulating calcium and phosphorus homeostasis (10–13).

A secreted midregional PTHrP fragment, PTHrP(38–94)amide, which is generated along with several other PTHrP species through posttranslational processing, appears to interact with a novel receptor that is distinct from the cloned PTH/PTHrP receptor and that mediates its actions through changes in intracellular free calcium rather than through the second messenger cAMP (14,15). It is plausible that this receptor also mediates the actions of PTHrP(38–94)amide and PTHrP(67–86)amide, which were recently shown to stimulate the transplacental transfer of calcium in fetal lambs and PTHrP-ablated murine fetuses, respectively (15,16). These findings confirmed earlier studies that had provided the first evidence of the importance of PTHrP in the regulation of fetal calcium homeostasis (17). Other secreted fragments, for example PTHrP(107–139), which was shown to inhibit osteoclastic bone resorption and to activate hippocampal neurons (18,19), are also generated through posttranslational cleavage of intact PTHrP (15). The actions of these and possibly other PTHrP fragments are likely to be mediated through additional still uncharacterized receptors.

The importance of PTHrP as the PTH-like factor responsible for most cases of the humoral hypercalcemia of malignancy syndrome is now well established (20–22). However, PTHrP is expressed in a remarkable variety of normal fetal and adult tissues, which suggests that it has additional biological roles and that these as yet undefined roles are distinct from those mediated by PTH. The exploration of these PTHrP-specific functions required novel experimental approaches and continues to be incomplete. The most revealing new insights were obtained from mice in which the PTHrP gene had been ablated through homologous recombination (23). The biochemical and histologic analysis of these genetically engineered animals, which lack either one or both copies of the PTHrP gene, provided a much improved understanding of the peptide's physiological functions.

Ablation of only one copy of the PTHrP gene resulted in mice that are normal at birth, show normal behavior and fertility, but develop osteopenia later in life, despite an apparently normal regulation of calcium and phosphorus homeostasis (24). In contrast, animals that lack both alleles of the PTHrP gene die at birth or shortly after despite their grossly normal size and appearance (23). Further examination revealed that these mice have striking skeletal changes, which include misshapen skulls, short snouts and mandibles, and disproportionately short extremities, but no obvious effects on the morphologic development of other major organs. These findings, although surprising at first, provided compelling evidence for an important role of PTHrP in chondrocyte differentiation and bone elongation.

From these and subsequent studies, it now appears likely that PTHrP facilitates the continuous proliferation of chondrocytes in the growth plate and that it postpones their programmed differentiation into hypertrophic chondrocytes. Consistent with this presumed role of PTHrP in endochondral bone formation, it has been long known that PTH (used in all earlier studies instead of PTHrP, which had not yet been discovered) affects chondrocyte maturation and activity *in vitro* (25,26). Recent studies confirmed these previous findings by showing that PTH and PTHrP stimulate the proliferation of fetal growth plate chondrocytes, presumably through cAMP-dependent mechanisms (27), inhibit the differentiation of these cells into hypertrophic chondrocytes, and stimulate the accumulation of cartilage-specific proteoglycans, which are thought to act as inhibitors of mineralization (28–30). Because of the lack of these cartilage-specific functions of PTHrP, growth plates of homozygous PTHrP gene-ablated mice have a thinner layer of proliferating chondrocytes, whereas the layer of hypertrophic chondrocytes is relatively normal in thickness but somewhat disorganized. These findings suggest that the lack of PTHrP accelerates the normal differentiation process of growth plate chondrocytes; that is, resting and proliferating chondrocytes undergo fewer cycles of cell division and differentiate prematurely into hypertrophic cells, which then undergo apoptosis before being replaced by invading osteoblasts.

Further evidence for an important role of PTHrP in chondrocyte proliferation and differentiation was also derived from recent studies with transgenic mice that overexpress PTHrP under the control of the mouse type II procollagen promoter (31). At birth these animals were already smaller in size and showed a marked disproportionate foreshortening of limbs and tail. The transgenic animals grew at a rate comparable to that of their normal littermates but maintained their phenotypic abnormalities throughout life. Further analysis of their skeleton revealed that this unusual form of short-limbed dwarfism was most probably caused by a severe delay in chondrocyte differentiation and endochondral ossification. In fact, these growth plate abnormalities may well represent the opposite of those found in PTHrP-ablated mice, which show an acceleration of the differentiation program that leads to a premature development of hypertrophic chondrocytes and a premature initiation of endochondral ossification (23).

THE PTH/PTHrP RECEPTOR

The actions of amino-terminal PTH and PTHrP fragments are mediated through the common PTH/PTHrP receptor, which belongs to a distinct family of G-protein-coupled receptors (32). When expressed in one of several clonal cell lines, PTH/PTHrP receptors from different mammalian species bind amino-terminal fragments of PTH and PTHrP with similar or indistinguishable affinity, and both ligands stimulate with similar potency the formation of two second messengers, cAMP and inositol phosphate (8,9,33–35). Similar to the widely expressed PTHrP, the mRNA encoding the PTH/PTHrP receptor is found in a surprisingly large variety of fetal and adult tissues. However, PTH/PTHrP receptor expression appears to be most abundant at three sites (36–40): in renal tubular cells and in osteoblasts, where it mediates the endocrine actions of PTH, and in prehypertrophic chondrocytes of the metaphyseal growth plate, where it mediates—as suggested from gene ablation and targeting experiments (23,31)—the autocrine/paracrine actions of locally synthesized PTHrP.

Mice in which both alleles encoding the PTH/PTHrP receptor were ablated showed growth plate abnormalities that are similar to, but more severe than, those observed in PTHrP-ablated animals (41). These findings further confirmed that the PTH/PTHrP receptor mediates the effects of PTHrP in the growth plate (Fig. 2). Moreover, the PTH/PTHrP receptor also mediates, although indirectly, actions of *Indian hedgehog (Ihh),* which belongs to the hedgehog family of secreted proteins that are important for embryonic patterning (42). *Ihh* mediates its actions through *Patched (Ptc)* (or a closely related protein), a receptor with 12 membrane-spanning helices that interacts physically with *Smoothened (Smo)* and thereby suppresses the constitutive activity of this latter protein (43,44). In contrast to the mRNA encoding the closely related *Sonic hedgehog (Shh),* the mRNA encoding *Ihh* is found only in later stages of embryonic limb development, and its expression is restricted to the transition zone within the growth plate, where proliferating chondrocytes differentiate into hypertrophic cells (45).

The ectopic expression of *Ihh* in chicken wing cartilage through a replication-competent retroviral vector blocked the normal chondrocyte differentiation program and prevented the appearance of hypertrophic chondrocytes that express collagen type X and *bone morphogenic protein-6 (Bmp).* The aberrant expression of *Ihh* thus led to similar changes to those observed in transgenic mice that overexpress PTHrP under the control of the collagen type II promoter (31) but are the opposite of those

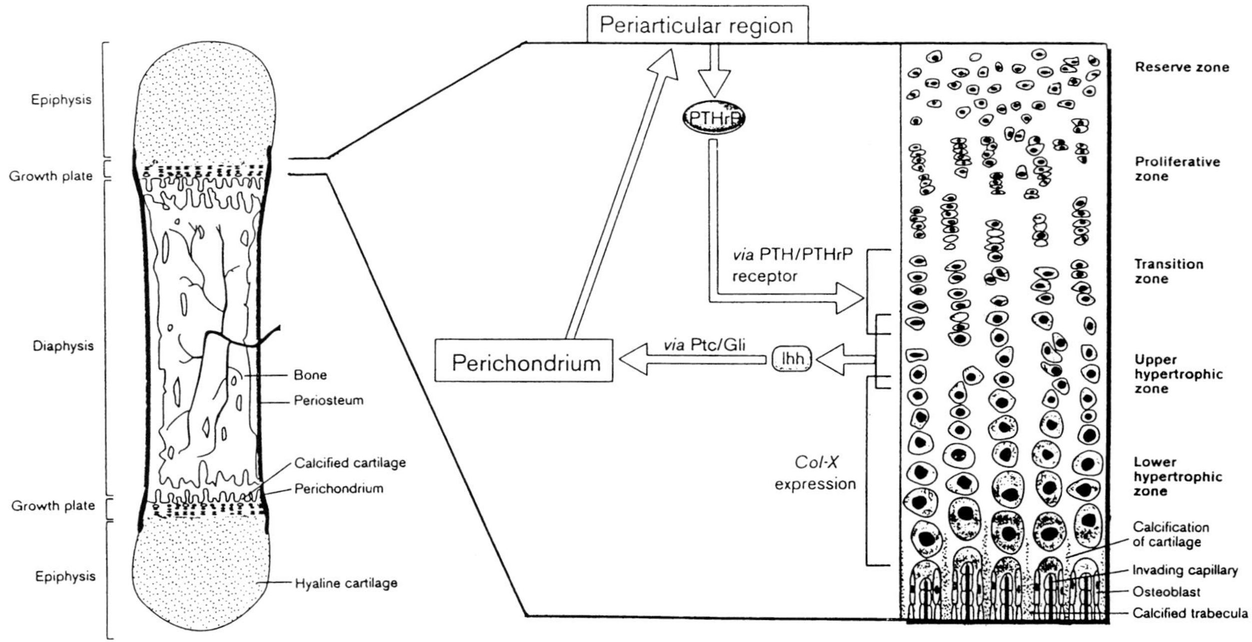

FIG. 2. Regulation of chondrocyte proliferation and differentiation by parathyroid hormone-related peptide (PTHrP) and *Indian hedgehog (Ihh).* Modified from Wallis (59).

found in mice in which the genes encoding PTHrP or its PTH/PTHrP receptor had been disrupted through homologous recombination (23,41). Interestingly, the perichondrium of the *Ihh*-infected growth plates revealed a strong up-regulation of the message encoding *Ptc,* and the PTHrP mRNA was up-regulated in the periarticular regions of infected limbs (45). This finding provided initial evidence for a negative feedback loop within the growth plate that involves PTHrP and its PTH/PTHrP receptor as well as *Ihh* and its receptor *Ptc.*

To explore these local regulatory mechanisms further, bone explants from either PTHrP-ablated or PTH/PTHrP receptor-ablated mice were treated with either PTHrP or *Shh* (which has biological properties that are indistinguishable from those of *Ihh*). Both ligands were able to repress the differentiation into hypertrophic chondrocytes in bone explants from normal mice. PTHrP treatment also repressed the differentiation into hypertrophic chondrocytes in bone explants from PTHrP-ablated animals, whereas *Shh* had no effect in these bones. This indicated that PTHrP is required to mediate the actions of *Shh/Ihh* in the growth plate (45). Similar experiments with bone explants from PTH/PTHrP receptor-ablated mice showed that neither PTHrP nor *Ihh* was able to repress the chondrocyte differentiation program (41), indicating that the PTH/PTHrP receptor mediates the actions of PTHrP directly and those of *Ihh* indirectly.

PTH2 RECEPTOR

In contrast to the common PTH/PTHrP receptor, the closely related PTH2 receptor interacts almost exclusively with PTH but not with PTHrP (46–48) (Fig. 1). This suggests that PTH mediates its actions through two distinct receptors, the PTH/PTHrP receptor and the PTH2 receptor. However, it may well be that another peptide, which has not yet been discovered, is the natural ligand for the PTH2 receptor (46,49). Expression of the PTH2 receptor is restricted to relatively few tissues, and its mRNA levels are typically much less abundant than those encoding the PTH/PTHrP receptor (46,49). Because of this ligand specificity and the low levels of expression in only a few tissues, it appears unlikely that the PTH2 receptor mediates any of the PTHrP-specific autocrine/paracrine effects on chondrocyte differentiation or proliferation. This conclusion is also supported by the findings cited above in mice that lack both alleles encoding the PTH/PTHrP receptor (41). Because these animals have a phenotype similar to that observed in PTHrP-ablated mice (23), the PTH2 receptor must be unable to mediate PTHrP-specific functions in growth plate chondrocytes and is therefore unlikely to play an important biological role in the endochondral bone formation process.

JANSEN'S METAPHYSEAL CHONDRODYSPLASIA

The sharing of a single receptor mediating the activity of two distinct ligands that have entirely different biological functions is unusual. This made it difficult to search for disorders in humans, or other mammals, that are caused by either activating or inactivating mutations in the PTH/PTHrP receptor. In fact, pseudohypoparathyroidism type Ib was long thought to be caused by inactivating mutations in the PTH/PTHrP receptor (50,51). However, recent studies led to the conclusion that this disorder must be caused by a molecular defect in a gene other than that encoding the PTH/PTHrP receptor (52–54). In retrospect, these negative findings are in agreement with our current understanding of the biological importance of the PTH/PTHrP receptor, which mediates the functions of PTH and of PTHrP. Consequently, inactivating PTH/PTHrP receptor mutations should lead to abnormalities in calcium and phosphorus homeostasis and to abnormalities in the metaphyseal growth plates.

PTH/PTHrP receptor mutations were, however, identified as the cause of Jansen's metaphyseal chondrodysplasia, an autosomal dominant disease that is characterized by short-limbed dwarfism and severe hypercalcemia and hypophosphatemia despite normal or undetectable levels of PTH and PTHrP in the blood circulation (55–58). As outlined above, PTH/PTHrP receptors are abundantly expressed in kidney and bone, and they mediate the endocrine actions of PTH in these tissues to maintain the concentrations of extracellular calcium and phosphate within narrow limits. PTH/PTHrP receptors are, furthermore, abundantly expressed in growth plate chondrocytes, where they mediate the autocrine/paracrine actions of PTHrP and regulate the normal process of endochondral bone formation. The most abundant expression of PTH/PTHrP receptors is thus observed in those tissues that show the most striking functional abnormalities in patients with Jansen's disease. Recently, two different heterozygous mutations were identified in the genomic DNA of several patients with this interesting disorder, but not in the DNA of their unaffected siblings and parents (55–57). Expression of the mutant PTH/PTHrP, receptors in COS-7 cells resulted in constitutive, ligand-independent accumulation of cAMP; the basal accumulation of inositol phosphates was not increased. These findings provided a plausible explanation for the severe changes in mineral ion homeostasis and growth plate development. Furthermore, these data support the notion that the common PTH/PTHrP receptor mediates the actions of PTH and PTHrP and that PTHrP is an important regulator of chondrocyte proliferation and differentiation and, consequently, of bone elongation and growth.

CONCLUSIONS

In summary, recent experimental data suggest that bone elongation and thus growth is regulated through a complicated autocrine/paracrine system that includes *Ihh,* a mammalian homolog of a developmentally important protein in *Drosophila,* PTHrP, and its PTH/PTHrP receptor. Furthermore, Jansen's metaphyseal chondrodysplasia, a rare disorder of mineral ion homeostasis and growth, is caused by activating mutations in the PTH/PTHrP receptor. This latter finding reemphasizes the importance of this G-protein-coupled receptor in the regulation of calcium and phosphate homeostasis, and in cartilage and bone development.

REFERENCES

1. Kronenberg HM, Bringhurst FR, Nussbaum S, *et al.* Parathyroid hormone: biosynthesis, secretion, chemistry, and action. In: Mundy GR, Martin TJ, eds. *Handbook of experimental pharmacology: physiology and pharmacology of bone.* Heidelberg: Springer-Verlag, 1993: 185–201.
2. Nutley MT, Parimi SA, Harvey S. Sequence analysis of hypothalamic parathyroid hormone messenger ribonucleic acid. *Endocrinology* 1995; 136: 5600–5607.
3. Stewart AF, Horst R, Deftos LJ, Cadman EC, Lang R, Broadus AE. Biochemical evaluation of patients with cancer-associated hypercalcemia. Evidence for humoral and non-humoral groups. *N Engl J Med* 1980; 303: 1377–1381.
4. Moseley JM, Kubota M, Diefenbach-Jagger H, *et al.* Parathyroid hormone-related protein purified from a human lung cancer cell line. *Proc Natl Acad Sci USA* 1987; 84: 5048–5052.
5. Suva L, Winslow GA, Wettenhall RE, *et al.* A parathyroid hormone-related protein implicated in malignant hypercalcemia: cloning and expression. *Science* 1987; 237: 893–896.
6. Strewler GJ, Stern PH, Jacobs JW, *et al.* Parathyroid hormone-like protein from human renal carcinoma cells. Structural and functional homology with parathyroid hormone. *J Clin Invest* 1987; 80: 1803–1807.
7. Mangin M, Webb AC, Dreyer BE, *et al.* Identification of a cDNA encoding a parathyroid hormone-like peptide from a human tumor associated with humoral hypercalcemia of malignancy. *Proc Natl Acad Sci USA* 1988; 85: 597–601.
8. Jüppner H, Abou-Samra AB, Freeman MW, *et al.* A G protein-linked receptor for parathyroid hormone and parathyroid hormone-related peptide. *Science* 1991; 254: 1024–1026.
9. Abou-Samra AB, Jüppner H, Force T, *et al.* Expression cloning of a common receptor for parathyroid hormone and parathyroid hormone-related peptide from rat osteoblast-like cells: a single receptor stimulates intracellular accumulation of both cAMP and inositol triphosphates and increases intracellular free calcium. *Proc Natl Acad Sci USA* 1992; 89: 2732–2736.
10. Kemp BE, Mosely JM, Rodda CP, *et al.* Parathyroid hormone-related protein of malignancy: active synthetic fragments. *Science* 1987; 238: 1568–1570.
11. Horiuchi N, Caulfield MP, Fisher JE, *et al.* Similarity of synthetic peptide from human tumour to parathyroid hormone *in vivo* and *in vitro. Science* 1987; 238: 1566–1568.
12. Fraher LJ, Hodsman AB, Jonas K, *et al.* A comparison of the *in vivo* biochemical responses to exogenous parathyroid hormone-(1–34) [PTH-(1–34)] and PTH-related peptide-(1–34) in man. *J Clin Endocrinol Metab* 1992; 75: 417–423.
13. Everhart-Caye M, Inzucchi SE, Guinness-Henry J, Mitnick MA, Stewart AF. Parathyroid hormone (PTH)-related protein(1–36) is equipotent to PTH(1–34) in humans. *J Clin Endocrinol Metab* 1996; 81: 199–208.
14. Orloff JJ, Ganz MB, Nathanson H, *et al.* A midregion parathyroid hormone-related peptide mobilizes cytosolic calcium and stimulates formation of inositol trisphosphate in a squamous carcinoma cell line. *Endocrinology* 1996; 137: 5376–5385.
15. Wu TL, Vasavada RC, Yang K, *et al.* Structural and physiological characterization of the mid-region secretory species of parathyroid hormone-related protein. *J Biol Chem* 1996; 271: 24371–24381.
16. Kovacs CS, Lanske B, Hunzelman JL, Guo J, Karaplis AC, Kronenberg HM. Parathyroid hormone-related peptide (PTHrP) regulates fetal placental calcium transport through a receptor distinct from the PTH/PTHrP receptor. *Proc Natl Acad Sci USA* 1996; 93: 15233–15238.
17. Rodda CP, Kubota M, Heath JA, *et al.* Evidence for a novel parathyroid hormone-related protein in fetal lamb parathyroid glands and sheep placenta: comparison with a similar protein implicated in humoral hypercalcemia of malignancy. *J Endocrinol* 1988; 117: 261–271.
18. Fenton AJ, Kemp BE, Kent GN, *et al.* A carboxyl-terminal peptide from the parathyroid hormone-related protein inhibits bone resorption by osteoclasts. *Endocrinology* 1991; 129: 1762–1768.
19. Fukayama S, Tashjian AH, Davis JN. Signaling by N- and C-terminal sequences of parathyroid hormone-related protein in hippocampal neurons. *Proc Natl Acad Sci USA* 1995; 92: 10182–10186.
20. Burtis WJ, Brady TG, Orloff JJ, *et al.* Immunochemical characterization of circulating parathyroid hormone related protein in patients with humoral hypercalcemia of cancer. *N Engl J Med* 1990; 322: 1106–1112.
21. Martin JT, Moseley JM, Gillespie MT. Parathyroid hormone-related protein: biochemistry and molecular biology. *Crit Rev Biochem Mol Biol* 1991; 26: 377–395.
22. Broadus AE, Stewart AF. Parathyroid hormone-related protein: structure, processing, and physiologi-

cal actions. In: Bilzikian JP, Levine MA, Marcus R, eds. *The parathyroids. Basic and clinical concepts.* New York: Raven Press, 1994; 259–294.

23. Karaplis AC, Luz A, Glowacki J, *et al.* Lethal skeletal dysplasia from targeted disruption of the parathyroid hormone-related peptide gene. *Genes Dev* 1994; 8: 277–289.
24. Amizuka N, Karaplis AC, Henderson JE, *et al.* Haploinsufficiency of parathyroid hormone-related peptide (PTHrP) results in abnormal post-natal bone development. *Dev Biol* 1996; 175: 166–176.
25. Lebovitz HE, Eisenbarth GS. Hormonal regulation of cartilage growth and metabolism. *Vitam Horm* 1975; 33: 575–648.
26. Smith DM, Roth LM, Johnston CC. Hormonal responsiveness of adenylate cyclase activity in cartilage. *Endocrinology* 1976; 98: 242–246.
27. Jikko A, Murakami H, Yan W, *et al.* Effects of cyclic adenosine 3′,5′-monophosphate on chondrocyte terminal differentiation and cartilage–matrix calcification. *Endocrinology* 1996; 137: 122–128.
28. Takano T, Takigawa M, Shirai E, Suzuki F, Rosenblatt M. Effects of synthetic analogs and fragments of bovine parathyroid hormone on adenosine 3′,5′-monophosphate level, ornithine decarboxylase activity, and glycosaminoglycan synthesis in rabbit costal chondrocytes in culture: structure activity relations. *Endocrinology* 1985; 116: 2536–2542.
29. Koike T, Iwamoto M, Shimazu A, Nakashima K, Suzuki F, Kato Y. Potent mitogenic effects of parathyroid hormone (PTH) on embryonic chick and rabbit chondrocytes. Differential effects of age on growth, proteoglycan, and cyclic AMP responses of chondrocytes to PTH. *J Clin Invest* 1990; 85: 626–631.
30. Iwamoto M, Jikko A, Murakami H, *et al.* Changes in parathyroid hormone receptors during chondrocyte cytodifferentiation. *J Biol Chem* 1994; 269: 17245–17251.
31. Weir EC, Philbrick WM, Amling M, Neff LA, Baron R, Broadus AE. Targeted overexpression of parathyroid hormone-related peptide in chondrocytes causes skeletal dysplasia and delayed endochondral bone formation. *Proc Natl Acad Sci USA* 1996; 93: 10240–10245.
32. Jüppner H. Molecular cloning and characterization of a parathyroid hormone (PTH)/PTH-related peptide (PTHrP) receptor: a member of an ancient family of G protein-coupled receptors. *Curr Opin Nephrol Hypertens* 1994; 3: 371–378.
33. Abou-Samra AB, Jüppner H, Khalifa A, *et al.* Parathyroid hormone (PTH) stimulates adrenocorticotropin release in AtT-20 cells stably expressing a common receptor for PTH and PTH-related peptide. *Endocrinology* 1993; 132: 801–805.
34. Schipani E, Karga H, Karaplis AC, *et al.* Identical complementary deoxyribonucleic acids encode a human renal and bone parathyroid hormone (PTH)/PTH-related peptide receptor. *Endocrinology* 1993; 132: 2157–2165.
35. Smith DP, Zang XY, Frolik CA, *et al.* Structure and functional expression of a complementary DNA for porcine parathyroid hormone/parathyroid hormone-related peptide receptor. *Biochim Biophys Acta* 1996; 1307: 339–347.
36. Tian J, Smorgorzewski M, Kedes L, Massry SG. Parathyroid hormone parathyroid hormone related protein receptor messenger RNA is present in many tissues besides the kidney. *Am J Nephrol* 1993; 13: 210–213.
37. Urena P, Kong XF, Abou-Samra AB, *et al.* Parathyroid hormone (PTH)/PTH-related peptide (PTHrP) receptor mRNA are widely distributed in rat tissues. *Endocrinology* 1993; 133: 617–623.
38. Lee K, Deeds JD, Chiba S, Un-no M, Bond AT, Segre GV. Parathyroid hormone induces sequential *c-fos* expression in bone cells *in vivo: in situ* localization of its receptor and *c-fos* messenger ribonucleic acids. *Endocrinology* 1994; 134: 441–450.
39. Lee K, Deeds JD, Segre GV. Expression of parathyroid hormone-related peptide and its receptor messenger ribonucleic acid during fetal development of rats. *Endocrinology* 1995; 136: 453–463.
40. Lee K, Brown D, Urena P, *et al.* Localization of parathyroid hormone/parathyroid hormone-related peptide receptor mRNA in kidney. *Am J Physiol* 1996; 270: F186–F191.
41. Lanske B, Karaplis AC, Luz A, *et al.* PTH/PTHrP receptor in early development and Indian hedgehog-regulated bone growth. *Science* 1996; 273: 663–666.
42. Bitgood MJ, McMahon AP. Hedgehog and Bmp genes are coexpressed at many diverse sites of cell–cell interaction in the mouse embryo. *Dev Biol* 1995; 172: 126–138.
43. Stone DM, Hynes M, Armanini M, *et al.* The tumour-suppressor gene patched encodes a candidate receptor for *Sonic hedgehog*. *Nature* 1996; 384: 129–134.
44. Marigo V, Davey RA, Zuo Y, Cunningham JM, Tabin CJ. Biochemical evidence that *Patched* is the *Hedgehog* receptor. *Nature* 1996; 384: 176–179.

45. Vortkamp A, Lee K, Lanske B, Segre GV, Kronenberg HM, Tabin CJ. Regulation of rate of cartilage differentiation by *Indian hedgehog* and PTH-related protein. *Science* 1996; 273: 613–622.
46. Usdin TB, Gruber C, Bonner TI. Identification and functional expression of a receptor selectively recognizing parathyroid hormone, the PTH2 receptor. *J Biol Chem* 1995; 270: 15455–15458.
47. Gardella TJ, Luck MD, Jensen GS, Usdin TB, Jüppner H. Converting parathyroid hormone-related peptide (PTHrP) into a potent PTH-2 receptor agonist. *J Biol Chem* 1996; 271: 19888–19893.
48. Behar V, Nakamoto C, Greenberg Z, *et al.* Histidine at position 5 is the specificity switch between two parathyroid hormone receptor subtypes. *Endocrinology* 1996; 137: 4217–4224.
49. Usdin TB, Bonner TI, Harta G, Mezey E. Distribution of PTH-2 receptor messenger RNA in rat. *Endocrinology* 1996; 137: 4285–4297.
50. Silve C, Santora A, Breslau N, Moses A, Spiegel A. Selective resistance to parathyroid hormone in cultured skin fibroblasts from patients with pseudohypoparathyroidism type Ib. *J Clin Endocrinol Metab* 1986; 62: 640–644.
51. Levine MA, Aurbach GD. Pseudohypoparathyroidism. In: DeGroot LJ, ed. *Endocrinology*. Philadelphia: WB Saunders, 1989; 1065–1079.
52. Schipani E, Weinstein LS, Bergwitz C, *et al.* Pseudohypoparathyroidism type Ib is not caused by mutations in the coding exons of the human parathyroid hormone (PTH)/PTH-related peptide receptor gene. *J Clin Endocrinol Metab* 1995; 80: 1611–1621.
53. Fukumoto S, Suzawa M, Takeuchi Y, *et al.* Absence of mutations in parathyroid hormone (PTH)/PTH-related protein receptor complementary deoxyribonucleic acid in patients with pseudohypoparathyroidism type Ib. *J Clin Endocrinol Metab* 1996; 81: 2554–2558.
54. Ding CL, Usdin TB, Labuda M, Levine MA. Molecular genetic analysis of pseudohypoparathyroidism type Ib: exclusion of the genes encoding the type 1 and type 2 PTH receptors (abstract). *J Bone Miner Res* 1996; 11(Suppl 1): M483.
55. Schipani E, Kruse K, Jüppner H. A constitutively active mutant PTH–PTHrP receptor in Jansen-type metaphyseal chondrodysplasia. *Science* 1995; 268: 98–100.
56. Schipani E, Langman CB, Parfitt AM, *et al.* Constitutively activated receptors for parathyroid hormone and parathyroid hormone-related peptide in Jansen's metaphyseal chondrodysplasia. *N Engl J Med* 1996; 335: 708–714.
57. Yasuda T, Arakawa K, Minagawa M, Minamitani K, Niimi H. Jansen-type metaphyseal chondrodysplasia: examination of the PTH/PTHrP receptor by the RT-PCR (abstract). *J Bone Miner Res* 1996; 11(Suppl 1): S647.
58. Jüppner H. Jansen's metaphyseal chondrodysplasia: a disorder due to a PTH/PTHrP receptor gene mutation. *Trends Endocrinol Metab* 1996; 7: 157–162.
59. Wallis GA. Bone growth: coordinating chondrocyte differentiation. *Curr Biol* 1996; 6: 1577–1580.

DISCUSSION

Dr. Tsang: Would you expand a little bit on why the animals died?

Dr. Jüppner: As a result of the acceleration of mineralization of all the bones that are formed through an endochondral process, the rib cage is much more rigid, and we believe that because of this rigidity, air exchange cannot occur, and the animals die from asphyxiation. This has not been formally proven yet.

Dr. Tsang: But they die *in utero* too.

Dr. Jüppner: In the case of the PTH/PTHrP receptor knockout, that is true. We don't have the answer as to why they die. The time of death also depends to some extent on the genetic background of the mice. In some, one gets survival until birth, and some mice actually try a few attempts to breathe and then die.

Dr. Tsang: Could you say something about the other sites apart from bone in the Jansen model?

Dr. Jüppner: The three prominent sites where this abnormal receptor is functional are the kidney, the bone, and obviously cartilage, which leads to the severely impaired growth. Presumably the receptors are also important at other sites in the body, but we do not know yet what these other functions may involve and how they present in affected individuals. A possible clue may come from a family in which a mother and her daughter have the same mutation and therefore the same disease. The mother had problems breast-feeding the newborn, and because we know that PTHrP is very important in breast development it may well be that the problems with breast-feeding were related to this constitutively active receptor expressed in the breast, but that is speculation.

Dr. Tsang: What is the problem in lactation, no lactation or poor lactation?

Dr. Jüppner: Poor lactation, I understand.

Dr. Prentice: In the blots you showed there appeared to be relatively low levels of receptor expression in the breast. Was that a lactating mammary gland or from a virgin animal? The reason I ask is that there is a lot of PTHrP in the lactating mammary gland, so perhaps you could speculate as to whether it might have a local effect within the breast itself, or perhaps it is secreted into the mother's circulation to act on distant target organs—bone, for example—or even have a role in the suckling infant itself.

Dr. Jüppner: As you pointed out a lot of PTHrP is being expressed in the breast, in particular after the onset of lactation, and you may also know that PTHrP, when overexpressed locally in the breast, causes branching abnormalities of the ductular system. What happens with regard to PTHrP receptor expression with the initiation of lactation, we don't really know. The blots that I showed were from virgin animals. Presumably both the ligand and the receptor have an important role in the milk production or secretion.

Dr. Prentice: Is there any possibility of the PTHrP in the milk being absorbed by the infant and having a role in the body of the infant itself? Is it likely to survive the gut of the infant?

Dr. Jüppner: Gut closure probably doesn't occur until a couple of weeks after birth, so it is possible that significant amounts are being absorbed into the circulation of the newborn, and I think that in newborn calves this has been documented already, but nobody knows whether it has any biological role in that setting.

Dr. Guesry: Although there are many reasons for milk production deficiency, one could speculate that the PTHrP system could be responsible for the regulation of calcium in the milk, which is so important for the baby. Has anybody looked at the level of calcium in milk of these Jansen's mothers?

Dr. Jüppner: I cannot answer this question. But I think it is clear that PTHrP does have an important role on ductular differentiation within the breast. So overexpression of PTHrP under the control of breast-tissue-specific promoter results in severely impaired ductular differentiation and hypotrophy of the gland. It is conceivable that similar defects result from these constitutively active receptors, but I do not have any information as to whether there is an abnormal calcium content in the milk.

Dr. Pettifor: To take the issue of the Jansen's metaphyseal dysplasia further, is the actual bone histology that you see in the metaphyseal dysplasia typical of hyperparathyroidism? The radiologic features you show are those of widening of the endochondral bone, but you don't see the subperiosteal erosions that would be classical of hyperparathyroidism in a situation of PTH excess, as opposed to receptor turnoff.

Dr. Jüppner: In tetracycline-labeled bone specimens you clearly see increased bone turnover and also an increased number of osteoclasts, but you are right, you do not see these on plain x-ray films, so there must be a different homeostasis between resorption and formation, which starts during intrauterine life.

Dr. Pettifor: Have you an explanation for how the two mutations stimulate the receptor, as they are both intramembranous?

Dr. Jüppner: Again, we do not really know because the crystal structure of the receptor has not been worked out, and this will probably take several years. But the current model is that the receptor normally interacts with the ligand, and this interaction causes a change in the secondary structure of the receptor, which then allows this slightly modified receptor to interact with the stimulatory G protein. The hypothesis with regard to these mutations is that they induce the same conformational change in the receptor to allow it to interact with the G protein. The same hypothesis has been put forward for other activating mutations in other G-protein-coupled receptors, but of course this needs to be proven at some point. Interestingly, if you take these activated receptors and expose them not to the natural ligand, PTH or PTHrP, but to a truncated peptide that comprises only the residues 7 to 34, you can reduce the degree of constitutive activity, which implies that a ligand that is lacking the first six residues is good enough to bind to this mutant receptor and reverses the change in structural conformation. So I am pretty sure that there must be some shift in conformation.

Dr. Caverzasio: You mentioned that the functional role of PTHrP in the growth plate is to delay the entry of chondrocytes into the differentiation process. But when the PTHrP receptor is activated, bone length is reduced. This doesn't fit in very well with the concept. How do you explain that?

Dr. Jüppner: If you don't have any PTHrP or any PTH/PTHrP receptor, you end up with short limbs as a result of premature ossification of the growth plate. If you have activating receptors, or if you are overexpressing PTHrP under the control of the type II collagen promoters, you are inhibiting differentiation into hypertrophic cells, but you are also stimulating matrix production in the proliferation zone. Our current thinking is that this increase in the amount of cell matrix and the loss of cell-to-cell contact are contributing factors leading to growth plates that are less stable and prevent normal elongation from occurring; thus, both a lack of PTHrP and an excess of PTHrP can lead to a skeleton that is too short. You need the right balance between differentiation and inhibition of differentiation into hypertrophic cells.

Dr. Eisman: One of the interesting points that you made is that the PTHrP receptor is expressed in exactly the right place to be responsive to the PTHrP and to change the differentiation of the chondrocyte. How is that regulated? Are we now looking at one of the *Hox* genes?

Dr. Jüppner: Maybe not the *Hox* genes, but at a level below the *Hox* genes in the pyramid, where there are several different transcription factors. With the PTHrP receptor gene, the situation is fairly complicated in that it has several noncoding exons and, as far we know, two different promoters that are used for the expression of this receptor—one that is fairly specific for kidney and another that is probably expressed in all other tissues. So there may be a differential regulation of the receptor in kidney and bone as well as in the growth plate.

Dr. Mithal: Is there a lot of phenotypic heterogeneity in Jansen's disease? Or do you expect all patients to have similar mutations or similar types of mutations and similar clinical manifestations?

Dr. Jüppner: They certainly all have similar manifestations, and that is independent of the ethnic background. Patients in Japan or Singapore have a similar phenotype to those in North America or Europe. But it is striking that of the 12 patients whom we and others have studied up to now, ten—that is, the vast majority—have the identical H223R mutation.

Dr. Mithal: What about the regulation of PTHrP? Do you have any information presently on what regulates the PTHrP gene?

Dr. Jüppner: PTHrP gene expression is fairly complicated. There are at least three different promoters giving rise to at least three different gene products that are different in length, and on top of that you have quite extensive posttranslational processing giving rise to amino-terminal and C-terminal fragments.

Dr. Specker: I was wondering if you could speculate a little bit more about maybe the possible role of estrogen. Could that steroid be involved? The one person who lacked estrogen receptors did not have closure of the growth plates.

Dr. Jüppner: You are talking about this one male patient who grew indefinitely. At this point, I think it is too early to speculate whether estrogens have an effect on receptor expression in the growth plate. They do have an effect in bone-derived osteoblast-like cells.

Dr. Moya: In pseudohypoparathyroidism, are the mutations of the receptor similar to those in Jansen's disease?

Dr. Jüppner: Actually there are no mutations in the PTH/PTHrP receptor in pseudohypoparathyroidism type 1b. That was the disease where we initially thought that inactivating receptor mutations must be responsible. To elaborate on that, in pseudohypoparathyroidism type 1b, patients have only a single defect, and that results in impaired action of PTH at the level of the kidney. At the level of bone most patients have no resistance to PTH, and I currently believe that because of this lack of resistance at bone level, affected patients can have relatively normal blood calcium levels for prolonged periods of time. So in pseudohypoparathyroidism there are no inactivating mutations in the receptor, and the chromosomal locus has been excluded from being linked to the disease using large families with this disorder. I believe that the defect must be caused by a mutation in a factor, but one that is selective for regulating PTH receptor expression and/or activity in the kidney.

Dr. Alliet: In the Williams–Beuren syndrome, which is caused by deletion in the elastin gene and is mainly characterized by an elfin-like facial appearance, psychomotor retardation, and cardiovascular abnormalities, one finds impaired growth and transient episodes of hypercalcemia, especially in the neonatal period. Is something known about the underlying pathophysiological mechanisms, and if not, could it be a result of temporarily increased PTHrP secretion by residual fetal tissue?

Dr. Jüppner: I don't think that any of these possibilities apply. The locus of the Williams–Beuren syndrome is on chromosome 7, PTHrP is on chromosome 12, PTH on 11, and the PTH receptor on 3, so these three entities can be excluded from being responsible for the hypercalcemia. The calcitonin receptor is very close to the elastin gene locus on chromosome 7, but it is on a different cytogenetic band and so presumably a few million base pairs away from this locus. I therefore think that mutations in the calcitonin receptor could not be responsible for the hypercalcemia in this disorder.

Dr. Bonjour: I was interested in the experiments in which you show that PTHrP produced by the mother is important for fetal development. Could you elaborate a little about this role? Is it at the placenta level or at the bone level?

Dr. Jüppner: The issue arose because if you take out the receptor gene, you have a more severe phenotype than if you take out just the gene encoding the PTHrP ligand. Possible explanations for this are either that the mother is supplying the growing fetus with some PTHrP, and therefore you get a partial rescue if only the PTHrP gene is deleted, or that adjacent fetuses that share some of the membranes supply the deficient fetus with some of the ligand. This is only speculation at present.

Nutrition and Bone Development, edited by
Jean-Philippe Bonjour and Reginald C. Tsang,
Nestlé Nutrition Workshop Series, Vol. 41, Nestec Ltd.,
Vevey/Lippincott–Raven Publishers,
Philadelphia © 1999.

Calcium Transport Across the Placenta

M. Zulf Mughal and *Shahid M. Husain

*Department of Paediatric Medicine, St. Mary's Hospital, Manchester M13 0JH, United Kingdom; and *Department of Child Health, St. Bartholomew's and the Royal London School of Medicine and Dentistry, Homerton Hospital, Homerton Row, London E9, United Kingdom*

In all mammalian species that have been studied so far, the rate of calcium accretion in the fetal skeleton increases dramatically during the last third of pregnancy. The placenta, therefore, has the task of transporting large amounts of calcium and other minerals from mother to the fetus to meet this requirement. For obvious ethical reasons, our somewhat patchy knowledge of placental calcium transport comes mainly from animal experiments.

ACTIVE CALCIUM TRANSPORT

In late pregnancy, the concentration of total, ultrafiltrable, and ionized calcium in the fetal plasma is higher than that in maternal plasma; in the human, this maternofetal gradient is present as early as 20 to 26 weeks of gestation (1). It is likely, therefore, that active transcellular mechanisms are involved in the maternofetal transfer of calcium in order to overcome the concentration gradient across the placenta. This notion is supported by data from animal experiments in which the fetal circulation of the *in situ* placenta has been perfused and the maternofetal transfer of calcium measured. In the rat, Štulc and Štulcová (2) found that the maternofetal clearance of ^{45}Ca (37.4 ± 0.8 ml/min) across the *in situ* perfused placenta was much greater than that of inert, electrically neutral, hydrophilic molecules such as sucrose (2.6 ± 0.3 ml/min), which are believed to cross the placenta by passive diffusion. Using the same technique, Shaw *et al.* (3) found that the unidirectional maternofetal clearance of ^{45}Ca across the *in situ* perfused rat placenta was significantly reduced when the perfusate temperature was lowered (Fig. 1). Both studies reported that maternofetal placental calcium transport was significantly reduced when the perfusate contained cyanide, which suggests that placental calcium transport is dependent on placental metabolism (2,3) (Fig. 2). Using a method in which a human placental lobule is perfused *in vitro,* Štulc (4) has provided evidence that the transcellular component of maternofetal calcium flux across the isolated human placental cotyledon is saturable and sensitive to cyanide.

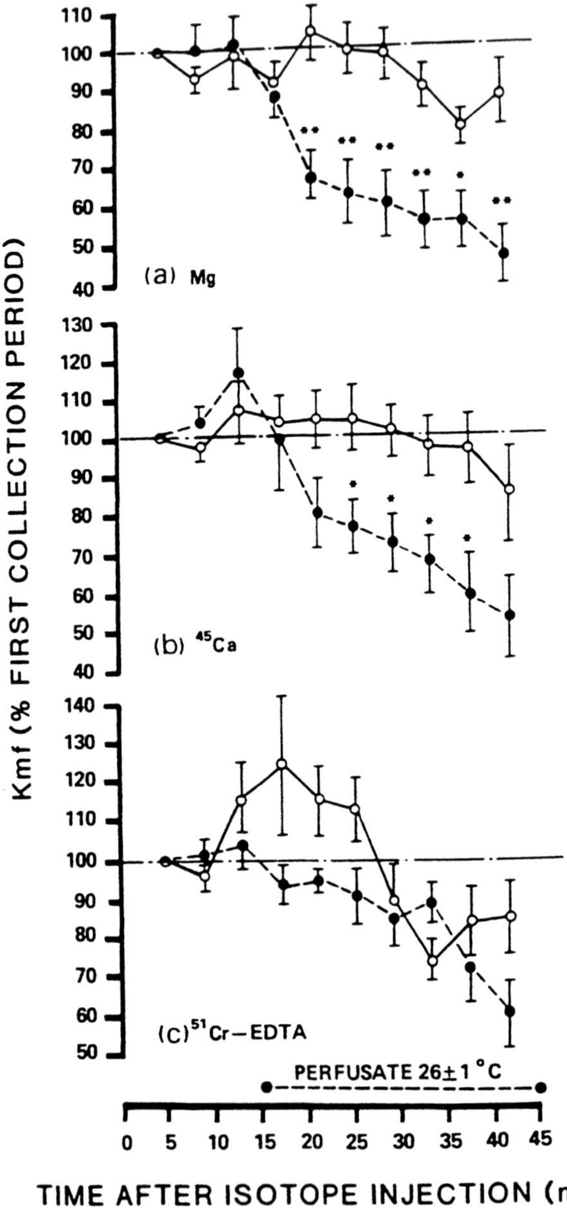

FIG. 1. Effects of addition of KCN (1 mmol/l final concentration) to perfusate fluid on maternofetal clearance (K_{mf}) of **A:** Mg, **B:** ^{45}Ca, and **C:** ^{51}Cr-EDTA across *in situ,* fetally perfused rat placentas ($n = 6$/group). Mean K_{mf} values ± SEM are normalized to that for the first 4-min perfusate collection period. Statistical significance between treated (●—●) and control (○—○) groups: $^{*}p < 0.05$; $^{**}p < 0.01$; $^{***}p < 0.001$ (Student's *t*-test, two-tailed). Reproduced with permission from Shaw *et al.* (3).

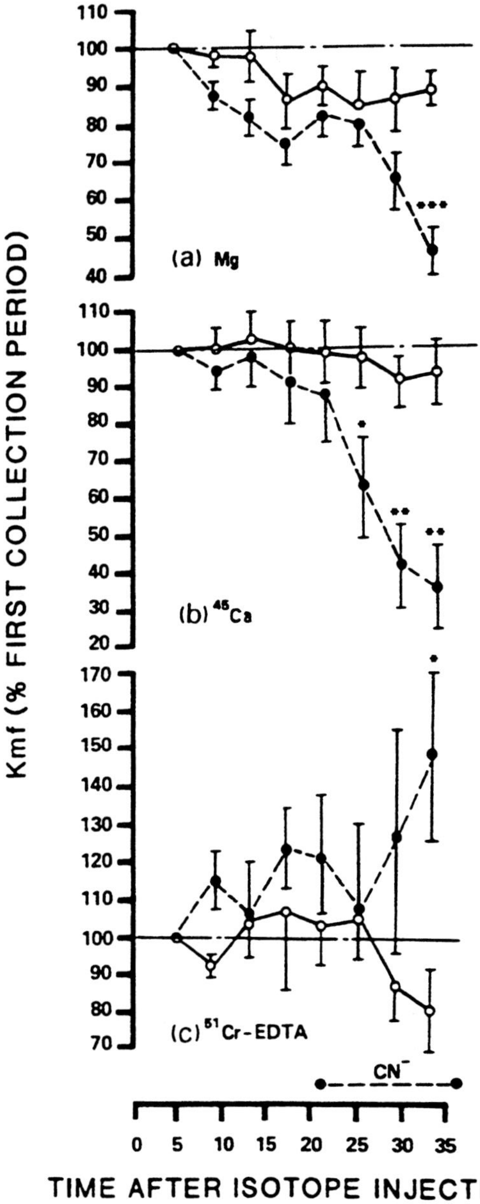

FIG. 2. Effects of lowering of temperature of perfusate fluid from 37 ± 1°C to 26 ± 1°C on maternofetal clearance (K_{mf}) of **A:** Mg, **B:** ^{45}Ca, and **C:** ^{51}Cr-EDTA across *in situ,* fetally perfused rat placentas ($n = 6$/group). Mean K_{mf} values ± SEM are normalized to that for the first 4-min perfusate collection period. Statistical significance between treated (•—•) and control (○—○) groups: $^{*}p < 0.05$, $^{**}p < 0.01$, $^{***}p < 0.001$ (Student's *t*-test, two-tailed). Reproduced with permission from Shaw *et al.* (3).

Thus, maternofetal transport of calcium across the placenta takes place against a concentration gradient, is temperature dependent, is inhibited by metabolic inhibitors such as cyanide, and is considerably greater than that of molecules that cross the placenta by simple diffusion. Taken together, these studies indicate that placental calcium transport involves active transfer processes by a transcellular route.

BIDIRECTIONAL PLACENTAL CALCIUM TRANSPORT

Placental transport of calcium occurs both in the maternofetal and fetomaternal directions. The algebraic sum of these bidirectional fluxes determines the rate of net placental flux. There is a marked species variation in the rate of unidirectional maternofetal and fetomaternal fluxes. In the sheep, at near term, Ramberg *et al.* (5) reported unidirectional maternofetal flux of 212 mg/kg fetal weight per day and unidirectional fetomaternal flux of 12 mg/kg per day. A similar situation probably prevails in the rat, as the value for the estimated net calcium flux (100 ± 4 nmol/min) between day 20 and day 21 of gestation (term = 22 days) is similar to the unidirectional maternofetal calcium flux (100 ± 7 nmol/min) on day 21 of gestation (2). By contrast, in the rhesus monkey, unidirectional maternofetal and fetomaternal fluxes are similar (390 mg/kg fetal weight per day and 325 mg/kg per day, respectively) (5). These fluxes are considerably higher than the rate of daily fetal calcium accumulation or the net flux, which at term has been estimated to be 40 mg Ca/kg fetal body weight per day (6). In the human, bidirectional clearances of calcium as measured across the perfused cotyledon are also similar (unidirectional maternofetal clearance = 40.9 ± 14.7 l/g placenta per minute; unidirectional fetomaternal clearance = 39.1 ± l/g per minute) magnitude (4).

MECHANISMS OF PLACENTAL CALCIUM TRANSPORT

In isolated placental cells, the cytosolic concentration of free calcium is reported to be in the nanomolar range (7). Therefore, the large traffic of calcium ions across the trophoblast poses a threat to normal cellular function, and efficient mechanisms for intracellular calcium buffering and translocation from the maternal facing cytosol to the fetal facing cytosol must exist. Although bidirectional movements may occur by diffusion through water-filled paracellular channels, asymmetric active transport requires a transcellular route. Very little is known about passage of calcium ions through the trophoblastic cytosol but is likely to involve three steps:

1. Influx of calcium ions from maternal plasma, across maternal facing placental membrane into the trophoblastic cytosol. There is evidence that calcium enters the trophoblast as a charged ion down an electrochemical gradient (8). This process is saturable (9), and therefore, it is likely to involve a specific carrier or a channel.
2. Movement of calcium through the cytosol without causing large fluctuations in the cytosolic calcium concentration. This may involve an important role for cal-

cium-binding proteins,[1] which may serve as an intracellular calcium buffer or an intracellular shuttle or both, facilitating transcellular calcium transport. There is a temporal relationship between calcium-binding protein mRNA expression and unidirectional maternofetal flux of calcium in the placenta of the rat (10). Intracellular organelles such as mitochondria, Golgi, and endoplasmic reticulum membranes may also serve as cytosolic calcium buffers and reservoirs in the placenta (8).

3. Efflux of calcium ions from cytosol across the fetal facing trophoblastic membranes to fetal plasma. In analogy with other transporting epithelia (for example, intestine), this step involves transport against a steep chemical gradient and therefore an energy-generating mechanism such as calcium- and magnesium-dependent adenosine triphosphatase (Ca-ATPase) is probably involved. Using a monoclonal antibody raised against the human erythrocyte plasma membrane Ca-ATPase (calcium pump) and immunohistochemistry, Borke *et al.* (11) have shown greater specific staining in the fetal facing membranes of the human and rat placentas. Furthermore, they also reported a 50% inhibition of calcium transport in fetal facing membrane vesicles from human placenta by polyclonal antibodies raised against the erythrocyte calcium pump. Present evidence suggests that the Ca^{2+}/Na^{+} exchange system does not play a role in transplacental calcium movement (2,8).

Finally, it is possible that calcium is transported across the trophoblast by endocytosis/exocytosis, that is, calcium uptake through formation of pinocytic vesicle at the maternal-facing placental membrane, which then travels through the cytosol to the opposite pole of the trophoblast, followed by fusion to fetal-facing placental membrane and release of calcium ions into fetal plasma. Although endocytosis is the major mechanism for IgG transport across the human placenta, there is no proof at present of placental calcium transport by this mechanism.

CONTROL OF PLACENTAL CALCIUM TRANSPORT

Factors that might influence the supply of calcium to the fetus include maternal and fetal plasma calcium concentrations, maternal and fetal blood flow, and the capacity and efficiency of placental transport mechanisms. As mentioned above, the rate of net placental calcium transport (or the rate of calcium accretion in fetal skeleton) increases rapidly during the last third of pregnancy. In the rat, the maternofetal clearance of calcium per gram of placental tissue increases 70-fold in the last 6 days of gestation (10), far more than could be expected by an increase in placental surface area or blood flow; uterine horn blood flow increases fivefold per placenta by day 21 of gestation compared to the virgin state (12). However, Mughal *et al.* (13) observed a marked decrease in the unidirectional maternofetal clearance of ^{45}Ca

[1] The term *calcium-binding proteins* includes a family of proteins involved in the transport and binding of calcium. We have not attempted either to describe these proteins in detail or to highlight differences in these proteins between species.

(but not of ^{51}Cr-EDTA, the reference diffusional marker) in growth-retarded rat fetuses induced by uterine artery ligation compared with that across placentas of control fetuses. We speculated that placental ischemia from chronic reduction in uteroplacental blood flow might result in depletion of the necessary energy supply for active placental calcium transport. Thus, transcellular active transport and not flow-limited transport is likely to be important for placental calcium transport.

THE INFLUENCE OF MATERNAL CALCIUM CONCENTRATION

There is indirect evidence from human studies that the maternal plasma calcium concentration may influence placental calcium transport. Maxwell (14) observed that in pregnant Chinese women, dietary deficiencies were associated with maternal plasma calcium concentrations as low as 1.0 mmol/l. These mothers gave birth to infants with congenital rickets, whose plasma calcium concentrations were around 1.6 mmol/l. Transient congenital hyperparathyroidism has been reported in infants born to mothers with hypocalcemia secondary to poorly treated hypoparathyroidism (15). It is postulated that under these conditions there is reduced net placental calcium transport, which leads to fetal hypocalcemia, and this in turn leads to fetal hyperparathyroidism. Conversely, transient neonatal hypoparathyroidism caused by untreated hyperparathyroidism has been reported in infants born to hypercalcemic mothers (16). Thus, in the pregnant human, placental calcium transport appears to be dependent on the maternal plasma calcium concentration. Furthermore, the placental calcium pump does not appear to be saturated even when the mother is hypercalcemic. Similar observations have been made in the guinea pig (17), pig (18), and rabbit (19); however, this is not the case in the sheep (20), cow (21), and rat (22). Thus, there is clearly a marked species variation in the fetal response to maternal hypocalcemia or hypercalcemia.

HORMONAL REGULATION OF PLACENTAL CALCIUM TRANSPORT

The placenta has no nerve supply. Therefore, the factors that increase placental calcium transport capacity as gestation proceeds must be either genetically preprogrammed or hormones produced by the mother, fetus, or the placenta itself. Hormonal signals controlling placental calcium transfer might act on either the maternal or the fetal sides of the placenta. Possible regulatory hormonal candidates include vitamin D, 1,25-dihydroxycholecalciferol (1,25-dihydroxyvitamin D, the biologically active metabolite of vitamin D), parathyroid hormone (PTH), parathyroid-hormone-related peptide (PTHrP), and calcitonin.

Vitamin D and 1,25-Dihydroxyvitamin D

There are anecdotal clinical reports of maternal vitamin D deficiency causing neonatal rickets (23), which is consistent with the thesis that maternal vitamin D may be important for placental calcium transfer. The presence of receptors for 1,25-

dihydroxyvitamin D in human and rat placentas (24) and calcium-binding protein in human (25), rat (26), and mouse (27) placentas supports the idea that this hormonal form of vitamin D might indeed regulate placental calcium transport. Potential sources of 1,25-dihydroxyvitamin D available to the fetus include that transferred from maternal plasma across the placenta (28), that synthesized by the fetal kidneys (29), and the placenta itself (30).

Animal experiments have provided conflicting data regarding the role of maternal vitamin D in placental calcium transfer. In the sheep, Durand *et al.* (31) noted that maternal treatment with 1α-hydroxycholecalciferol (which is converted to 1,25-dihydroxyvitamin D by the liver) for 12 days led to a significant increase in the fetal content of calcium as well as maternofetal calcium transfer. In contrast, Brommage and De Luca (32) did not observe any effect of maternal vitamin D deficiency on the maternofetal calcium gradient or the total fetal calcium content of the rat. Mughal *et al.* (33) found that the total fetal calcium content and the maternofetal clearance of ^{45}Ca across *in situ* perfused rat placenta were not affected by maternal vitamin D deficiency and thyroparathyroidectomy. Thus, it is unclear whether maternal vitamin D regulates placental calcium flux.

Fetal nephrectomy in the rat had no effect on the maternofetal total calcium gradient (34), although injection of a pharmacologic dose of 1,25-dihydroxyvitamin D (2 ng per fetus) into 19-day rat fetuses did increase the fetal calcium concentration on day 21 of gestation, compared with that in control fetuses (35). These studies provide only indirect evidence for the effect of fetal 1,25-dihydroxyvitamin D on placental calcium transport and do not rule out the possibility that this hormone may influence fetal plasma calcium concentrations by a different mechanism, such as by causing fetal bone resorption. The observation by Robinson *et al.* (36) that 1,25-dihydroxyvitamin D stimulates maternofetal calcium flux across *in situ* perfused placentas of rat fetuses parathyroidectomized by gross decapitation but not across placentas of intact fetuses supports a direct permissive effect of the hormone on placental calcium transfer. Because parathyroid hormone is an important trophic stimulator of 1,25-dihydroxyvitamin D synthesis, it is likely that parathyroidectomized rat fetuses have lower plasma concentrations of the hormone than intact fetuses. Therefore, 1,25-dihydroxyvitamin D probably stimulates placental calcium transfer only when fetal plasma concentrations are low to start with.

Ross *et al.* (37) observed a marked decrease in the fetal plasma concentration of 1,25-dihydroxyvitamin D following fetal nephrectomy in sheep, which was associated with reversal of the usual maternofetal calcium gradient. The maternofetal calcium gradient was restored by infusion of 1,25-dihydroxyvitamin D into the fetal circulation. It is not clear whether this finding represents evidence for control of placental calcium transport by 1,25-dihydroxyvitamin D synthesized by fetal kidneys or whether it represents the short-term dependence of fetal plasma calcium concentrations on mobilization from fetal bone. Moore *et al.* (38), using a similar experimental protocol, obtained identical results, but they also observed a rise in fetal plasma phosphorus concentrations following fetal nephrectomy, which was prevented by daily intravenous injections of 1,25-dihydroxyvitamin D into these fetuses. These investigators suggested that the fall in fetal plasma ionized calcium concentrations occurs as a result of fetal hyperphosphatemia following fetal nephrectomy.

Parathyroid Hormone

In the rat, fetal parathyroidectomy by decapitation leads to a fall in the plasma total calcium concentration, which is restored by administration of PTH (36). Similarly, in the sheep, fetal thyroparathyroidectomy with thyroxin replacement results in a precipitate fall in fetal ionized calcium concentration within 24 hours (39). As previously mentioned, Robinson *et al.* (36) observed a significant fall in maternofetal clearance of ^{45}Ca across the *in situ* perfused placentas of decapitated rat fetuses. The clearance was increased (but not returned to normal levels) by subcutaneous administration of bovine PTH(1–84) to the fetuses. This stimulatory effect of PTH(1–84) on maternofetal ^{45}Ca clearance may be caused by its direct action on the placental calcium pump or, alternatively, may increase fetal 1,25-dihydroxyvitamin D production. Perfusion of the fetal circulation of intact and decapitated rat fetuses with perfusion media containing forskolin (an activator of adenylate cyclase) stimulated maternofetal clearance of ^{45}Ca. However, synthetic rat parathyroid hormone amide [r(Nle^{8,21}, Tyr^{34})PTH(1–34)] had no effect under these conditions, and because this amide can also increase placental cyclic adenosine monophosphate (cAMP) release (40), the role of placental adenylate cyclase in calcium transfer is not clear.

Parathyroid Hormone-Related Peptide

The fetal plasma concentration of immunoreactive PTH is lower than that observed in maternal plasma (41). By contrast, in the rat (42) and human (41), the concentration of bioactive PTH in fetal plasma, measured using a cytochemical assay, was higher than in maternal plasma. Furthermore, Loveridge *et al.* (43) observed that extracts of ovine fetal parathyroid glands contained a substance in addition to parathyroid hormone which could not be neutralized by antiserum against PTH in a cytochemical bioassay. This substance reacted similarly to human parathyroid hormone-related peptide (PTHrP) in the bioassay. Based on these observations the authors concluded that fetal parathyroid glands were producing a second PTHrP like substance that acts functionally but not immunochemically as PTH. Using a radioimmunoassay based on an antiserum to human PTHrP(1–16), Abbas *et al.* (44) detected material resembling PTHrP in fetal parathyroid glands and placental membranes. Addition of fetal parathyroid extract or PTHrP, but not of bovine PTH(1–84) or rat PTH(1–34), to autologous blood used to perfuse placentas of thyroparathyroidectomized sheep fetuses *in situ* led to an increase in the rate of calcium accumulation in the fetal blood reservoir (45). These investigators suggested that fetal parathyroid glands produced an oncofetal peptide, similar to the hypercalcemic PTHrP expressed by some solid tumors, that stimulated placental calcium in this species. Recent work in the sheep (46) and the mouse (47) suggests that midmolecule fragments of PTHrP might be responsible for the stimulation of placental calcium transport. However, PTHrP has no effect on calcium transport by the rat placenta (40), which may reflect method or species differences.

Calcitonin

In sheep, Barlet *et al.* (48) showed that chronic maternal calcitonin deficiency achieved by maternal thyroparathyroidectomy and thyroxin replacement led to a significant increase in the total fetal calcium content and fetal accumulation of ^{45}Ca in late pregnancy. Calcitonin replacement in these ewes led to normalization of both the fetal calcium content and the maternofetal transfer of ^{45}Ca. Thus, in this species, maternal calcitonin appears to decrease the maternofetal calcium flux.

CONCLUSION

Our knowledge of placental calcium transport is rudimentary with many unanswered questions:

- What are the precise mechanisms of placental transfer and how are they controlled?
- How do these factors interact to satisfy the demand of the fetal skeletal mineralization?
- What switches on the increased rate of net calcium flux across the placenta during the latter part of gestation?

These are some of the issues that need to be addressed before a comprehensive understanding of fetal growth and mineralization can be achieved. Such knowledge is crucial because epidemiologic studies by Barker (49) suggest that poor fetal growth *in utero* is associated with a later increased risk of developing coronary heart disease, hypertension, and diabetes during adult life. Calcium accretion by the fetus is an important element of such growth. Growth *in utero* and during the first year may also have an important influence on development of low bone mineral density in adult life (50). Thus, it is plausible that factors influencing fetal bone mineralization, together with genetic factors, may affect the attainment of an adequate peak bone mass, an important factor in the subsequent development of postmenopausal osteoporosis.

REFERENCES

1. Forestier F, Daffos F, Rainaut M, Bruneau M, Trivin F. Blood chemistry of normal human fetuses at midtrimester of pregnancy. *Pediatr Res* 1987; 21: 579–583.
2. Štulc J, Štulcová B. Transport of calcium by the placenta of the rat. *J Physiol* 1986; 371: 1–16.
3. Shaw AJ, Mughal MZ, Mohammed T, Maresh MJ, Sibley CP. Evidence for active maternofetal transfer of magnesium across the *in-situ* perfused rat placenta. *Pediatr Res* 1990; 27: 622–625.
4. Štulc J, Štulcová B, Smid M, Sach I. Parallel mechanisms of Ca^{2+} transfer across the perfused human cotyledon. *Am J Obstet Gynecol* 1994: 170: 162–167.
5. Ramberg CF Jr, Delivoria-Papadopoulos M, Crandall ED, Kronfeld DS. Kinetic analysis of calcium transport across the placenta. *J Appl Physiol* 1973; 35: 662–668.

6. MacDonald NS, Hutchinson D L, Hepler M, Flynn E. Movement of calcium in both directions across the primate placenta. *Proc Soc Exp Biol Med* 1965; 119: 476–481.
7. Hellman P, Ridefelt P, Juhlin C, Akerstrom G, Rastad J, Gylfe E. Parathyroid-like regulation of parathyroid-hormone-related protein release and cytoplasmic calcium in cytotrophoblast cells of human placenta. *Arch Biochem Biophys* 1992; 293: 174–180.
8. van Kreel BK, van Dijk JP. Mechanisms involved in the transfer of calcium across the isolated guinea pig placenta. *J Dev Physiol* 1983; 5: 155–165.
9. Štulc J, Štulcová A. Transport of calcium across the dually perfused placenta of the rat. *J Physiol* 1990; 420: 295–311.
10. Glazier JD, Atkinson DE, Thornburg KL, Sharpe PT, Edwards D, Boyd RD, Sibley CP. Gestational changes in Ca^{2+} transport across rat placenta and mRNA for calbindin$_{9K}$ and Ca^{2+}-ATPase. *Am J Physiol* 1992; 263: R930–R935.
11. Borke JL, Caride A, Verma AK, Kelley LK, Smith CH, Penniston JT, Kumar R. Calcium pump epitopes in placental trophoblast basal plasma membranes. *Am J Physiol* 1989; 257: C341–C346.
12. Lasunción MA, Lorenzo J, Palacin M, Herrera E. Maternal factors modulating nutrient transfer to fetus. *Biol Neonate* 1987; 51: 86–93.
13. Mughal MZ, Ross R, Tsang RC. Clearance of calcium across *in-situ* perfused placentas of intrauterine growth retarded rat fetuses. *Pediatr Res* 1989; 25: 420–422.
14. Maxwell JP. Further studies of adult rickets (osteomalacia) and fetal rickets. *Proc R Soc Med* 1934; 28: 265–300.
15. Landing BH, Kamoshita S. Congenital hyperparathyroidism secondary to maternal hypoparathyroidism. *J Pediatr* 1970; 77: 842–847.
16. Jacobson BB, Terslev E, Lund B, Sorensen H. Neonatal hypocalcemia associated with maternal hyperparathyroidism. *Arch Dis Child* 1978; 53: 308–311.
17. Durand D, Dalle M, Barlet JP. Plasma calcium homeostasis in the guinea pig during the perinatal period. *Biol Neonate* 1982; 42: 120–126.
18. Care AD, Ross R, Pickard DW, *et al.* Calcium homeostasis in the fetal pig. *J Dev Physiol* 1982; 4: 85–106.
19. Graham RW, Porter GP. Fetal maternal plasma calcium relationships in the rabbit. *Q J Exp Physiol* 1971; 56: 160–168.
20. Bawden JW, Wolkoff AS. Fetal blood calcium responses to maternal calcium infusion in sheep. *Am J Obstet Gynecol* 1967; 99: 55–60.
21. Barlet J-P, Davicco MJ, Lefaivre J, Carrillo BJ. Fetal blood calcium response to maternal hypercalcemia induced in the cow by calcium infusion or by *Solanum glucophyllum* ingestion. *Horm Metab Res* 1979; 11: 57–60.
22. Chalon S, Garel J-M. Plasma calcium control in the rat fetus. II. Influence of fetal hormones. *Biol Neonate* 1985; 48: 323–328.
23. Park W, Paust H, Kaufmann HJ, Offermann G. Osteomalacia of the mother rickets of the newborn. *Eur J Pediatr* 1987; 146: 292–293.
24. Pike JW, Gooze LL, Haussler, MR. Biochemical evidence for 1,25-dihydroxyvitamin D receptor macromolecules in parathyroid, pancreatic, pituitary and placental tissues. *Life Sci* 1980; 26: 407–414.
25. Tuan RS. Calcium-binding protein of the human placenta: characterization, immunohistochemical localization and functional involvement in Ca^{2+} transport. *Biochem J* 1985; 227: 317–326.
26. Bruns MEH, Fausto A, Avioli L V. Placental calcium binding protein in rats. Apparent identity with vitamin D-dependent calcium binding protein from the rat intestine. *J Biol Chem* 1978; 253: 3186–3190.
27. Bruns MEH, Wallshein V, Bruns DE. Regulation of calcium-binding protein in mouse placenta and intestine. *Am J Physiol* 1982; 242: E47–E52.
28. Ron M, Levitz M, Chuba J, Dancis J. Transfer of 25-hydroxyvitamin D_3 and 1,25-dihydroxyvitamin D_3 across the perfused human placenta. *Am J Obstet Gynecol* 1984; 148: 370–374.
29. Fenton E, Britton HG. 25-Hydroxycholecalciferol 1α-hydroxylase activity in the kidney of the foetal, neonatal and adult guinea pig. *Biol Neonate* 1980; 37: 254–256.
30. Whitsett JA, Ho M, Tsang RC, Norman EJ, Adams KG. Synthesis of 1,25-dihydroxyvitamin D_3 by human placenta *in vitro. J Clin Endocrinol Metab* 1981; 53: 484–488.
31. Durand D, Bartlet JP, Braithwaite GD. The effect of 1α-hydroxycalciferol on the placental transfer of calcium and phosphate in sheep. *Br J Nutr* 1983; 49: 475.
32. Brommage R, DeLuca HF. Placental transport of calcium and phosphorus is not regulated by vitamin D. *Am J Physiol* 1984; 246: F526–F529.

33. Mughal MZ, Robinson NR, Sibley CP. Materno-fetal calcium (Ca) transfer across the *in situ* perfused rat placenta: relation to maternal 1,25-dihydroxyvitamin D (1,25D) administration (abstract). *Pediatr Res* 1987; 23: 433A.
34. Chalon S, Garel J-M. Plasma calcium control in the rat fetus. III. Influence of alterations in maternal plasma calcium on fetal plasma calcium levels. *Biol Neonate* 1985; 48: 329–335.
35. Chalon S, Garel J-M. 1,25-Dihydroxyvitamin D_3 injections into rat fetuses: effects on fetal plasma calcium, plasma phosphate and mineral content. *Reprod Nutr Dev* 1983; 23: 567–573.
36. Robinson NR, Sibley CP, Mughal MZ, Boyd RD. Fetal control of calcium transport across the rat placenta. *Pediatr Res* 1989; 26: 109–115.
37. Ross R, Care AD, Robinson JS, Pickard DW, Weatherley AJ. Perinatal 1,25-dihydroxycholecalciferol in the sheep and its role in the maintenance of the transplacental calcium gradient. *J Endocrinol* 1980; 87: 17.
38. Moore ES, Langman CB, Favus MJ, Coe FL. Role of fetal 1,25-dihydroxyvitamin D production in intrauterine phosphorus and calcium metabolism. *Pediatr Res* 1985; 19: 566–569.
39. Care AD, Ross R. Fetal calcium homeostasis. *J Dev Physiol* 1984; 6: 59–66.
40. Shaw AJ, Mughal MZ, Maresh MJ, Sibley CP. Effects of two synthetic parathyroid hormone-related protein fragments on maternofetal transfer of calcium and magnesium and release of cyclic AMP by the *in-situ* perfused rat placenta. *J Endocrinol* 1991; 129: 399–404.
41. Rubin LP, Posillico JT, Anast CS, Brown EM. Circulating levels of biologically active and immunoreactive intact parathyroid hormone in human newborns. *Pediatr Res* 1991; 29: 201–207.
42. Bourdeau A, Manganella G, Thil-Trubert CL, Sachs C, Cournot G. Bioactive parathyroid hormone in pregnant rats and fetuses. *Am J Physiol* 1990; 258: E549.
43. Loveridge N, Caple IW, Rodda C, Martin TJ, Care AD. Further evidence for a parathyroid hormone-relatedprotein in fetal parathyroid glands of sheep. Q J Exp Physiol 1988; 73: 781–784.
44. Abbas SK, Pickard DW, Illingworth D, *et al.* Measurement of parathyroid hormone-related protein in extracts of fetal parathyroid glands and placental membranes. *J Endocrinol* 1990; 124: 319–325.
45. Rodda CP, Kubota M, Heath JA, *et al.* Evidence for a novel parathyroid hormone-related protein in fetal lamb parathyroid glands and sheep placenta: comparisons with a similar protein implicated in humoral hypercalcaemia of malignancy. *J Endocrinol* 1988; 117: 261–271.
46. Care AD, Abbas SK, Pickard DW, *et al.* Stimulation of ovine placental transport of calcium and magnesium by mid-molecule fragments of human parathyroid hormone-related protein. *Exp Physiol* 1990; 75: 605–608.
47. Kovacs CS, Lanske B, Hunzelman JL, Guo J, Karaplis AC, Kronenberg HM. Parathyroid hormone-related peptide (PTHrP) regulates fetal-placental calcium transport through a receptor distict from the PTH/PTHrP receptor. *Proc Natl Acad Sci USA.* 1996; 93: 15233–15238.
48. Barlet J-P. Calcitonin may modulate placental transfer in ewes. *J Endocrinol* 1985; 104: 17–21.
49. Barker DJ. Outcome of low birthweight. *Horm Res* 1994; 42: 223–230.
50. Cooper C, Fall C, Egger P, Hobbs R, Eastell R, Barker D. Growth in infancy and bone mass in later life. *Bone and Tooth Society.* 1997; 56: 17–21.
51. Husain SM, Mughal MZ. Fetal calcium and magnesium metabolism. In: Tsang RC, ed. *Calcium and Magnesium Metabolism in Early Life.* Boca Raton: CRC Press, 1995.

DISCUSSION

Dr. Tsang: How relevant are the findings to the human placenta *in situ?*

Dr. Mughal: Once you deliver the placenta, you are dealing with a dying organ. However, histology of placentas that have been perfused does not show evidence of massive destruction, though perfusion could create artificial channels through the organ. All you can do is get some insight into what might be happening in life, but I don't think these experiments provide the true quantitative data on ion fluxes *in vivo.* However, there does seem to be a Ca^{2+} flux in both directions, and that has been confirmed *in vivo* in the rhesus monkey.

Dr. Klish: I was curious that there appeared to be no net accretion of calcium, at least in the human and maybe in the rhesus monkey. However, I wonder whether there might be an alternative mechanism. We know that in the human species, many other nutrients such as glucose and amino acids are first secreted into the amniotic fluid and then absorbed into the fetus through the fetal intestinal tract. Does this happen in the case of calcium, and could that be one of the reasons why these vascular flux studies seem to be somewhat in error?

Dr. Mughal: I think the amount of calcium that would be secreted in the amniotic fluid is very small, but I don't know whether it would be ingested by the gut *in vivo*. Massive bidirectional fluxes have been found for other ions as well, and this just shows that there is a flow of ions in both directions. It seems that a small, gradual accretion takes place in the human and human-type placentas in monkeys.

Dr. Seeman: Are there any diseases in childhood or adolescence that can be directly attributed to disorders of calcium flux, and if so, would these be primarily abnormalities of the skull, as I presume that is one of the largest or most rapidly growing organs during that time?

Dr. Mughal: I don't know of any. The reason we studied intrauterine growth retardation was that the studies done in Professor Tsang's laboratory showed that bone densities of IUGR babies were lower than those of appropriate for gestation infants. We wanted to find out whether placental calcium transport mechanisms were affected across the IUGR placentas. We did find evidence for that in the rat, and also in diabetic pregnancy, where maternal fetal calcium transport is also reduced. I am not sure whether this results in any adolescent diseases, but there is a lot of interest in osteoporosis. There are studies from Southampton, UK (49,50), that have shown that if you are lighter and grow poorly in the first year of life, your bone density when you finish growing tends to be lower. This suggests that there might be some kind of metabolic imprinting going on in the intrauterine environment, whether it be placental calcium transfer or other factors, that also perhaps continues in the first year of life and affects the acquisition of peak bone density.

Dr. Seeman: I guess you would expect bone density to be lower in premature infants because they are smaller. Was adjustment for bone size done in those children? Would they still have a low bone density?

Dr. Tsang: In infants who are small for gestational age, there are varying degrees of reduced bone density, depending on the size of the baby. Correcting for size blunts the reduction in density, but in severe cases it still seems to be reduced.

Dr. Guesry: According to studies you have reviewed, it seems that the fetus is in the driving seat with regard to calcium homeostasis. As you know, quite large numbers of babies are born with severely atrophic kidneys. I wonder whether anybody has looked at bone mass in those babies at birth?

Dr. Mughal: One study looked at babies with Potter syndrome (absent kidneys) and found that the level of 1,25-dihydroxyvitamin D in the circulation was very low. I don't think they looked at bone density, but the 1,25-dihydroxyvitamin D normally produced by the fetal kidney may well play an important role in regulating maternal–fetal calcium transport and perhaps in mineralization of the fetal skeleton.

Dr. Prentice: I was interested in your observation about the low bone mineral density in children born in Manchester to mothers who were seasonally vitamin D deficient. Could you give us some more information on the degree of vitamin D deficiency? There is quite a lot of pressure in the United Kingdom at the moment to remove the 10 μg (400 I.U.) per day recommendation that we make for vitamin D for pregnant mothers, and I just wondered if you would like to comment on that.

Dr. Mughal: We have studied only four mothers so far, but they were all very deficient, with 25-hydroxyvitamin D levels that were either undetectable or definitely less than 5 ng/ml. They had secondary hyperparathyroidism, and some of them were hypocalcemic, even allowing for the fact that calcium levels fall in pregnancy. In the United Kingdom it is suggested that all mothers during pregnancy with inadequate exposure to sunshine should be supplemented with 400 I.U. of vitamin D (10 μg), but in the large perinatal center where I work, which has a large at-risk population, hardly anybody gets supplemented. This is an area that definitely needs further study now that we have better technology to address the problem. These babies often have neonatal convulsions, and they occasionally have rachitic changes, including ping-pong-ball skull—you can actually depress the hypomineralized parietal bone with the index finger.

Dr. Tsang: Could you comment on phosphate transport in the clinical setting? Some studies in northern China have shown reduced phosphate in the cord blood, so maybe there is a phosphate transport problem, perhaps only because of hypophosphatemia in the mother.

Dr. Mughal: There is some evidence that the uptake of phosphate is saturable and may be under some degree of control. I recall that some studies were done 20 or 30 years ago where maternal phosphate status was manipulated in experimental animals, and this did seem to affect fetal phosphate indices.

Dr. Alliet: Are you aware of any maternal drugs taken during pregnancy that can directly influence the placental calcium?

Dr. Mughal: If you regard vitamin D as a drug, yes! I am not aware of any pharmacologic agents.

Dr. Schanler: Magnesium is used in pregnancy. What effect does that have?

Dr. Mughal: Magnesium transport is similar to calcium transport: it is actively transported but not saturated as treatment of preeclampsia with intravenous magnesium sulphate leads to hypermagnesemia in the newborn infant. Placental perfusion studies in the rat suggest that the sodium–magnesium exchanger system is involved in magnesium transport. There is no evidence of its control by maternal hormones. We have not been able to perturb magnesium transport by altering fetal or maternal vitamin D or parathyroid hormone status.

Dr. Pohlandt: Do you have any information about the time in human pregnancy when the gradient is built up between the mother and the fetus? I would suggest that the massive transport begins only when the formation of bones starts.

Dr. Mughal: The maternal–fetal calcium gradient is certainly present at 20 weeks.

Dr. Pohlandt: So we have first a gradient between mother and fetus, and the system on the fetal side may be saturated. Then when bone is formed, calcium is drawn into the bone, and the system is no longer saturated. Transport then has to be increased further to saturate the newly forming bone.

Dr. Mughal: That sounds like an interesting sequence of events.

Nutrition and Bone Development, edited by
Jean-Philippe Bonjour and Reginald C. Tsang,
Nestlé Nutrition Workshop Series, Vol. 41, Nestec Ltd.,
Vevey/Lippincott–Raven Publishers,
Philadelphia © 1999.

Phosphate, Osteogenic Factors, and Bone Growth

Joseph Caverzasio, Gaby Palmer, and Jean-Philippe Bonjour

WHO Collaborating Center for Osteoporosis and Bone Diseases, Department of Internal Medicine, University Hospital, 1211 Geneva 14, Switzerland

The main physiological function of the structure and shape of bone is to act as a mechanical support. This function is achieved by the mineralization of an extracellular matrix formed by specialized cells. Inorganic phosphate (Pi) is an essential element for the physiological functioning of osteogenic cells because it is an integral component of apatite crystal. Phosphate homeostasis is mainly controlled in the kidney by several regulatory processes that determine its concentration in the extracellular fluid (1–3). From this compartment, Pi is used for intracellular energy production in all cell types and for the mineralization of the bone matrix. Plasma Pi is higher during growth than in adult life, probably to match the increased demands of the growing organism for phosphate. The mechanisms responsible for adjusting Pi homeostasis during growth are not yet completely understood. They probably involve growth factors that also directly or indirectly affect bone growth. A major role of Pi for normal bone development is suggested by the impairment of bone growth and mineralization that occurs in physiological and pathophysiological conditions associated with low plasma Pi (4,5). The importance of Pi homeostasis during growth is best shown by X-linked hypophosphatemic metabolic bone disease, which occurs in both humans and mice. The disorder is characterized by impaired renal reabsorption of filtered phosphate, hypophosphatemia, inappropriate serum concentration of 1,25-dihydroxyvitamin D_3, and skeletal abnormalities including short stature, femoral and tibial bowing, rickets, and osteomalacia (6).

INORGANIC PHOSPHATE HOMEOSTASIS DURING GROWTH

During the development and maturation of vertebrates, selective regulatory mechanisms maintain the extracellular concentration of Pi at a relatively high level compared with that prevailing in the adult. This homeostatic process is probably essential to fulfill the increased Pi needs resulting from cellular growth and net mineral deposition in the skeleton.

Two important factors that positively influence the Pi balance of the organism during growth have been identified (7). First, a high tubular Pi reabsorptive capacity is thought to play a major role in the increased phosphate retention required for growth. Second, a raised plasma concentration of 1,25-dihydroxyvitamin D_3 (calcitriol) is also considered to be an important controlling element in Pi homeostasis.

The observation that both the tubular Pi reabsorptive capacity and the circulating concentration of 1,25-dihydroxyvitamin D_3 are stimulated during growth suggests the existence of a common factor regulating the activity of both variables. Among the factors that could either directly or indirectly be involved in the control of the tubular phosphate transport capacity and the metabolism of vitamin D during growth, growth hormone was obviously considered as the first potential candidate. In human and experimental animals, the administration of growth hormone increased both the tubular reabsorption and the plasma Pi concentration by a parathyroid hormone (PTH)-independent mechanism (8,9). This observation supported the view that growth hormone was involved in the enhanced tubular reabsorption of Pi during development. However, in acute animal experiments, growth hormone administration failed to stimulate renal Pi reabsorption within hours (10). Such a delayed response suggested that growth hormone stimulation of renal Pi transport could be indirectly induced by insulin-like growth factor 1 (IGF-1), the mediator of some of its anabolic effects.

The possible role of IGF-1 in mediating the stimulatory effect of growth hormone on both tubular Pi transport and 1,25-dihydroxyvitamin D_3 was tested in hypophysectomized rats (11). In these animals the very low concentration of circulating IGF-1 is associated with a decrease in the tubular reabsorption of Pi, decreased plasma 1,25-dihydroxyvitamin D_3, and hypophosphatemia. Chronic administration of recombinant human IGF-1, at a dose that restored the circulating level of IGF-1 and enhanced growth, increased these three variables (11). The IGF-1-induced stimulation of tubular Pi reabsorptive capacity was not associated with any significant change in the plasma concentration of calcium. It was also observed in the absence of parathyroid glands. From these observations, it was concluded that IGF-1 plays a critical role in phosphate homeostasis in relation to growth by stimulating Pi transport capacity and 1,25-dihydroxyvitamin D_3 production by the renal epithelium (12).

In addition to its renal effects on the tubular reabsorption of Pi and the production of 1,25-dihydroxyvitamin D_3, experimental evidence suggests that this growth factor is also involved in the regulation of bone growth. *In vivo* and *in vitro* studies have shown that growth hormone and IGF-1 have important regulatory roles in the rates of differentiation and proliferation of chondrocytes in the specialized region of long bones known as the epiphyseal growth plate (13). It has been suggested that local production of IGF-1 is an important mediator of growth hormone action at this tissue level. The IGF-1 also plays a role in trabecular and cortical bone formation. This factor can stimulate both proliferation and differentiation of cultured osteoblasts. For instance, it increases type 1 collagen synthesis, alkaline phosphatase activity,

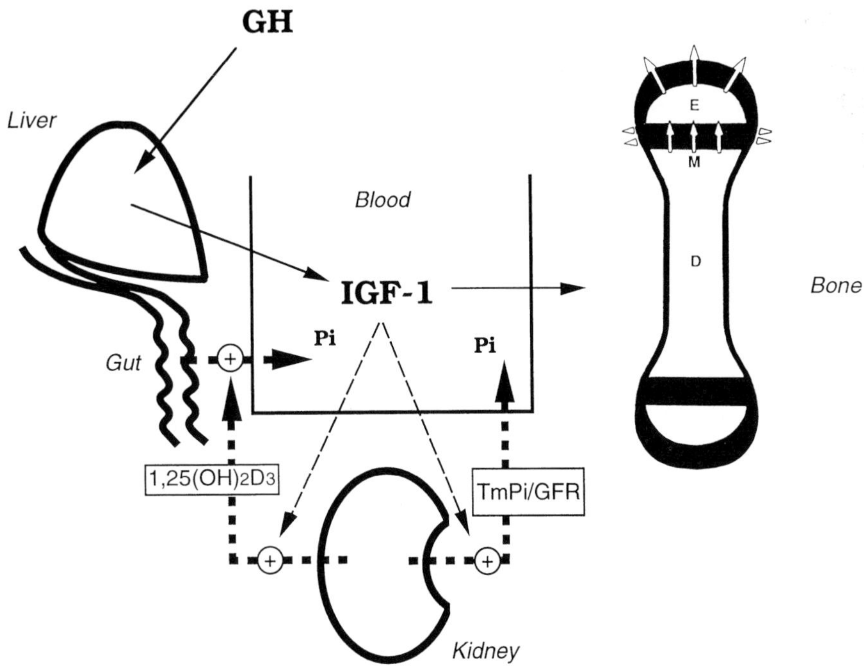

FIG. 1. Role of insulin-like growth factor 1 (IGF-1) in inorganic phosphate homeostasis. Two renal controlling elements, tubular inorganic phosphate (Pi) transport and 1,25-dihydroxyvitamin D_3 [$1,25(OH)_2D_3$] production systems, are positively influenced by IGF-1. By modulating Pi fluxes at renal, intestinal, and skeletal levels, IGF-1 represents an important factor in orchestrating essential events in inorganic phosphate homeostasis for bone growth and development.

and osteocalcin production. As depicted in Fig. 1, this information suggests that IGF-1 is an important factor in orchestrating essential events in Pi homeostasis for bone growth and development.

FUNCTIONAL ROLE OF INORGANIC PHOSPHATE IN BONE-FORMING CELLS

In vivo, a direct effect of Pi on bone metabolism has been difficult to assess, mainly because of alterations in hormonal factors with changes in plasma Pi concentrations. In organ culture experiments, however, it has been shown that Pi can directly affect bone growth, the production rate of collagen, and the mineralization of bone matrix (14). How Pi influences bone growth and the production of collagen by osteogenic cells is not known, but the mechanism whereby it participates in the process of calcification of bone matrix has recently been examined and the main aspects are summarized below.

Characteristics of Inorganic Phosphate Transport in Bone-Forming Cells

Several observations suggest that the availability of Pi at mineralization sites is not dependent merely on its concentration in the systemic extracellular compartment. Therefore, the possibility that osteogenic cells may participate in the transfer of Pi from the systemic compartment to the bone matrix was considered.

The mechanism by which Pi enters epithelial and other cell types is well described. The plasma membrane of these cells is equipped with Na^+-coupled Pi symport systems that are driven by the inwardly directed Na^+ gradient. A similar transport system has been described in bone-forming cells (15). Analyses of the characteristics of Pi transport in ROS 17/2.8 osteoblast-like cells suggested that the Pi carriers of these cells could be different from those previously described in renal epithelial cells. Essentially, the Pi transport activity was greater at acidic extracellular pH, probably because of a greater affinity of the transport system for Pi at low pH. This finding contrasted with observations on renal and intestinal brush border membrane transport systems, where acidic pH was shown to inhibit Pi transport because of a lower affinity of the carrier for Na^+ (2).

Regulation of Inorganic Phosphate Transport in Osteogenic Cells by Calciotropic Factors

It was first demonstrated that PTH selectively stimulates Pi transport in UMR-106 osteoblast-like cells. The cellular mechanism probably involves an increase in cyclic adenosine monophosphate (cAMP) levels, and the effect is not dependent on *de novo* protein synthesis (16). A positive correlation was found between the increased Pi transport and the cAMP response to various concentrations of PTH. In addition, the stimulation of cAMP by forskolin reproduced the stimulatory effect of PTH on Pi transport. These data provided the first experimental evidence that a major calciotropic hormone could regulate the handling of Pi by osteoblastic cells. It is interesting to note that the stimulation of cellular cAMP by PTH in kidney epithelial cells induces an opposite response. Understanding the mechanisms whereby PTH either selectively stimulates or inhibits Pi transport in bone and kidney cells, respectively, would contribute to an understanding of the cellular system involved in the regulation of the diverse effects of this hormone on different target tissues.

Insulin-like growth factor 1 is also a stimulator of Pi transport in osteogenic cells. This effect was first described in primary cultures of epiphyseal growth plate chondrocytes (17). The characteristics of Pi transport stimulation by this growth factor in osteogenic cells are similar to those reported in kidney cells. The signal transduction mechanism responsible for the stimulation of Pi transport by IGF-1 is not yet known. However, the recent observation in kidney cells that this effect of IGF-1 is mimicked by vanadate, a strong inhibitor of tyrosine phosphatases, suggests that tyrosine phosphorylation mediates the change in Pi transport activity (18).

Fluoride is another osteogenic agent that affects Pi transport in osteoblasts. In both UMR-106 and MC3T3-E1 osteoblast-like cells, fluoride selectively induced a dose- and a time-related stimulation of Pi transport (19). Recently, it has been reported that traces of aluminum markedly enhance the stimulation of Pi transport induced by fluoride, suggesting that a fluoroalumino complex might be responsible for the change in transport activity (20). The characteristics of the stimulation of Pi transport by fluoride are quite similar to those of IGF-1 in kidney cells. Analysis of the role of tyrosine phosphorylation in mediating this cellular response, using various experimental approaches, indicated that this signal transduction pathway is also involved in the stimulation of Pi transport activity induced by fluoride (20).

A fourth important growth factor of osteogenic cells, platelet-derived growth factor (PDGF), was recently found to be a potent stimulator of Pi transport in osteoblast-like cells (21). The essential signaling events responsible for this hormone response involved tyrosine phosphorylation of phospholipase Cγ and activation of protein kinase C.

Inorganic Phosphate Transport in Matrix Vesicles and Its Role in Mineralization

Matrix vesicles are small organelles with diameters of 100 to 200 nm that have been observed in mineralizing tissues and cultures of osteogenic cells, often in contact with initial mineral crystals. It is generally accepted on the basis of histologic evidence that matrix vesicles arise from bone-forming cells through a process of budding from the elongated tubular extensions that project from the plasma membrane of these cells (22). In some instances, calcified cartilage and woven bone seem to mineralize via matrix vesicles. The mechanism of matrix-mediated calcification is not yet fully understood. Several lines of evidence indicate that uptake of mineral ions by matrix vesicles from the extracellular environment is required for initiation of the calcification of these organelles. There is experimental evidence that matrix vesicles are endowed with a Na^+/Pi cotransport system (23). Analysis of the characteristics of Na^+-coupled Pi uptake in matrix vesicles established that these structures contain a Na^+/Pi cotransport system with properties similar to those of the Pi transport system present in the plasma membrane of bone-forming cells (Fig. 2). The role of Na^+/Pi cotransport activity in the initiation of matrix vesicle calcification was then investigated. Radioisotopic accumulation of Ca^{2+} and Pi by these organelles, determined in a synthetic lymph medium containing either NaCl or choline chloride, indicated that the presence of Na^+ was required for the uptake of Pi and Ca^{2+} by matrix vesicles. Furthermore, Pi accumulation in matrix vesicles preceded the accumulation of Ca^{2+} by several hours (Fig. 3) (23). These observations suggested an important role of a Pi transport system in matrix vesicles for initiation of matrix vesicle calcification.

Possible Functional Role of Inorganic Phosphate Transport in Osteogenic Cells

The notion that a sodium-coupled Pi transport system is involved in the initial events of matrix vesicle calcification, and the origin of these structures from the plasma membrane of bone forming cells, suggested that there might be specific processes through which these cells might control the initial events involved in mineralization of their extracellular matrix. Indeed, there is compelling evidence that osteogenic cells do not simply secrete extracellular organic molecules for the formation of a calcified matrix but actively participate in the control of these events. Among the various possible systems involved in the development of this complex function, the expression of Pi transport activity in matrix vesicles during the differentiation of bone-forming cells was investigated in MC3T3-E1 osteoblast-like cells (24). Phos-

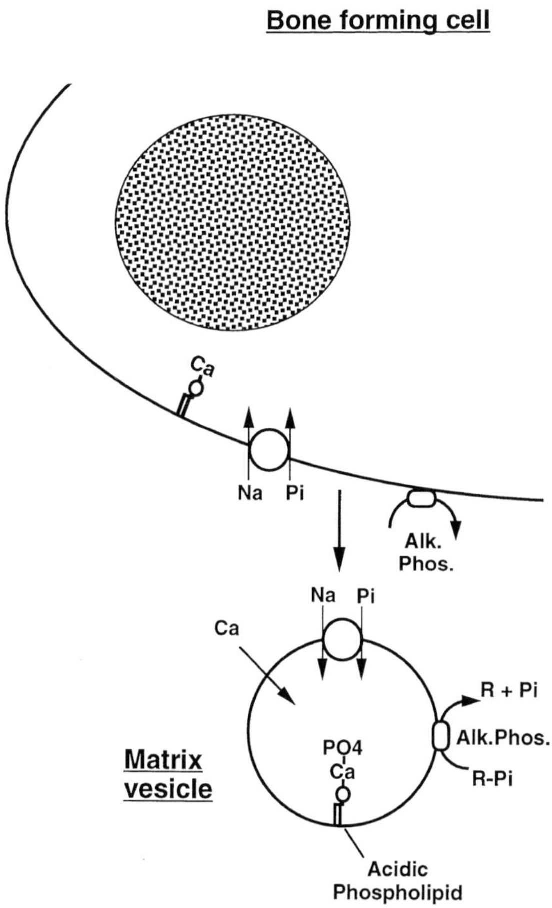

FIG. 2. Schematic representation of essential matrix vesicle elements involved in calcification and their origin from plasma membrane of bone-forming cells. Among these elements are Ca^{2+}-bound phospholipids, alkaline phosphatase (Alk Phos) attached to external surface of plasma membrane, and the Na^{+}-coupled inorganic phosphate (Pi) transport system that probably plays an important role in initial events responsible for matrix calcification.

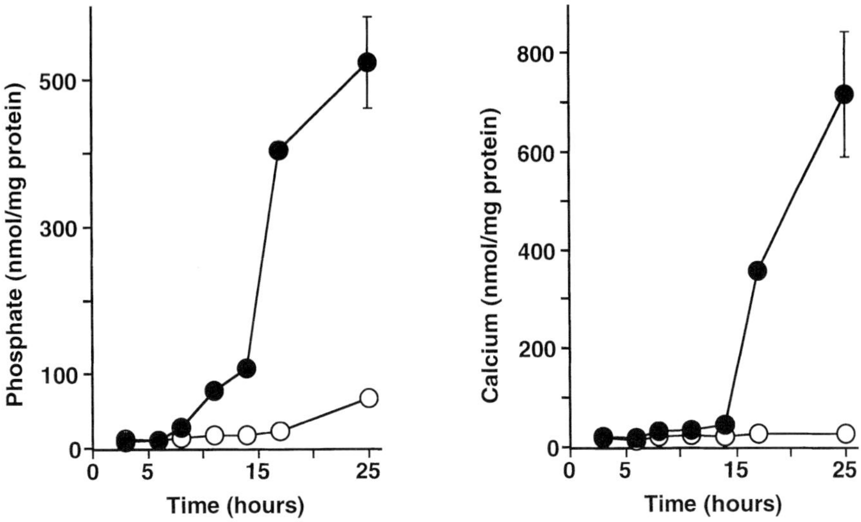

FIG. 3. Accumulation of inorganic phosphate (Pi) **(left)** and Ca^{2+} **(right)** in matrix vesicles isolated from chicken growth plate cartilage. In the presence of NaCl *(black circles)* in synthetic cartilage lymph medium, Pi first accumulates over several hours before rapid uptake of both Ca^{2+} and Pi. These events are not observed in the presence of choline chloride *(white circles)*. Data from Montessuit (23).

phate transport activity was found to be low in matrix vesicles released during the proliferative phase. During the phase of differentiation, which corresponds to the synthesis of a collagenous matrix, Pi transport activity in released matrix vesicles was significantly expressed. After completion of bone matrix formation, the activity gradually returned to initial baseline values (Fig. 4).

This observation strongly suggests that there is a specific mechanism for enhanced Pi transport activity in matrix vesicles released during the formation of the collagenous matrix. This could function either through enrichment of Pi carriers in released matrix vesicles or through the formation of specific matrix vesicles with a high Pi transport activity during that period of the differentiation process. In addition to this mechanism, the possibility that changes in Pi transport activity in the plasma membrane of osteogenic cells induced by calciotropic factors might be transferred to matrix vesicles was also considered. In the MC3T3-E1 experimental system, exposure of osteoblast-like cells to growth factors enhanced Pi transport in both the plasma membrane and the released matrix vesicles (24). These observations suggest that there is a process for insertion of active Pi carriers into the membrane of matrix vesicles. In addition, the number or activity of these transport systems in released matrix vesicles can be regulated by osteogenic cells (Fig. 5).

The physiological importance of this transfer of Pi transport activity from the osteogenic cell to the matrix vesicles in response to stimulatory factors remains to be explored. However, it is conceivable that during rapid bone growth, rate-limiting

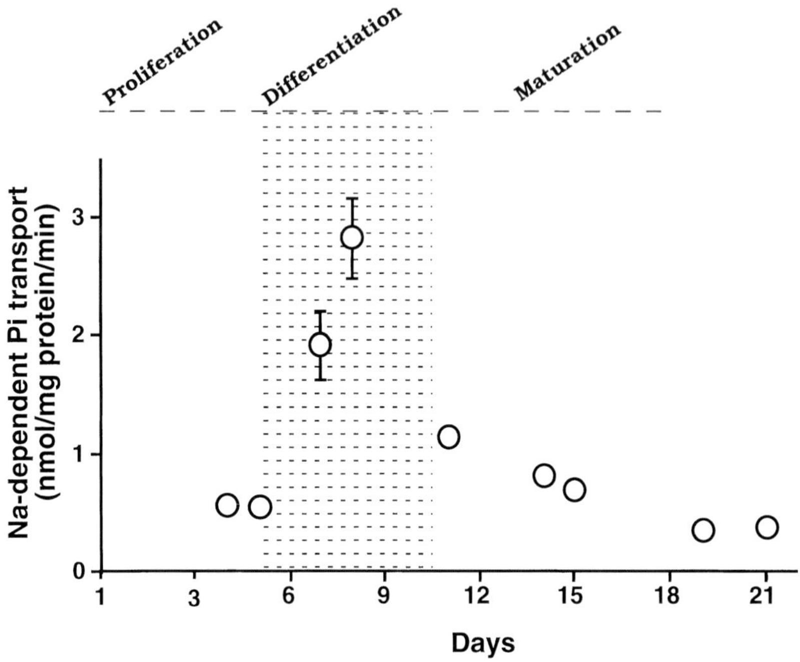

FIG. 4. Expression of Na^+-dependent inorganic phosphate (Pi) transport activity in matrix vesicles isolated from cultured MC3T3-E1 osteoblast-like cells. A low Pi transport activity is recorded during the proliferating phase. At time of cell differentiation, when osteoblast-like cells lay down an extracellular matrix, Pi transport activity is markedly increased, with a gradual return to baseline activity with time in culture. Data from Montessuit (24).

mechanisms responsible for initiation and development of matrix calcification could operate more efficiently. In this context, a higher Pi transport activity in matrix vesicles would accelerate initial events for Ca^{2+} and Pi accumulation and allow bone matrix mineralization to proceed more rapidly.

PERSPECTIVES

Recent work on the characteristics and the functional aspects of Pi transport in bone-forming cells and matrix vesicles suggests that, among the various processes responsible for the differentiation of bone-forming cells, the development of the bone matrix calcification is likely to be influenced by Pi. The activity of the Pi transport system in osteogenic cells can be regulated by several calciotropic factors, and change in Pi transport activity induced by growth factors is also observed in matrix vesicles. If alteration in Pi transport activity modulates the process of calcification in these structures, a relationship that remains to be demonstrated, one might speculate that this activity represents a mechanism whereby osteogenic cells regulate the calcification of their extracellular matrix. If this relationship can be demonstrated, it is likely that potential hormonal or local factors are involved in this regulatory process by acting on specific cellular mechanisms (Fig. 5). Important information is expected when the molecular structure of bone Pi transport systems becomes known. Significant progress has recently been made by the observation of a newly identified phosphate transporter/retrovirus receptor expressed in osteosarcoma cells and its regulation by IGF-1 (25). Finally, whether other important functions of bone-

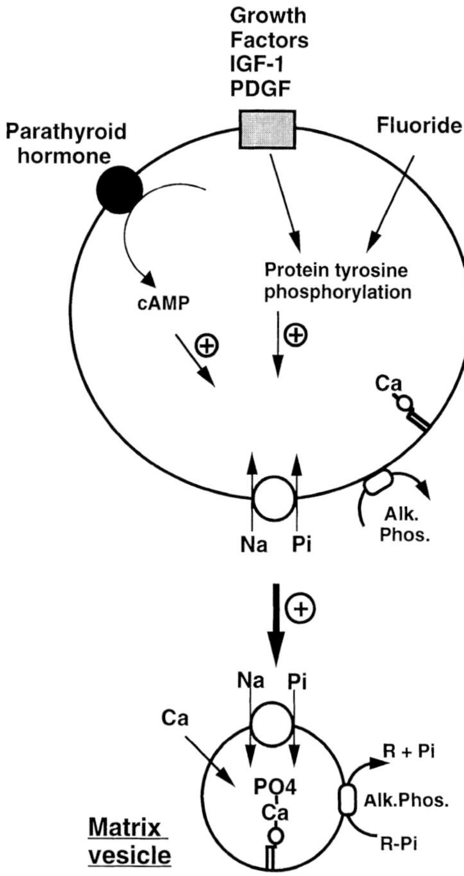

FIG. 5. Schematic representation of regulatory factors and their signal transduction mechanisms known to stimulate Na-coupled inorganic phosphate (Pi) transport in osteoblast-like cells. As mentioned in the text, experimental evidence has been obtained suggesting parallel regulation of Pi transport activity in the plasma membrane of bone-forming cells and in their derived matrix vesicles. Because Pi transport activity in matrix vesicles is probably important for accumulation of mineral ions, it is hypothesized that the regulation of Pi transport activity in matrix vesicles by osteogenic cells might play a significant role in the control of processes involved in the calcification of the bone matrix.

forming cells such as their responses to mitogenic factors or the formation of the bone matrix are also influenced by Pi are interesting questions which remain to be investigated.

REFERENCES

1. Bonjour J-P, Caverzasio J. Phosphate transport in the kidney. *Rev Physiol Biochem Pharmacol* 1984; 100: 161–214.
2. Murer H, Werner A, Reshkin SJ, Wuarin F, Biber J. Cellular mechanisms in proximal tubular reabsorption of inorganic phosphate. *Am J Physiol* 1991; 260: C885–C899.
3. Berndt TJ, Knox FG. Renal regulation of phosphate excretion. In: Seldin DW, Giebisch G, eds. *The kidney: physiology and pathophysiology, 2nd ed, vol 1.* New York: Raven Press, 1992: 2511–2532.
4. Albright F, Butler AM, Bloomberg E. Rickets resistant to vitamin D therapy. *Am J Dis Child* 1937; 54: 529–547.
5. Baylink DJ, Wergedal JS, Stauffer M. Formation, mineralization, and resorption of bone in hypophosphatemic rats. *J Clin Invest* 1971; 50: 2519–2530.
6. Rasmussen H, Tenenhouse HS. Hypophosphatemia. In: Scriver CR, Baudet Al, Sly WS, Valle D, eds. *The metabolic basis of inherited disease.* New York: McGraw-Hill, 1989: 2581–2601.
7. Caverzasio J, Bonjour J-P, Fleisch H. Tubular handling of inorganic phosphate in young growing and adult rats. *Am J Physiol* 1982; 242: F705–F710.
8. Corvilain J, Abramow M. Some effects of human growth hormone on renal hemodynamics and on tubular phosphate transport in man. *J Clin Invest* 1962; 41: 1230–1235.
9. Corvilain J, Abramow M. Effect of growth hormone on tubular transport of phosphate in normal and parathyroidectomized dogs. *J Clin Invest* 1964; 43: 1608–1612.
10. Westby GR, Goldfarb M, Goldberg M, Agus ZS. Acute effects of bovine growth hormone on renal calcium and phosphate excretion. *Metabolism* 1977; 26: 525–530.
11. Caverzasio J, Montessuit C, Bonjour J-P. Stimulatory effect of insulin-like growth factor-1 on renal inorganic phosphate transport and plasma 1,25-dihydroxyvitamin D_3. *Endocrinology* 1990; 127: 453–459.
12. Caverzasio J, Bonjour J-P. IGF-1, a key regulator of renal phosphate transport and 1,25-dihydroxyvitamin D_3 production during growth. *News Physiol Sci* 1991; 6: 206–210.
13. Caverzasio J, Theintz G, Ammann P, Slosman D, Rizzoli R, Bonjour J-P. Role of IGFs in bone development. In: Sizonenko PC, Aubert ML, Vassalli JD, eds. *Frontiers in endocrinology, vol 6. Developmental endocrinology.* Rome: Ares-Serono Symposia, 1994: 239–241.
14. Bingham PJ, Raisz LG. Bone growth in organ culture: effects of phosphate and other nutrients on bone and cartilage. *Calcif Tissue Res* 1974; 14: 31–48.
15. Caverzasio J, Selz T, Bonjour J-P. Characteristics of inorganic phosphate transport in osteoblast-like cells. *Calcif Tissue Int* 1988; 43: 83–87.
16. Selz T, Caverzasio J, Bonjour J-P. Regulation of Na-dependent inorganic phosphate transport by parathyroid hormone in osteoblast-like cells. *Am J Physiol* 1989; 256: E93–E100.
17. Montessuit C, Bonjour J-P, Caverzasio J. Inorganic phosphate transport regulation by chicken growth plate chondrocytes. *Am J Physiol* 1994; 267: E24–E31.
18. Caverzasio J, Bonjour J-P. Tyrosine phosphorylation selectively regulates renal cellular phosphate transport. Evidence that it mediates the stimulatory effect of insulin-like growth factor-1. *Endocrinology* 1992; 130: 373–380.
19. Selz T, Caverzasio J, Bonjour J-P. Fluoride selectively stimulates Na-dependent phosphate transport in osteoblast-like cells. *Am J Physiol* 1991; 260: E833–E838.
20. Imai T, Burgener D, Zhen X, Bonjour J-P, Caverzasio J. Aluminum potentiates inorganic phosphate transport induced by fluoride in osteoblast-like cells. *Am J Physiol* 1996; 34: E694–E701.
21. Zhen X, Bonjour J-P, Caverzasio J. Platelet-derived growth factor stimulates sodium-dependent inorganic phosphate transport in osteoblast-like cells via phospholipase C and phosphatidylinositol 3-kinase. *J Bone Miner Res* 1997; 12: 36–44.
22. Anderson HC. Matrix vesicle calcification: review and update. In: Peck WA, ed. *Bone and mineral research, vol 3.* Amsterdam: Elsevier Science Publishers, 1985: 109–149.
23. Montessuit C, Caverzasio J, Bonjour J-P. Characterization of a inorganic phosphate transport system in cartilage matrix vesicles. *J Biol Chem* 1991; 266: 17791–17797.

24. Montessuit C, Bonjour J-P, Caverzasio J. Expression and regulation of Na-dependent inorganic phosphate transport in matrix vesicles produced by osteoblast-like cells. *J Bone Miner Res* 1995; 10: 625–631.
25. Palmer G, Kavanaugh MP, Bonjour J-P, Caverzasio J. Expression of a newly identified phosphate transporter/retrovirus receptor in SaOS-2 osteosarcoma cells and its regulation by insulin-like growth factor 1. *Endocrinology* 1997; 138: 5202–5209.

DISCUSSION

Dr. Pettifor: Obviously this whole area of phosphate homeostasis is an exploding field. One group working in this field has been unable to find expression of the *pex* gene in the kidney. Does that not worry you in relation to its role in phosphate handling by the kidney? And what do you believe is the role of so-called phosphatonin? Do you believe in that substance or in the oncogenic phosphaturic factor that is produced from a lot of fibroblastic-type tissues?

Dr. Caverzasio: It is true that *pex* gene expression has not been found in the kidney, but Brigitte Ecarrot (Genetic Unit, Shriners Hospital, Montreal, Canada) has found it to be expressed in bone tissue in mice. This suggests regulation of this putative factor at the bone level: it would be activated if it is a stimulatory factor or inactivated if it is a phosphaturic factor. Because it has been suggested that this factor can circulate, I am not worried that it is not expressed in the kidney.

Many factors derived from the liver or from bone-forming cells have been suggested to be the phosphaturic factor. Until now there has been no critical analysis of these data.

Dr. Klish: Could you elaborate on the effect of fluoride on tyrosine phosphorylation, the effect it might have on crystallization, and whether or not that is the cause of fluorosis with fluoride overdose?

Dr. Caverzasio: We have found that fluoride probably interacts with a G protein mechanism. This particular G protein activates a tyrosine phosphorylation process, but we don't know yet which tyrosine kinase is involved. However, because fluoride interacts with a G protein, and it is well known that it can stimulate different G protein subtypes, it is possible that in addition to stimulating the right G protein, it may also activate other G proteins, leading to actions that are not specific for the stimulation of bone-forming cells.

Dr. Specker: Do you feel that phosphate in the diet during growth could ever be a limiting factor in bone mass accretion.

Dr. Caverzasio: At least in the studies that have been done with experimental animals, there has always been excess calcium and phosphate in the diets, so I cannot refer to those analyses. So far as human phosphate intake is concerned, Dr. Garabédian may be able to answer.

Dr. Garabédian: There are two examples of decreased phosphate in the human: one is the premature baby, who is prone to phosphate deficiency, which causes osteopenia, and the other is parenteral nutrition, where there is also phosphate deficiency, which causes bone problems. I have a question. How do you explain the fact that children or adults with hypophosphatemic rickets have increased bone density. They have osteomalacia, but if you measure bone mineral density, you find it increased, and if you look at x-rays you see increased cortical bone. Do you have any explanation?

Dr. Caverzasio: I have no explanation.

Dr. Gilsanz: I could suggest an explanation. Suppose for a moment that you have optimal bone with a certain degree of mineralization. Now suppose that you have increased osteoid.

Whatever the cause—rickets, hyperparathyroidism—you have poor bone. These children need more bone to be able to tolerate the stress and the load. So the fact that you have an increased bone mass is not against the concept that you could have decreased intrinsic mineral density. As a matter of fact, osteosclerosis is very commonly seen in older patients with renal failure.

Dr. Pettifor: I think the other issue is the problem of osteoclastic activity for bone resorption in a bone surface that is covered by osteoid. I don't think that you have the same amount of bone resorption that you have in normal bone, and therefore, there is an accumulation of bone plus osteoid. When you mineralize eventually, you will have an increase in bone mass.

Dr. Eisman: It is intriguing to me that the sodium phosphate cotransporter is one that was originally identified as a retroviral receptor. Was that originally defined in bone cells, or is it widely distributed?

Dr. Caverzasio: It is widely distributed in many tissues, including the kidney. We don't know yet whether it has a specific regulating function at the bone level.

Dr. Eisman: If it is a receptor for the retroviruses, is this just a cell surface protein that they can bind to and then subvert, or is it something to do with their sodium- and phosphate-transporting activity that is important to the retrovirus?

Dr. Caverzasio: No, because there are other transport systems, such as the amino acid transport systems, that also serve as receptors for certain viruses. Probably this is because they are well conserved and are always expressed to a certain degree, so the viruses have adapted to these molecules.

Dr. Mughal: In hypophosphatemic rickets, it is a puzzle that the lowered plasma phosphate concentration, which is usually an important stimulator for 1,25-dihydroxyvitamin D synthesis, is associated in these children with relatively low $1,25(OH)_2D$ levels. Is that a separate problem in this condition, or is it all linked with the *pex* genes?

Dr. Caverzasio: So far we don't know what factor regulates the expression of either $1,25(OH)_2D$ or renal Pi transport during growth. There appears to be a defect in both the expression of the phosphate transport system and the regulation of production of $1,25(OH)_2D$ in *Hyp* patients. But we don't know what mechanism is involved in this regulation.

Dr. Mughal: Isn't it interesting that one disease could have two defects: in the synthesis of $1,25(OH)_2D$ and in phosphate handling by the kidney?

Dr. Caverzasio: I do not think there are two different factors here. It is well documented that with growth you have increased $1,25(OH)_2D$ and increased renal reabsorption of phosphate. So we believe there is a common factor that regulates these two variables.

Dr. Jüppner: To expand on that a little, in tumor-induced rickets where you presumably have the circulating phosphatonin, you are secreting vast amounts of phosphate into the urine and at the same time suppressing the 1-hydroxylase; and in the X-linked type of phosphatemic rickets, where the *pex* gene is presumably defective and can't degrade the normal circulating levels of phosphatonin, you would expect the same defect. So as with PTH, which has multiple functions at the kidney level, we now presumably have a new hormone that on the one hand secretes phosphate into the urine and on the other hand suppresses $1,25(OH)_2D$.

Dr. Mughal: That doesn't explain everything because in tumor-induced hypophosphatemia, you get marked muscular weakness, whereas children with hypophosphatemic rickets have normal muscle function. The muscles seem to work very well in this condition, even with very low phosphate levels. This suggests that there are things going on at multiple levels.

Dr. Bonjour: From a study we did about 15 years ago (1–3), we were quite convinced that the defect was not a problem of the phosphate transporter but that it was a regulator of tubular phosphate reabsorption that was deficient, and this regulator could have a simultaneous impact on $1,25(OH)_2D$ production. The *pex* gene story fits in very well, in that you have a system like the renin–angiotensin system where there is an enzyme, an endopeptidase for the *pex* gene, that generates the product, which is a hormone that acts on the proximal tubule and stimulates both $1,25(OH)_2D$ and phosphate transport.

Dr. Pettifor: Do you believe that dietary control of phosphate handling by the kidney may be through the same mechanism?

Dr. Bonjour: Yes, because the hallmark of X-linked hypophosphaturic rickets is not reduced phosphate transport *per se*—you can increase phosphate transport in X-linked hypophosphatemic mice by just removing the parathyroids—but the fact that affected individuals cannot adapt to phosphate restriction. So I am sure that we will find that the *pex* product is involved in adaptation to the supply of phosphate from the diet.

Dr. Caverzasio: It is not so much the *pex* product, it is the phosphatonin.

Dr. Bonjour: It could be phosphatonin. Whatever it is, I would predict it would stimulate phosphate reabsorption.

REFERENCES

1. Tröhler U, Bonjour J-Ph., Fleisch H. Inorganic phosphate homeostasis: Renal adaptation to the dietary intake in intact and thyroparathyroidectomized rats. *J Clin Invest* 1976; 57: 264–273.
2. Mühlbauer RC, Bonjour JP, Fleisch H. Abnormal tubular adaptation to dietary Pi restriction in X-linked hypophosphatemic mice. *Am J Physiol* 1982; 242: F353–F359.
3. Bonjour JP, Caverzasio J, Mühlbauer R, Trechsel U, Tröhler U. Are $1,25(OH)_2D_3$ production and tubular phosphate transport regulated by one common mechanism which would be defective in X-linked hypophosphatemic rickets? In: Norman AW, Schaefer K, Herrath DV, Grigoleit HQ, eds. *Vitamin D, chemical, biochemical and clinical endocrinology of calcium metabolism.* Berlin: Walter de Gruyter, 1982: 427–433.

Nutrition and Bone Development, edited by
Jean-Philippe Bonjour and Reginald C. Tsang,
Nestlé Nutrition Workshop Series, Vol. 41, Nestec Ltd.,
Vevey/Lippincott–Raven Publishers,
Philadelphia © 1999.

Phosphorus Metabolism and Physiology in the Newborn

Ketan C. Mehta and Reginald C. Tsang

Department of Pediatrics and Pediatric Bone Research Center, Division of Neonatology, Children's Hospital Medical Center, The University of Cincinnati Medical Center, Cincinnati, Ohio 45267, USA

Phosphorus is an important constituent for mineralization of bone, for tissue structure and function, and for metabolism. The phosphorus content of human milk is exceptionally low compared with other mammalian milks (1); nonetheless, from all available evidence it is optimal for normal growth and mineralization of bone in human infants. In this review we summarize phosphorus metabolism in relation to phosphorus intake during infancy.

PHYSIOLOGY

During fetal life, the majority of phosphorus accretion occurs during the third trimester of pregnancy. After birth, the most rapid rate of phosphorus accretion occurs during the infant period (2). Total body phosphorus is divided into three compartments: (a) bone, which contains 89%, (b) skeletal muscle, which contains 9%, and (c) extracellular fluid, which contains the remaining 2% (3). Only 1% of total body phosphorus is in the blood in the form of organic ester phosphates, inorganic phosphates, or phospholipids. Serum concentration of inorganic phosphate, although not a precise reflection of total body phosphorus, may provide insight to phosphorus deficiency or excess.

Absorption

In early infancy, dietary phosphorus is provided largely by human milk, cow's milk-based formulas, or soy-based formulas. The phosphorus content of cow's milk formulas is generally lower (28 to 38 mg/dl) than soy milk formulas (42 to 51 mg/dl). In comparison, human milk contains significantly less phosphorus (14 mg/dl). Approximately, 59% to 90% of dietary phosphorus is absorbed (4). Most phosphorus absorption probably occurs by passive diffusion. However, there is evidence to support an active, facilitated diffusion process by 1,25-dihydroxyvitamin D (5,6).

Other than vitamin D, several factors may influence absorption of phosphorus. Total calcium intake may theoretically influence phosphorus absorption. Calcium is absorbed less efficiently than phosphorus; therefore, the presence of high calcium concentrations in the intestine may result in salt formation and decreased net phosphorus absorption. The presence of dietary phytic acids also interferes with phosphorus absorption. Phytic acids cannot be hydrolyzed by the human gastrointestinal tract; therefore, much of the phosphorus contained in phytic acids is unavailable for absorption. A small amount of phosphorus may be absorbed after the hydrolysis of phytic acid by colonic bacteria. The concentration of phytic acids is low in human milk (7) compared with cow's milk- or soy-derived formulas. Phosphorus absorption is high in human milk relative to cow's milk or soy formulas; soy formulas contain the highest concentration of phytic acids. The higher content of phosphorus in cow's milk- and soy-based formulas compensates for the lower absorption of phosphate in these formulas.

Excretion

Phosphorus excretion occurs through renal regulation. Serum phosphorus is filtered by the glomerulus, and homeostasis is maintained by variation in tubular phosphorus reabsorption. Parathyroid hormone (PTH) affects the renal clearance of phosphorus by influencing the rate of proximal tubular reabsorption. In the full-term newborn, phosphorus excretion may be significantly limited by the low glomerular filtration rate (GFR). The GFR rises from 32 ml/min per 1.73 m^2 at 1 week to 87 ml/min per 1.73 m^2 at 4 to 6 months of age (8). In infants, low GFR may result in increased serum phosphorus concentration and promotion of bone mineralization. The presence of lactose may also influence urinary excretion of phosphorus. The consumption of lactose-containing cow's milk formula compared to sucrose and corn starch hydrosylate formulas increases calcium absorption by an unknown mechanism but does not alter absorption of phosphorus (9,10). Infants consuming a lactose-containing cow's milk formula have a lower urinary excretion and increased retention of phosphorus (9). This enhanced phosphorus retention is most likely to be secondary to increased calcium retention rather than being a direct renal effect on the renal clearance of phosphorus.

HIGH PHOSPHORUS INTAKE, HYPOCALCEMIA, AND SECONDARY HYPERPARATHYROIDISM

"Late" (5 to 10 days of age) infantile hypocalcemia has been associated with the high phosphorus load in cow's milk-based formula compared to human milk (11,12). Infants fed cow's milk-based formula have been found to have hyperplastic parathyroid glands when compared to infants fed human milk (13). This most probably represents parathyroid hyperplasia in response to the high phosphorus intake during the neonatal period. Infants fed a standard cow's milk-based formula have low blood calcium and magnesium concentrations and high blood phosphorus and PTH concentrations compared to infants fed human milk (14–17). A study examining infants fed either cow's milk-based formula with calcium/phosphorus weight ratios equal to 1.2, 1.5, and 1.75, or human milk (with calcium/phosphorus ratio equal to 2.2) showed there was not a dose–response relationship between increasing serum calcium concentrations and formulas with increasing calcium/phosphorus ratios (16). However, there was a positive relation between higher phosphorus intake in the first 6 days of life and higher serum PTH concentration. We suggest that a high phosphorus intake rather than the calcium/phosphorus ratio may be responsible for the lower serum calcium concentration and higher serum phosphorus and PTH concentration in these term infants.

Despite a phosphorus content in modern cow's milk-based formulas that is lower than that in earlier formulas, the phosphorus content of most current cow's milk formulas is still higher than that of human milk (15,17). This may result in a secondary hyperparathyroid state and, theoretically, may disrupt mineral homeostasis and bone formation and turnover. Osteocalcin, a marker of osteoblast activity and bone turnover, was found to be lower in infants fed cow's milk-based formula compared to human milk at 2 and 6 months of age (18). We speculate that the lower osteocalcin concentration is related to high serum PTH, which can theoretically retard osteoblastic activity.

PHOSPHORUS INTAKE AND BONE MINERAL CONTENT

In general, bone mineral content is similar among infants fed human milk, standard cow's milk formula, or recent modified soy formulas during the first 6 months of life (19–21). The urinary excretion of phosphorus is higher in infants fed cow's milk formula or soy formula than in human-milk-fed infants (21). The higher urinary excretion of phosphorus most probably represents the higher total phosphorus intake of infants fed cow's milk formula. This supports the notion that current cow's milk or soy formula may have too high a phosphorus content, at least when compared to the gold standard of human-milk-fed infants.

There has been a recent trend toward the development of cow's milk formulas with a lower phosphorus content. A recent study performed at the University of Cincinnati Medical Center examined the effect on infant bone mineral content of low phosphorus compared to conventional phosphorus in term cow's milk-based formulas (22). At 6 months, infants fed on a low-mineral formula (Carnation Good Start, Ca = 430 mg/l, P = 240 mg/l) had a lower total bone mineral content than infants fed on a high-mineral formula (Similac, Ca = 510 mg/l, P = 390 mg/l). However, the value in infants fed on the lower-mineral formula was similar to that in human-milk-fed infants, and by 1 year of age there were no differences in bone mineral content. We suggest that, although a lowered phosphorus content in a cow's milk-based formula may result in a transient lowering of bone mineral content compared to a standard phosphorus formula, the resulting lowered value will be similar to the gold standard of the human-milk-fed infant.

HYPOPHOSPHATEMIA

Dietary phosphorus deficiency is unusual because the phosphorus content of cow's milk-based formula, soy formulas, and human milk provides sufficient phosphorus for the physiological needs of the full-term infant. In the preterm infant, neither human milk nor standard cow's milk nor soy-based formula supplies sufficient phosphorus and calcium for the mineralization of bone (23). Rickets of prematurity occurs because of an insufficient intake of phosphorus and calcium, resulting in decreased linear growth (24). Hypophosphatemia, hypercalcemia, hypophosphaturia, and hypercalciuria are salient features in very-low-birth-weight infants with rickets of prematurity, especially in those fed human milk (25). The clinical findings are consistent with a phosphate deficiency condition. This metabolic derangement of phosphorus and calcium homeostasis may be alleviated, in part, by feeding the preterm infant human milk fortified with phosphorus and calcium or a preterm cow's milk-based formula with higher phosphorus and calcium content than term cow's milk-based formula (26).

In the full-term infant, hypophosphatemia and rickets may occur as a result of vitamin D deficiency, renal tubular acidosis, Fanconi's syndrome, or familial hypophosphatemia. The common feature of these diseases is an inordinately high renal clearance of phosphorus, resulting in total body phosphorus depletion. Clinically, severe hypophosphatemia may manifest itself as anemia, bone pain, fatigue, or ataxia.

OTHER METABOLIC EFFECTS OF ALTERATIONS IN PHOSPHATE INTAKE

A high dietary phosphorus intake may theoretically result in the development of metabolic acidosis because of the newborn infant's low renal capacity to excrete acid in association with a high urinary phosphorus (1). In addition, a low phosphorus intake promotes a low residual phosphorus content in the large intestine, as occurs in human-milk-fed infants (1). A low phosphorus in the intestinal environment is thought to retard mutarotation of β-lactose to α-lactose; the increased concentration of β-lactose reaching the colon is associated with the proliferation of bifidus bacteria, which produce short-chain organic acids and a low stool pH (1,25). Low stool pH decreases the proliferation of pathogenic bacteria and might decrease the risk of infective gastroenteritis (27,28).

CONCLUSIONS

Human milk provides sufficient phosphorus for growth and bone mineralization. Historically, "humanized" cow's milk formulas have been created to simulate human milk. However, the phosphorus content of cow's milk-based formulas may still be unduly high in relation to physiological needs. If human milk is chosen as the gold standard with regard to infant feeding, then a lower-phosphorus-containing cow's milk-based formula may be prudent to maintain a phosphorus homeostasis similar to that observed in human-milk-fed infants.

REFERENCES

1. Manz F. Why is the phosphorus content of human milk exceptionally low? *Monatsschr Kinderheilkd* 1992; 140 (Suppl): 35S–39S.
2. Trotter M, Hixon BB. Sequential changes in weight, density, and percentage ash weight of human skeletons from early fetal period through old age. *Anat Rec* 1974; 179: 1–18.
3. Bainbridge RR, Koo WWK, Tsang RC. Neonatal calcium and phosphorus disorders. In: Lifshitz F, ed. *Pediatric Endocrinology*. New York: Marcel Dekker, 1996: 473–496.
4. Ziegler EE, Fomon SJ. Lactose enhances mineral absorption in infancy. *J Pediatr Gastroenterol Nutr* 1983; 2: 228–294.
5. Chen TC, Castillo L, Korycka-Dahl, DeLuca HF. Role of vitamin D metabolites in phosphate transport of rat intestine. *J Nutr* 1974; 104: 1056–1060.
6. Cramer CF. Progress and rate of absorption of radiophosphorus through the intestinal tract of rats. *Can J Biochem Physiol* 1961; 39: 499–503.
7. Williams ML, Rose CS, Morrow G, Sloan SE, Barness LA. Calcium and fat absorption in neonatal period. *Am J Clin Nutr* 1970; 23: 1322–1330.
8. Brodehl J, Gellissen K, Weber H-P. Postnatal development of tubular phosphate reabsorption. *Clin Nephrol* 1982; 17: 163–171.
9. Ziegler EE, Fomon SJ. Lactose enhances mineral absorption in infancy. *J Pediatr Gastroenterol Nutr* 1983; 2: 228–294.
10. Moya M, Cortes E, Ballest MI, Vento M, Juste M. Short-term polycose substitution for lactose reduces calcium absorption in healthy term babies. *J Pediatr Gastroenterol Nutr* 1992; 14: 57–61.
11. Bakwin H. Tetany in newborn infants. *Am J Dis Child* 1937; 54: 1211–1226.
12. Gittleman IF, Pincus JB. Influence of diet on occurrence of hyperphosphatemia in newborn infants. *Pediatrics* 1951; 8: 778–787.
13. Gardner LI. Tetany and parathyroid hyperplasia in the newborn infant: influence of dietary phosphate load. *Pediatrics* 1952; 9: 534.
14. Greer FR, Tsang RC, Lein RS, Searcy JE, Wu R, Steichen JJ. Increasing serum calcium and magnesium concentrations in breast-fed infants: longitudinal studies of minerals in human milk and in sera of nursing mothers and their infants. *J Pediatr* 1982; 100: 59–64.
15. Specker BL, Lichtenstein P, Mimouni F, Gormley C, Tsang RC. Calcium-regulating hormones and minerals from birth to 18 months of age: a cross-sectional study. II. Effects of sex, race, age, season and diet on serum minerals, parathyroid hormone, and calcitonin. *Pediatrics* 1986; 77: 891–896.
16. Specker BL, Tsang RC, Ho ML, Landi TM, Gratton TL. Low serum calcium and high parathyroid hormone levels in neonates fed humanized cow's milk based formula. *Am J Dis Child* 1991; 145: 941–945.
17. Venkatamaran PS, Tsang RC, Greer FR, Noguchi A, Laskarzewsky P. Late infantile tetany and secondary hyperparathyroidism in infants fed humanized cow's milk formulas: longitudinal follow-up. *Am J Dis Child* 1985; 139: 664–668.
18. Michaelsen KF, Johansen JS, Samuelson G, Price PA, Christiansen C. Serum bone-carboxyglutamic acid protein in a longitudinal study of infants: lower values in formula-fed infants. *Pediatr Res* 1992; 341: 401–405.
19. Greer FR, Searcy JE, Levin RS, Steichen JJ, Asch PS, Tsang RC. Bone mineral content and serum 25-hydroxyvitamin D concentration in breast-fed infants with and without supplemental vitamin D. *J Pediatr* 1981; 98: 696.
20. Steichen JJ, Tsang RC. Bone mineralization and growth in term infants fed soy-based or cow's milk based formula. *J Pediatr* 1987; 110: 687.
21. Hilman LS, Chow W, Salmons SS, Weaver E, Erickson M, Hansen J. Vitamin D metabolism, mineral homeostasis, and bone mineralization in term infants fed human milk, cow's milk-based formula, or soy-based formula. *J Pediatr* 1988; 112: 864–874.
22. Specker BL, Beck A, Kelkwarf H, Ho M. Randomized trial of varying mineral intake on total body bone mineral accretion during the first year of life. *Pediatrics* 1997; 99(6): e12.
23. Steichen JJ, Gratton TL, Tsang RC. Osteopenia of prematurity: the cause and possible treatment. *J Pediatr* 1980; 96: 528–534.

24. Lucas A, Brooke OG, Baker BA, Bishop N, Morley R. High alkaline phosphatase activity and growth in preterm neonates. *Arch Dis Child* 1989; 64: 902–909.
25. Koo WWK, Tsang RC. Calcium, magnesium, phosphorus, and vitamin D. In: Tsang RC, Lucas A, Uauy R, Zlotkin S, eds. *Nutritional needs of the preterm infant.* Baltimore: Williams & Wilkins, 1993: 135–155.
26. Langhendries JP, Detry J, Van Hees J, *et al.* Effect of a fermented infant formula containing viable bifidobacteria on the fecal flora composition and pH of healthy full-term infants. *J Pediatr Gastroenterol Nutr* 1995; 21: 177–181.
27. Jason JM, Nieburg P, Marks JS. Mortality and infectious disease associated with infant feeding practices in developing countries. *Pediatrics* 1984; 74 (Suppl): 702–707.
28. Howie PW, Forsyth JS, Ogston SA, Clark A, du V Florey C. Protective effect of breast feeding against infection. *Br Med J* 1990; 300: 11–16.

DISCUSSION

Dr. Guesry: In spite of what you say, I must remind you that for the past 10 years the Nestlé infant formulas have been low in phosphate, with a level of phosphorus that is not two or three times higher than in human milk but only 50% higher, and they have a calcium-to-phosphorus ratio of 1.8, not 1.3 to 1.5.

Dr. Tsang: I am in favor of that.

Dr. Haschke: The last picture that you showed referred to the increased calcium excretion in the urine, and you interpreted this as a tubular defect, or did I misunderstand you?

Dr. Tsang: In at least some physiological studies of phosphate depletion, there does appear to be a tubular defect in terms of calcium reabsorption.

Dr. Haschke: But if we need to incorporate calcium and phosphorus into the bone, it must always be in a 2:1 ratio. If there is not enough phosphorus, calcium has to be lost. This is surely a regulatory mechanism, not really a defect.

Dr. Tsang: It is a regulatory issue. I don't mean that it is a genetic defect. And of course, part of the problem is that there is hypercalcemia, which is an adaptive phenomenon, so you have losses with that as well.

Dr. Marini: You showed that phosphate concentration diminishes in the breast milk in the first week and later, but the increase in the milk intake of the baby should compensate for the lower levels of phosphate.

Dr. Tsang: There is partial compensation, but if you calculate from typical intakes, there is still a progressive decrease in phosphorus intake, especially relative to the weight of the baby.

Dr. Eisman: The implication of what you are saying is that all the phosphate is going into the bone, but of course a lot of it is going into growing muscle and other tissues. Is it possible, particularly for the preterm infant, where we really don't have a gold standard, to try to calculate what is necessary for the growth of the soft tissues as well?

Dr. Tsang: I think so. Ricardo Uauy did a series of studies in which he made those calculations. They are, of course, extrapolated guesses, and you would have to factor a certain amount that would go into soft tissue on that basis. The general message is, I think it is not much affected, even after that calculation; but I agree one really should calculate the soft tissue growth as well.

Dr. Prentice: I wonder if you would like to speculate on what might be happening in the African situation. In The Gambia and Zaire, the phosphorus levels in breast milk remain at about 16 mg/100 ml right through to 2 years of lactation, whereas the calcium content falls, so the ratio (mg/mg) falls from about 1.6 down to 1.0 by about 6 months of lactation. I wonder what you think might be happening at the biological level in the children with that difference in breast milk composition.

Dr. Tsang: There are very few studies looking at calcium/phosphate metabolism after 6 to 12 months, especially on human milk feeding. In North America, we sometimes see babies with rickets who have been on prolonged breast feeding, typically from vegetarian or African-American families. In those instances where the phosphate concentration has been measured in the blood and in the breast milk, it is extremely low. In that situation there is not just vitamin D deficiency but also a degree of phosphate deficiency relating to the fact that the phosphate has fallen so far. But you are telling me that in The Gambia the phosphate concentrations do not fall very low, so I suppose they will be protected from rickets. Is the incidence of rickets low in that population?

Dr. Prentice: In the part of The Gambia that I work in, infantile rickets is not seen except secondary to scurvy. We don't tend to see it, even though the infants have extremely low calcium intakes. Why we don't see it in the same way it is seen in South Africa I don't know, but this is something we need to work on. I wonder whether the high phosphate levels might help those children to cope with their very low calcium intakes by enabling them to retain as much calcium as possible. Is that a likely hypothesis?

Dr. Tsang: That sounds like a possibility. I would guess that in a prolonged breast-feeding situation, it might be protective. Would John Pettifor like to comment?

Dr. Pettifor: I don't think we would see calcium deficiency in that age group. They are still getting a fair amount of calcium from breast milk, even if it isn't adequate to meet the normal requirements, and they are also getting some from the complementary foods they are being provided with as well.

Dr. Tsang: Do you get the same high phosphate concentrations in breast milk in South Africa?

Dr. Pettifor: I don't have data up to 1 or 2 years. But the question I was going to ask was that if one looks at the biochemical changes that occur during infancy in breast-fed infants, they are very much like those of a phosphate depletion syndrome. There tends to be low PTH, hypercalcemia, hypercalciuria, low phosphate, and high $1{,}25(OH)_2D$, and one wonders whether in fact that isn't what the normal values are. So what I was going to ask, and perhaps I could ask Nestlé to comment, is that I am worried that we are overconcerned about the phosphate content of formula preparations and that these have been reduced and reduced to an extent that might be deleterious rather than to the advantage of the infant.

Dr. Tsang: You have a good point, but I don't think most companies are doing that, at least not aggressively, though as with anything else there could be problems if one goes to extremes. At this time the amount of phosphorus being used in most infant formulas is really quite high, and I think it makes sense to reduce it. How far we should reduce it will, I think, become an issue. Absorption of phosphorus is very good, as high as 90%, so we are not invoking any problems there.

Dr. Guesry: We are still supplying 50% more phosphorus than human milk on average, so our phosphate levels are not very low, as you imply. Secondly, we have done a study in Brussels showing that bone density on our formula was slightly higher than that in human milk.

Dr. Rigo: Using metabolic balance studies, we showed that in term infants the limited content of phosphorus in human milk also limited calcium retention. We observed very low levels of phosphorus and quite high levels of calcium in the urine in term infants. Do you have any comment about this limited calcium retention during the first week of life, even in term infants, in terms of bone mineralization?

Dr. Tsang: I don't know why you call it limited. I would say that the amount of calcium excreted is appropriate in term infants. However, when we look at preterm infants, as you and others have demonstrated, calcium excretion reaches 25% of the intake, which I would consider huge. In the term infant it is less than 5%, and the amount excreted is physiologically determined by the phosphate content, which I think is a reasonable concept. It is only the preterm infant who dumps so much calcium. But you also point out something that perhaps we did not emphasize strongly enough, which is that in a term or a preterm infant the ability to conserve phosphorus is phenomenal: in the term infant phosphorus absorption is very high, and excretion is very low; in the preterm infant absorption is also extremely high, and excretion almost zero. The body knows that it needs phosphate, so it totally shuts down phosphate excretion by the kidney. Experimental studies in preterm infants who were given aluminum hydroxide as a phosphate-binding agent showed that within 12 hours the urinary excretion of phosphate fell to zero, so the babies knew there was a potential threat to their existence. As you imply, the phosphate issue is a key one.

Dr. Rigo: In utero, up to the end of pregnancy, calcium retention is very high. By contrast, calcium retention decreases sharply after birth in breast-fed infants. It is not only because of the limited calcium supply or absorption rate during this period; it may also be the results of the limited phosphorus supply provided by human milk.

Dr. Tsang: In utero there is a certain need, and in postnatal life there is a certain other need. There is no necessity for there to be a continuum. There are many things that adjust themselves quite differently after birth. After all, *in utero* the fetus is hypercalcemic, with calcium concentrations that would make us very nervous in the postnatal infant. So I do not think we can translate intrauterine life to extrauterine life that readily, especially in a term infant. One might argue that the preterm infant is still supposed to be *in utero,* but once the baby is born, all the other hormones and receptors and so on are changed totally. Obviously there are different needs after birth.

Dr. Pohlandt: But Dr. Rigo observed a reduction of urinary phosphate to near zero and hypercalciuria in term babies fed breast milk. We have to think about how to explain that. In the preterm baby you accepted this finding as a consequence of relative phosphate deficiency. Why shouldn't the same be valid for the term baby? We don't have any other explanation. No phosphate in the urine along with hypercalciuria indicates a relative phosphate deficiency, even in the term baby.

Dr. Tsang: You could argue that way. But in general, most human-milk-fed babies are assumed to be normal. So what you call hypercalciuria in the urine could be defined as normal for a breast-fed infant. You refer to it as high only relative to an adult or childhood reference standard. Who is to say that the adult is normal? Maybe the baby is normal.

Dr. Pohlandt: But Dr. Rigo wanted to emphasize that even the term baby has, for a time, a relative deficiency of phosphate. That is the point he wanted to make.

Dr. Tsang: I understand that, but I think it is a "half-full or half-empty" kind of argument. If we view it from the point of view that a term-sized baby having breast milk and with no obvious insult is considered normal, then all the measurements that we have made on him are relatively normal. Your reference point of calciuria was an arbitrary one, an adult one. Who is to say the adult is normal?

Dr. Pohlandt: I didn't use the term normal or abnormal.

Dr. Tsang: But "deficiency" is "abnormal."

Dr. Pohlandt: We observed no phosphate in the urine, and the question is, why does the term baby on breast milk not excrete any phosphate?

Dr. Tsang: Because that is normal!

Dr. Moya: I would like to know whether your normal newborn babies on breast-feeding were supplemented with vitamin D, and if they weren't, do you think that the administration of normal amounts of vitamin D might change the level of plasma phosphate?

Dr. Tsang: In the prospective study, the infants were given vitamin D. The effect has not been studied directly, but from other kinds of studies we have looked at I don't think it has a big effect.

Dr. Seeman: Have there been randomized trials where the only variable is the differing level of phosphate? Everything else is the same, so then you can make some inferences about bone density, size of the animal, serum calcium and phosphate, and so forth. Have there been those randomized trials, or are all of the inferences you are making basically little observational studies done in different countries, so we can infer nothing?

Dr. Tsang: The studies that were done were the prospective studies that I showed you. You cannot randomize between breast and formula because it is unethical. Calcium and phosphate contents have been varied, but unfortunately there has been more variation in the calcium content than in the phosphate content. A formula study varying the phosphate would be the right study to do.

Dr. Haschke: Have you an explanation for the declining concentration of phosphorus but stable calcium in breast milk? I would suggest that it reflects the decline in the cellular elements of breast milk, phosphorus being in the cells and calcium extracellular.

Dr. Tsang: That is an intriguing possibility.

Dr. Eisman: When you look at a preterm infant, what is the gold standard? How are you going to know that you have done the best and most appropriate thing for the infant? Until you know that, you can do any study you like, but you don't know which answer is the right answer.

Dr. Tsang: The conventional approach has been to use the full-term breast-fed baby as the norm for nearly everything that we do in infant nutrition. So that if the bone mineral content of a preterm infant normalized at the level found in the full-term baby, that would be one happy ending. Another happy ending would be if the blood calcium and phosphate concentrations were to be in the same normal range of the full-term breast-fed infant. One also has to consider the long-term imprinting effects because there are recent studies that seem to imply an imprinting element. Thus, if the infant was deprived for a while at a critical time, this might cause irreversible effects in the long term, on bone mass for example. Balance studies are done, but their interpretation is fraught with problems. They are necessary for our understanding of physiology, but they don't necessarily provide one with the endpoints that one really wants.

Dr. Schanler: You forgot to add the intrauterine equation. That is the gold standard on which we interpret body composition changes in the premature infant. We use the old carcass analysis data, but we now have corroboration for some of the minerals from neutron activation analysis, and those old numbers derived from chemistry seem quite accurate. If anything is to be a gold standard in terms of nutrition, I think we should use those data for the premature infant.

Dr. Pettifor: I have a question in relation to your neonatal hypocalcemia story, with normal full-term infants fed on artificial milk formula. Many infants get fed on such formulas, and yet very few present with symptomatic neonatal hypocalcemia. What is specific about those four or five children you presented that separates them from the vast majority of the other children who take the formula without any problems at all? Is there any evidence that they have an end-organ resistance to PTH, and if so what would be the mechanism for that resistance?

Dr. Tsang: I tend to view that as just the end of a normal curve, the tail-end phenomenon. You could imply that maybe there was something else involved, such as a kidney problem, but there have never been any studies looking at renal function *per se* in this situation.

Dr. Pettifor: But to follow on, these infants behave very much like some children with vitamin D deficiency in the early infant period, who present with hypocalcemia and often hyperphosphatemia; they have hyperparathyroidism, but they have not yet been able to respond appropriately to the vitamin D deficiency. Yet there are a large number of other children who go through that phase without developing the hypocalcemia and the hyperphosphatemia. What is it specifically in those children that prevents them from responding appropriately?

Dr. Tsang: The babies have normal vitamin D status. Most of the babies do show a fall in serum calcium, so it is a real change. I still believe this is a matter of degree: infants at the far end of the curve are different from the infants in the middle of the curve, but I agree there could be other factors involved.

Nutrition and Bone Development, edited by
Jean-Philippe Bonjour and Reginald C. Tsang,
Nestlé Nutrition Workshop Series, Vol. 41, Nestec Ltd.,
Vevey/Lippincott–Raven Publishers,
Philadelphia © 1999.

Factors Affecting Bone Mass at Birth

Ran Namgung

Department of Pediatrics, Yonsei University College of Medicine, Seoul, Korea

Very little is known about factors that affect fetal bone mineralization. Theoretically it should be determined by placental mineral transfer, fetal bone mineral accretion rate, and fetal bone resorption rate. Studies of calcium-regulating hormones and indices of bone metabolism in cord blood may allow an understanding of the factors that influence calcium and bone metabolism in the human fetus.

Season of birth, low weight relative to gestation, and having a diabetic mother have been found recently to have a significant impact on the skeleton of newborn infants. Though the possible mechanisms associated with these alterations in newborn bone mineralization are unclear, it is evident from our findings that major influences on bone metabolism occur *in utero.* Because effects on fetal bone are often mediated through the mother, any disturbance in maternal mineral metabolism, for example nutrient deficiency or disease, or conditions affecting placental mineral transfer could be factors affecting fetal bone mineralization.

SEASON

Season could influence fetal bone metabolism, possibly through changes in vitamin D metabolism. Vitamin D is essential for mineral homeostasis and adequate bone mineralization. The lack of vitamin D in pregnancy may adversely affect fetal bone development. Normal fetal mineral accretion may be derived from maternal skeleton (1), and thus, variations of maternal mineral metabolism could theoretically affect the fetus. We have proposed in several studies that season-related changes in vitamin D metabolism in pregnant women may affect fetal bone metabolism.

Many earlier studies have shown seasonal variations in serum 25-hydroxyvitamin D concentrations in both pregnant women and their newborn infants, with low values in winter (2,3). Severe vitamin D deficiency in pregnancy can lead to intrauterine growth retardation (4), adverse effects on neonatal ossification (5), and congenital rickets (6), confirming the potential impact of maternal vitamin D deficiency on fetal bone development.

Studies in adults have shown seasonal variations of forearm (7–9) and vertebral bone mineral content (BMC) (10,11), with lower BMC during winter than in summer.

Seasonal differences in adult BMC are thought to be caused by seasonal variations in bone-remodeling activity (8) or seasonal changes in vitamin D metabolism (7).

Thus, assuming that BMC variations may relate in part to vitamin D status, we hypothesized that BMC would be lower and serum osteocalcin higher (reflecting increased bone turnover) in winter-born than summer-born newborn infants. We tested our original *a priori* hypothesis in three separate studies of healthy term North American neonates (12–14) and found marked seasonal differences (8–12%) in newborn BMC at full term in both appropriately grown infants (12,13) and small-for-gestation (SGA) infants (14).

The BMC of the distal third of the radius was measured before 3 days of age in 140 winter-born (January through March) and 106 summer-born (July through September) newborn infants by single photon absorptiometry (Lunar Radiation, Madison, Wisconsin, USA). Significant seasonal differences were found: summer-born infants had significantly lower BMC (8%) than winter-born infants (mean ± SE: 82.7 ± 1.4 versus 89.9 ± 2.3 mg/cm, $p = 0.009$) (13) (Fig. 1). Summer-born infants had significantly higher cord serum osteocalcin (Fig. 2) and 1,25-dihydroxy-vitamin D concentrations than winter-born infants. In BMC data from SGA infants ($n = 42$) from a parallel study (14), we also found significantly lower BMC in summer-born than in winter-born infants (Fig. 3). The BMC findings are opposite to our original *a priori* hypothesis and to the findings in adults, and these are in sharp contrast to the differences of less than 2% by season in adults.

We speculated that the reversal of seasonal bone mass in newborns in the United

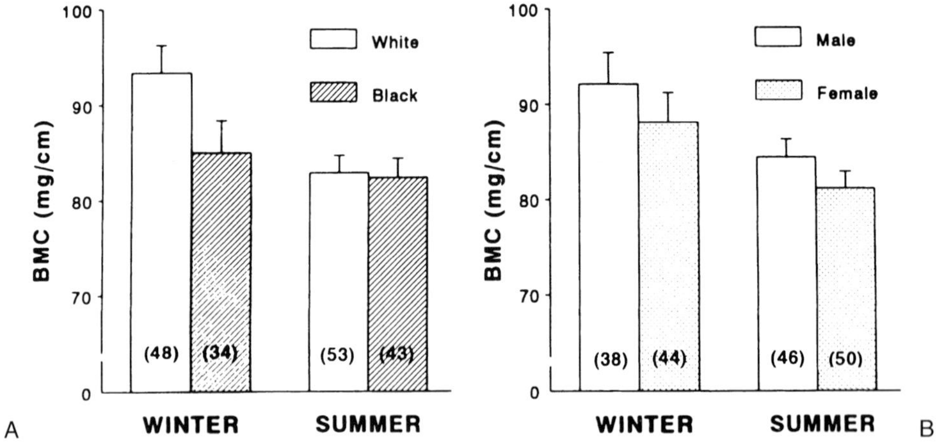

FIG. 1. Newborn BMC (mg/cm) in winter and summer by race and gender. Values are least-square means adjusted for birth weight ± SE with numbers of newborns in parentheses. Summer-born infants had significantly lower BMC than winter-born infants ($p = 0.009$). Race and sex differences in BMC corresponded to birth weight differences; after adjustment for birth weight, race and sex differences were $p = 0.09$ and $p = 0.17$, respectively. Seasonal differences in BMC remained significant after adjustment for race and sex effects ($p = 0.002$ and $p = 0.001$, respectively). From Namgung *et al.* (13) with permission.

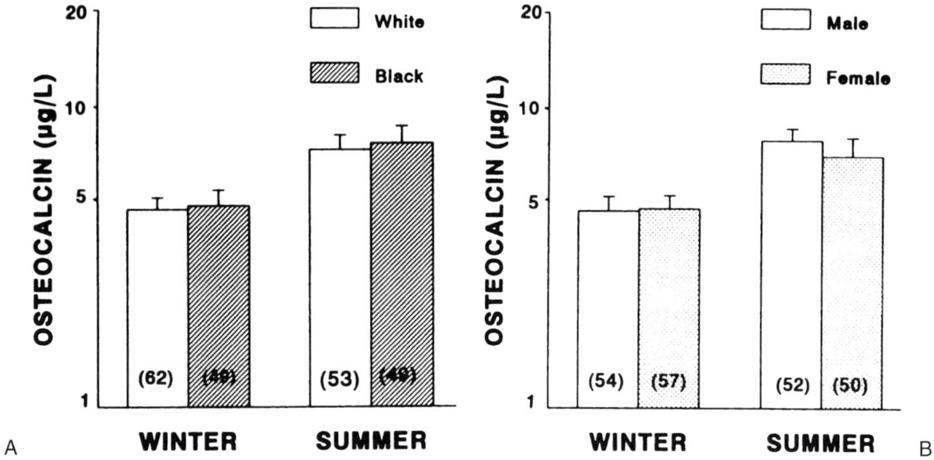

FIG. 2. Serum osteocalcin concentrations (g/l) were higher in summer-born than in winter-born infants ($p = 0.0001$) and did not differ by race or sex. Values are mean ± SE with numbers of newborns in parentheses. From Namgung *et al.* (13) with permission.

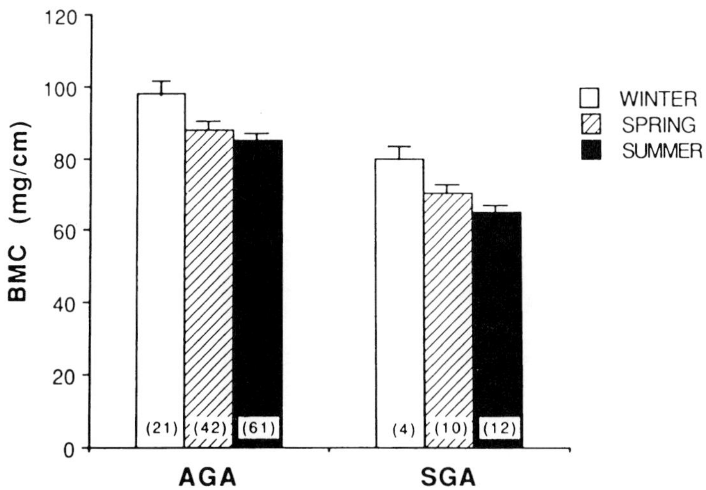

FIG. 3. Newborn BMC (mg/cm) in SGA versus AGA infants by season of birth. The BMC was significantly lower in SGA than in AGA infants ($p = 0.0001$) and differed by season of birth: spring or summer BMC values were lower than winter values in both SGA and AGA infants ($p = 0.003$). The BMC differences between groups remained significant after adjustment for season ($p = 0.0001$). Values are mean ± SE. Numbers of infants are shown in parentheses. From Namgung *et al.* (14) with permission.

States may occur because of the effect of maternal vitamin D status, particularly in the first trimester of pregnancy (that is, 6 months before the infant is born), thereby accounting for the time lapse and opposite seasonal results from those of the adults. During the first trimester of pregnancy, most women in the United States have not received much prenatal care and are less likely to be taking multivitamin pills that contain vitamin D. Thus, the mother is relatively unprotected (that is, not given vitamin D supplements), and seasonal changes of vitamin D status can occur. We suggest that these seasonal vitamin D status changes result in first-trimester bone alterations in winter that are evident 6 months later as reduced bone mass at birth in summer compared with winter. After the first trimester, most women receive vitamin D supplements. Generally, at the time of delivery in the United States, there are no differences in serum vitamin D concentrations by season, presumably because of vitamin D supplementation.

The period of vulnerability of the fetus to altered maternal vitamin D status, if any, is unclear. In the human fetus, bone is already well formed at 8 weeks of gestation, with gross features already evident in fetal limb structure (15). Though the amount of calcium accrued by the skeleton during the early fetal period is quantitatively small, this period is critical because most teratologic insults occur during this period, and many major teratologic syndromes involve malformations and maldevelopment of bone (for example, the thalidomide syndrome). The importance of first trimester bone development thus cannot be overemphasized.

We have suggested that the high serum osteocalcin concentrations in summer-born North American infants may be an adaptive response to the lower BMC of these infants, possibly secondary to the raised plasma 1,25-dihydroxyvitamin D concentrations. Based on our findings, we suggest that reduced bone mass in summer-born newborns in the United States is related to reduced maternal vitamin D status in the preceding winter. We speculate that sunshine deprivation in winter alters vitamin D metabolism in the mother and fetus during an important period of early fetal skeletal development, resulting in low BMC at birth 6 months later. Thus, season should be considered to be a factor affecting bone mass at birth.

SMALL FOR GESTATION

Low weight relative to gestation could be a factor influencing fetal bone metabolism, possibly through alterations in placental mineral transfer. Previous studies have showed evidence of alterations in bone mineralization and parathyroid hormone (PTH) in such infants (16–18). In experimental fetal growth retardation (modified Wigglesworth model in the rat), reduced placental blood supply causes reduced placental calcium transport proportional to the reduction in body size (19). The mechanism for the low BMC in SGA infants is not clear. In an earlier study (16), we found that the BMC of the distal radius, measured by single photon absorptiometry, was significantly lower and that serum PTH concentrations were higher in SGA than in appropriate-for-gestational-age (AGA) infants at birth. We suggested that the SGA fetus responds to possible *in utero* calcium deficiency with increased secretion of PTH.

In a recent study (14), we found evidence of decreased bone formation in SGA versus AGA infants. The BMC was measured in the distal one-third of the radius by photon absorptiometry in 42 term SGA infants and 126 term AGA infants, matched 1:3 specifically by gestation (± 1 week) and birth month. By design, gestational ages were similar, but birth weights were significantly lower in SGA than in AGA infants (mean ± SD: 2,419 ± 178 g versus 3,430 ± 339 g). The BMC was significantly lower (22%) in SGA than in AGA infants (mean ± SE: 69.3 ± 1.6 versus 88.3 ± 1.5 mg/cm, $p = 0.0001$). Differences in BMC between groups remained significant after the influence of season had been considered ($p = 0.0001$) (Fig. 3). Cord serum osteocalcin (Fig. 4) and 1,25-dihydroxyvitamin D concentrations were significantly lower in SGA than in AGA infants. There were no differences between groups in cord serum concentrations of intact PTH, 25-hydroxyvitamin D, and minerals. The BMC was negatively correlated with intact PTH.

On the basis of our findings, we suggest that a low uteroplacental blood flow in SGA infants may cause reduced fetal–placental production of 1,25-dihydroxyvitamin D, resulting in low serum osteocalcin, an index of bone formation, and low BMC; fetal serum parathyroid hormone values may be relatively increased because of a reduction in placental mineral supply. Reduced mineral supply across the placenta may have a direct effect on bone formation.

To determine whether low BMC in SGA infants is related to the alterations in

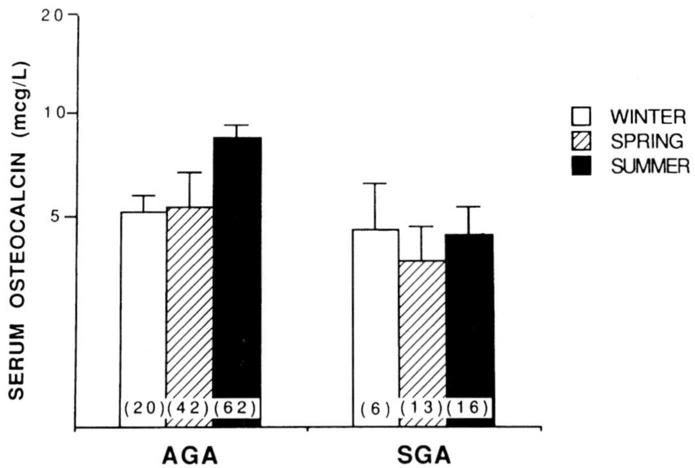

FIG. 4. Serum osteocalcin (g/l) concentrations were lower in SGA than in AGA infants ($p = 0.0005$). Osteocalcin differed by season of birth ($p = 0.001$): the osteocalcin concentration was higher in summer than in winter or spring in AGA infants ($p = 0.0003$), whereas in SGA infants it was not. Osteocalcin differences between groups remained significant after adjustment for season ($p = 0.0005$). Values are expressed as mean ± SE. Numbers of infants are shown in parentheses. From Namgung *et al.* (14) with permission.

bone collagen metabolism, we measured serum carboxy-terminal propeptide of type I procollagen (PICP) and cross-linked carboxy-terminal telopeptide of type I collagen (ICTP) concentrations, new markers of bone collagen type I biosynthesis and degradation (20,21), in 19 SGA and 38 AGA infants (22). There were no differences in serum PICP and ICTP concentrations between groups. These findings are not consistent with the thesis of altered fetal bone collagen type I biosynthesis or degradation in SGA. We suggest that the reduced BMC in SGA infants is predominantly related to a reduced supply of minerals across the placenta rather than to defective regulation of bone collagen type I metabolism.

INFANTS OF DIABETIC MOTHERS

Maternal diabetes could be a factor influencing fetal bone metabolism through alterations in maternal mineral metabolism or limited mineral availability in diabetic pregnancy. In a diabetic pregnant rat model, fetal BMC was significantly lower than in control fetuses (23). Decreased BMC has been reported in diabetic patients (24) and might be related to insulin deficiency because insulin treatment improves BMC in juvenile diabetes. Neonatal hypocalcemia and neonatal hypomagnesemia occur frequently in infants of insulin-dependent diabetic mothers; the incidence and severity of hypocalcemia are directly related to the severity of maternal diabetes and related to the urinary magnesium losses in diabetes (25).

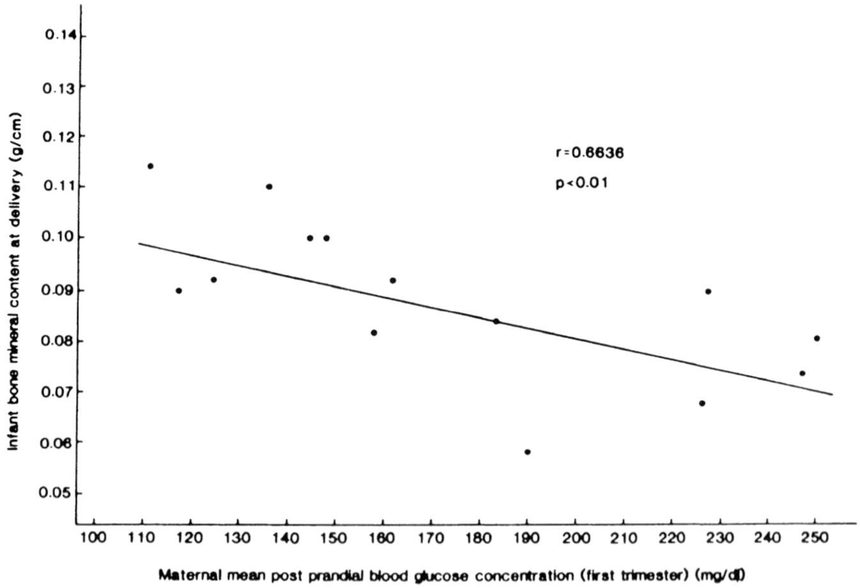

FIG. 5. Infant bone mineral content values plotted against mean first trimester postprandial blood glucose concentration. There is a significant inverse correlation between these two variables ($r = -0.6636$, $p < 0.01$). From Mimouni *et al.* (27) with permission.

We theorized that infants of diabetic mothers (IDM) have decreased BMC at birth, correlating with poor control of diabetes during pregnancy. Because an increase in 1,25-dihydroxyvitamin D concentration has been reported in IDM (26), raised 1,25-dihydroxyvitamin D may contribute to decreased BMC in such infants through increased bone resorption. The BMC was measured by single photon absorptiometry in 45 diabetic women (class B-RT) during pregnancy and at birth in their infants as well as in 55 normal term newborn infants born of nondiabetic mothers. The BMC at birth was significantly decreased in IDM compared with control infants and correlated inversely with mean first trimester maternal capillary blood glucose (Fig. 5), implying that factors early in pregnancy might have an effect on fetal BMC (27). The low BMC in IDM may be related to the decreased mineral transfer across the placenta, possibly secondary to the decreased mineral availability in diabetic pregnancy caused by the absence of a physiological increase in maternal PTH in diabetic pregnancies.

A recent study from our group (28) found evidence of increased intrauterine bone resorption in term infants of mothers with insulin-dependent diabetes: cord serum ICTP concentrations, a marker of bone resorption, were higher in IDM than in control subjects, indicating increased osteoclastic activity in IDM than in controls. However, serum PICP concentration, a marker of bone formation, was not different between groups.

RACE AND GENDER

In adults and adolescents, bone mass is greater in blacks (29) and in men (30) than in whites and women, respectively. In children at 1 to 6 years of age, blacks have higher BMC than whites, and males have higher BMC than females (31). Differences in BMC by race and gender in children are present even after controlling for the influence of body weight (31).

The higher bone mass in blacks may be caused in part by a larger body mass, which results in increased strain on the skeleton, which would then stimulate bone formation (32). The findings in children at 1 to 6 years, however, support a race difference in BMC independent of body weight (31).

In our recent study (13), we measured BMC in 101 white, 77 black, 84 male, and 94 female infants before 3 days of age by single photon absorptiometry. White infants had higher BMC and higher birth weight than black infants (mean $\pm$ SE: white versus black, 88.4 $\pm$ 1.8 versus 82.9 $\pm$ 1.9 mg/cm, $p = 0.04$, and mean $\pm$ SD: 3,398 $\pm$ 37.6 versus 3,244 $\pm$ 35.6 g, $p = 0.003$, respectively). These race differences in BMC corresponded to birth weight difference, and after adjustment for birth weight, there was no significant difference by race ($p = 0.09$). Seasonal differences in BMC remained after adjustment for race effects ($p = 0.002$) (Fig. 1).

Male infants had higher BMC and higher birth weight than female infants (male versus female, 88.8 $\pm$ 1.9 versus 83.6 $\pm$ 1.9 mg/cm, $p = 0.05$ and 3,381 $\pm$ 39.3 versus 3,273 $\pm$ 34.9 g, $p = 0.04$, respectively). Gender differences in BMC corresponded to birth weight differences, and after adjustment for birth weight, were not significant ($p = 0.17$). Seasonal differences in BMC remained after adjustment for gender effects ($p = 0.001$) (Fig. 1). No race or gender effects on cord serum biochemical measurements were found except for the expected lower serum 25-hydroxyvitamin D concentrations in blacks compared with whites.

Thus, season, weight relative to gestation, and having a diabetic mother are important factors affecting bone mass at birth; these factors should be considered as factors affecting newborn bone metabolism.

REFERENCES

1. Comar CL. Radiocalcium studies in pregnancy. *Ann NY Acad Sci* 1956; 64: 281–298.
2. Kuroda E, Okano T, Mizuno N. Plasma levels of 25-hydroxyvitamin D_2 and 25-hydroxyvitamin D_3 in maternal, cord and neonatal blood. *J Nutr Sci Vitaminol* 1981; 27: 55–65.
3. Verity CM, Burman D, Beadle PC, Holton JB, Morris A. Seasonal changes in perinatal vitamin D metabolism maternal and cord blood biochemistry in normal pregnancies. *Arch Dis Child* 1981; 56: 943–948.
4. Brooke OG, Brown IRF, Bone CDM, *et al.* Vitamin D supplements in pregnant Asian women: effects on calcium status and fetal growth. *Br Med J* 1980; 280: 751–754.
5. Specker BL, Ho ML, Oestreich A, *et al.* Prospective study of vitamin D supplementation and rickets in China. *J Pediatr* 1992; 120: 733–739.
6. Moncrieff M, Fadahunsi TO. Congenital rickets due to maternal vitamin D deficiency. *Arch Dis Child* 1974; 49: 810–811.
7. Aitken JM, Anderson JB, Horton PW. Seasonal variations in bone mineral content after the menopause. *Nature* 1973; 241: 59–60.
8. Hyldstrup L, McNair P, Jensen GF, Transbøl I. Seasonal variations in indices of bone formation precede appropriate bone mineral changes in normal men. *Bone* 1986; 7: 167–170.
9. Devogelaer JP, Depresseux G, Le Thi C, Nagant C. Seasonal variation in bone mineral content in postmenopausal women. In: Dequeker J, Geusens P, Wahner HW, eds. *Bone mineral measurements by photon absorptiometry: methodological problems.* Leuven, Belgium: Leuven University Press, 1988: 225.
10. Krølner B. Seasonal variation of lumbar spine bone mineral content in normal women. *Calcif Tissue Int* 1983; 35: 145–147.
11. Bergstralh EJ, Sinaki M, Offord KP, Wahner HW, Melton LJ. Effect of season on physical activity score, back extensor muscle strength, and lumbar bone mineral density. *J Bone Miner Res* 1990; 5: 371–377.
12. Namgung R, Mimouni F, Campaigne BN, Ho ML, Tsang RC. Low bone mineral content in summer-born compared with winter-born infants. *J Pediatr Gastroenterol Nutr* 1992; 15: 285–288.
13. Namgung R, Tsang RC, Specker BL, Sierra RI, Ho ML. Low bone mineral content and high serum osteocalcin and $1,25(OH)_2$vitamin D in summer- versus winter-born newborn infants: an early fetal effect? *J Pediatr Gastroenterol Nutr* 1994; 19: 220–227.
14. Namgung R, Tsang RC, Specker BL, Sierra RI, Ho ML. Reduced serum osteocalcin and 1,25-dihydroxyvitamin D concentrations and low bone mineral content in small for gestational age infants: evidence of decreased bone formation rates. *J Pediatr* 1993; 122: 269–275.
15. Moore KL, ed. *The developing human: clinically oriented embryology.* Philadelphia: WB Saunders, 1988.
16. Minton SD, Steichen JJ, Tsang RC. Decreased bone mineral content in small for gestational age infants: Normal serum 25-hydroxyvitamin D and decreasing parathyroid hormone. *Pediatrics* 1983; 71: 383–388.
17. Pohlandt F, Mathers N. Bone mineral content of appropriate and light for gestational age preterm and term newborn infants. *Acta Paediatr Scand* 1989; 78: 835–839.
18. Petersen G, Gotfredsen A, Knudsen FU. Total body bone mineral in light-for-gestational-age infants and appropriate-for-gestational-age infants. *Acta Paediatr Scand* 1989; 78: 437–450.
19. Mughal MZ, Ross R, Tsang RC. Clearance of calcium across *in situ* perfused placentas of intrauterine growth-retarded rat fetuses. *Pediatr Res* 1989; 25: 420–422.
20. Parfitt AM, Simon LS, Villanueva AR, Krane SM. Procollagen type I carboxy-terminal extension

peptide in serum as a marker of collagen biosynthesis in bone: correlation with iliac bone formation rates and comparison with total alkaline phosphatase. *J Bone Miner Res* 1987; 2: 427–436.
21. Eriksen EF, Charles P, Melsen F, Mosekilde L, Risteli L, Risteli J. Serum markers of type I collagen formation and degradation in metabolic bone disease: correlation with bone histomorphometry. *J Bone Miner Res* 1993; 8: 127–132.
22. Namgung R, Tsang RC, Sierra RI, Ho ML. Normal serum indices of bone collagen biosynthesis and degradation in small for gestational age infants. *J Pediatr Gastroenterol Nutr* 1996; 23: 224–228.
23. VerHaeghe J, Bouillon R, Nyomba BL, *et al.* Vitamin D and bone mineral homeostasis during pregnancy in the diabetic BB rat. *Endocrinology* 1986; 118: 1019–1025.
24. Levine ME, Boisseau VC, Avioli LV. Effects of diabetes mellitus on bone mass in juvenile and adult onset diabetes. *N Engl J Med* 1976; 294: 241–245.
25. Tsang RC, Kleinman L, Sutherland JM, *et al.* Hypocalcemia in infants of diabetic mothers: studies in Ca, P and Mg metabolism and in parathormone responsiveness. *J Pediatr* 1972; 80: 384–395.
26. Steichen JJ, Tsang RC, Ho M, *et al.* Perinatal magnesium, calcium and 1,25-dihydroxyvitamin D in relation to prospective randomized management of maternal diabetes. *Calcif Tissue Int* 1981; 33: 317.
27. Mimouni F, Steichen JJ, Tsang RC, Hertzberg V, Miodovnik M. Decreased bone mineral content in infants of diabetic mothers. *Am J Perinatol* 1988; 5: 339–343.
28. Demarini S, Specker BL, Sierra RI, Miodovnik M, Tsang RC. Evidence of increased intrauterine bone resorption in term infants of mothers with insulin-dependent diabetes. *J Pediatr* 1995; 126: 796–798.
29. Cohn SH, Abesamis C, Yasumura S, Aloia JF, Zanzi I, Ellis KJ. Comparative skeletal mass and radial bone mineral content in black and white women. *Metabolism* 1977; 26: 171–178.
30. Mazess RB, Cameron JR. Bone mineral content in normal US Whites. In: Mazess RB, ed. *International conference on bone mineral measurement. DHEW Publication No. (NIH) 75–683.* Washington DC: US Department of Health, Education and Welfare, 1973: 228–237.
31. Li JY, Specker BL, Ho ML, Tsang RC. Bone mineral content in black and white children 1 to 6 years of age; early appearance of race and sex differences. *Am J Dis Child* 1989; 143: 1346–1349.
32. Bell NH, Greene A, Epstein S, Oexmann MJ, Shaw S, Shary J. Evidence for alteration of the vitamin D-endocrine system in blacks. *J Clin Invest* 1985; 76: 470–473.

DISCUSSION

Dr. Alliet: You said in your population the mothers had very poor medical control and did not get any vitamin supplements during the first trimester. Did you repeat your measurements in a group receiving vitamin D supplements in the first trimester?

Dr. Namgung: When we did the first prospective study, we took the vitamin D intake history from the mother, but we had no opportunity to measure maternal vitamin D status in the first trimester of pregnancy (more than 80% of pregnant mothers took prenatal vitamin supplements, but most of them started it in the second trimester of pregnancy). The estimated amount of vitamin D intake was not different by season. We are now designing another prospective trial of vitamin D supplementation, divided by trimesters of pregnancy.

Dr. Guesry: Calcium deposition is exponential during intrauterine life. This means that the amount deposited during the last month of pregnancy is as important as the amount deposited during the first 8 months, so I wonder whether your explanation relating to the synthesis of vitamin D by sun exposure is the correct one, or if there is another reason. And in the infant of a diabetic mother, is it not true that the placenta ages and deteriorates rapidly at the end of the pregnancy? So I wonder if calcium transfer is normal during the last month of pregnancy in this situation.

Dr. Namgung: To answer the first question, our mothers took vitamin D supplements from the second trimester onward, and when we measured cord serum 25-hydroxyvitamin D concentration, there was no significant difference by season (seasonal changes in vitamin D status can occur in the first trimester of pregnancy). This is the reason why we speculate that the effect may have occurred early in pregnancy (although the amount of calcium transferred from mother to fetus is greatest later in pregnancy, skeletal development occurs very early in pregnancy, and early adverse effects in D metabolism might theoretically have profound effects). As to your second question, as far as I know there are no published data.

Dr. Mughal: I can answer that in the rat model of diabetic pregnancy. We have induced diabetes by injecting streptozotocin in rats, then allowed them to become pregnant and perfused their placentas. There is no doubt that at term the maternal–fetal calcium transport across the diabetic placenta is reduced. One of the problems that we have with any bone density work in infants, particularly when growth is being affected, is to normalize it for changes in the growth. How can we be sure that changes in bone mineral density are true changes and not simply a reflection of whatever phenomena are causing alterations in growth?

Dr. Namgung: We adjusted for birth size in the analysis of the data. Birth weight is included in the statistical model.

Dr. Mughal: Is that an appropriate denominator to use when correcting for bone mineral content?

Dr. Namgung: It was significant when we adjusted for size.

Dr. Pohlandt: You are familiar with the study of Mazess (1), which you list in your references. This study emphasized that the best correlate of bone mineral content was not gestational age but birth weight. When they analyzed the small-for-gestational-age babies taking into account their reduced weight, they did not find any differences compared with appropriate-for-dates babies. You haven't broken down your data according to actual weight. Do you really find a difference in bone mineral content if you take into account the reduced weight of your babies?

Dr. Namgung: The birth weight in SGA group was around 2.4 kg, and in the AGA group it was around 3.4 kg; body size was thus significantly different. When we included body size in the statistical analysis, the difference in bone mineral content was no longer significant.

Dr. Pohlandt: So if the difference has gone, you shouldn't say that there is a reduced bone mineral content. The babies are small and light, and therefore, the bone mineral content is reduced appropriately to their reduced body size and weight.

Dr. Namgung: Your comment is right, I agree, bone mineral content is proportionate to weight. Thus, bone mineralization is reduced in porportion to weight reduction. We designed the study specifically to look at SGA infants. I think their pathophysiology is completely different from that of normal infants, and even though difference in the bone mineral content disappeared when we included the body size in the statistical analysis, the meaning is different I think. Actually, we found evidence of decreased bone formation in SGA versus AGA infants, as reflected by lower osteocalcin in SGA.

Dr. Bachrach: We could spend a whole day on what to correct for. Just correcting for body weight, particularly in the infant of a diabetic mother, can be very misleading because we know these babies have a much higher proportion of body fat than normal. We cannot assume that body fat and lean body mass are equal determinants of bone mass. So just to correct these infants of diabetic mothers for total body weight could be misleading. I hope that in the next study of infants of diabetic mothers, people will look at factors other than calcium and vitamin D and will take into account IGFs and so forth that we know may be affected as well.

Dr. Rigo: Recently, Winston Koo *et al.* reported normative data of whole body bone mineral content in American newborn infants. In this study, using multivariate analysis, he did not find any significant influence of gender, race, or season on whole body bone mineral content. Do you think that the discrepancy with your results could be related to methodology: radius versus whole body measurement?

Dr. Namgung: Dr. Specker and Dr. Tsang also measured serum 25-hydroxyvitamin D concentration by season in Cincinnati, and there was a striking threefold difference in winter versus summer, low in winter. So, I don't think the difference in our results resulted from the method of bone measurement. Dr. Koo's population was in the southern part of the United States, in the sunbelt area. So there would presumably be little seasonal variation in vitamin D metabolism.

Dr. Rigo: The study was performed in Memphis, Tennessee. Last year, at the ESPR meeting in Lyon, we reported data of whole body bone mineral content performed in infants of diabetic mothers (2). After adjustment for body weight, there was no significant difference in BMC between IDM and controls.

Dr. Namgung: I think the differences may depend on the criteria for subject selection, particularly whether the mothers are insulin dependent or not.

Dr. Tsang: I would like to clarify this a little more. I think that one of the issues was control of diabetes. The later study obviously had much better diabetic control. The first study involved subjects who were not nearly so well controlled, and you saw that the relationship was directly with glucose control. So I think it could represent a different population. The size issue we discussed with Dr. Koo's study. You may remember that in Mimouni's diabetes study (3), the babies were larger, but, nevertheless, their bone mineral content was less, as opposed to Koo's study, where the size of the baby wasn't that discrepant and therefore presumably reflected a better-controlled population.

Dr. Gilsanz: To try to make bone density measurements in newborns is extremely difficult. Not only do you have to correct for body size, you have to correct for the distribution of the soft tissues around the bone that you are going to analyze. In other words, not only do they have to have the same weight, but they have to have the same anthropomorphic configuration, and that is very difficult. These measurements are useful, but we should know their limitations. To really establish if infants of diabetic mothers have low bone mineral content at birth based on this technique is extremely difficult. This is obvious from the number of discrepant results that have been published.

Dr. Tsang: When you talk about fat interference in measurement of bone mass, what is the order of magnitude of the possible interference?

Dr. Gilsanz: The data are available. This has been investigated with phantoms by Dr. Engelke. He calculated that if you move 2 cm of fat from in front of a phantom representing a spine to laterally, the error on the value is 9% to 10%. Depending on whether the fat is to the side of the spine or in front of it, the bone density value can be decreased or increased.

REFERENCES

1. Mazess RB, Cameron JR. Bone mineral content in normal U.S. Whites. In: Mazess RB, ed. *International Conference on Bone Mineral Measurement. DHEW Publication No. (NIH) 75-683.* Washington, DC: US Department of Health, Education and Welfare, 1973: 228–237.
2. Rigo J, De Curtis M, Pieltain C, Nyamugabo K, Senterre J. Bone mineral density index (BMDI) determined by whole body dual energy x-ray absorptiometry (DEXA) in IDM, IUGR and preterm infants: comparison to intrauterine reference values. *Pediatr Res* 1996; 40(3): 548A.
3. Mimouni F, Steichen JJ, Tsang RC, Hertzberg V, Miodornik M. Decreased bone mineral content in infants of diabetic mothers. *Am J Perinatol* 1998; 5: 339–343.

Nutrition and Bone Development, edited by
Jean-Philippe Bonjour and Reginald C. Tsang,
Nestlé Nutrition Workshop Series, Vol. 41, Nestec Ltd.,
Vevey/Lippincott–Raven Publishers,
Philadelphia © 1999.

Premature Bone

Jacques Rigo, M. De Curtis, K. Nyamugabo, C. Pieltain, *P. Gerard, and J. Senterre

*Neonatology Unit and *Mathematics Department, University of Liège, CHR Citadelle, 4000 Liège, Belgium*

The goal of feeding regimens for low-birth-weight infants is to obtain a prompt postnatal resumption of growth at a rate approximating intrauterine growth (1). Human intrauterine growth and body composition have therefore received considerable attention over many years in order to obtain reference values and to define the most appropriate diet for preterm and term infants (2).

For bone formation, an adequate supply of protein and energy is required for collagen matrix synthesis, and ample provision of calcium and phosphorus is necessary for adequate mineralization (3). During development, nutrients are mainly transferred across the placenta. From carcass analysis of stillbirths and deceased neonates (2,4), it has been calculated that during the last trimester of gestation daily growth represents around 30 g of body weight, 23 g of fat-free mass, and 310 mg of calcium; after birth and during the first 2 months of life, the figures are 30 g body weight, 17 g fat-free mass, and 125 mg calcium (5). The use of the gastrointestinal tract to provide all nutrients for growth causes a large reduction in calcium availability for bone mineralization and leads to a relative decrease in bone mineral density, as suggested by the lower calcium-to-nitrogen ratio measured in human femur obtained in term neonates during the first month of life (6).

In preterm infants, daily growth may be similar or greater than that seen *in utero,* but daily calcium retention, accounting for about 50% of fetal accretion, leads to an increasing incidence of osteopenia (7). Therefore, it appears that bone mineralization in premature babies is one of the major challenges of neonatal nutrition and that the development of noninvasive techniques is required to allow collection of much needed information on bone growth and mineralization in preterm and term infants.

DUAL-ENERGY X-RAY ABSORPTIOMETRY

Dual-energy x-ray absorptiometry (DXA) is generally accepted as an accurate and precise noninvasive technique for assessing bone mineralization *in vivo* (8,9). Validation of its use in subjects with low body mass has supported its increasing use in

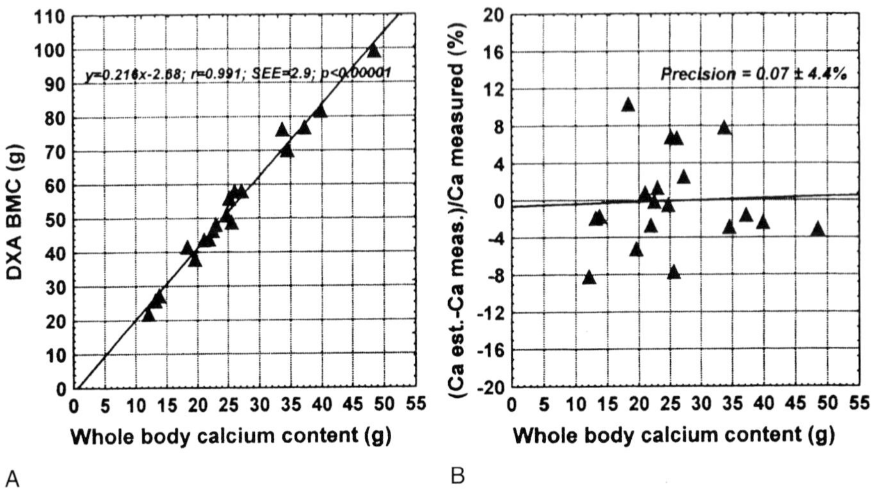

FIG. 1 A: Correlation between bone mineral content determined by DXA and chemically measured whole body calcium content in piglet carcass. **B:**Estimation of the precision of DXA measurement. Difference between DXA and chemical calcium values in percentage of the chemically measured value.

children. Recently we performed a validation study of whole body DXA in 13 newborn piglets ranging from 1,470 to 5,500 g using QDR2000 Infant Whole Body Software 5.65 (Hologic Inc., Waltham, Massachusetts, USA) (9). This new program with an infant table pad allows a substantially decreased threshold of bone detection in small subjects up to 50 to 150 mg/cm^2 (8). Reproducibility of DXA measurements was 0.09% for body weight and 1.95% for bone mineral content. Bone mineral content estimated by DXA was significantly correlated with whole body ash weight ($r = 0.96$) and whole body chemical calcium content ($r = 0.99$). An equation for conversion of bone mineral content into calcium was calculated (9). The precision of DXA measurement for calcium content was 4.4% (Fig. 1). Because radiation exposure during whole body scanning is low (<3 μSV), we concluded that DXA may be considered a noninvasive, safe, and accurate method for evaluating bone mineral content in preterm and term neonates, but that normative data for these subjects need to be acquired.

NORMATIVE VALUE OF BONE MINERALIZATION IN PRETERM AND TERM INFANTS

One hundred six appropriate-for-gestational-age preterm and term infants with birth weight ranging from 1,100 to 4,210 g and gestational age from 27 to 41 weeks were evaluated soon after birth (Table 1).

All infants were scanned in the first week of life with the exception of 20 preterm

TABLE 1. *Anthropometric characteristics of infants (mean ± 1 SD)*

	Intrauterine study	
	Preterm infants (n = 53)	Term infants (n = 53)
Gender	28 F, 25 M	30 F, 23 M
At birth		
Weight (g)	1,902 ± 434	3,243 ± 426
Length (cm)	42.9 ± 2.6	49.5 ± 2.0
Gestational age (weeks)	33.3 ± 2.4	39.0 ± 1.3
At DXA analysis		
Weight (g)	1,879 ± 425	3,144 ± 437
Length (cm)	43.5 ± 2.5	49.9 ± 2.0
Age (days)	8 ± 3	4 ± 2

infants who were analyzed during the second week. The delay was related to clinical condition or to the availability of the DXA apparatus. Body composition was measured using the same material as in the validation study (9). Infants were naked and swaddled in a paper sheet in order to avoid movement during the scan and to keep all four extremities apart from the body. They were aligned supine on the infant table pad. In order to assure area reproducibility, the upper extremities were separated from the trunk, the lower extremities were maintained extended in slight abduction, and the head was positioned facing to the side. No sedation was necessary, and scans with artifacts detected by discontinuity of the lateral edges of bones of the skeleton on the video monitor were excluded.

Whole body analysis allows measurements of body weight (g), bone mineral content (BMC) (g), bone area (BA) (cm^2), and bone mineral density (BMD = BMC/BA) (g/cm^2). Multiple linear regression analyses were performed to determine the explanatory ability of each of seven independent variables—birth weight, gestational age, postnatal age, gender, study weight, study length, and DXA weight—on each of three dependent variables (bone mineral content, bone area, and bone mineral density) separately. In this process, the most powerful individual predictor of bone mineralization was first determined, followed by other sets of independent variables that significantly augmented the explanatory ability of the single best predictor.

Because bone volume cannot be measured with DXA, the proportional relationship between bone mineral content and bone area was evaluated using the logarithmic regression between bone mineral content and bone area (10), and a bone mineral density index, $BMDI = BMC/(BA)^p$, was calculated, where p is the coefficient of bone area in this relationship. Multivariate analysis was also performed in order to determine independent variables that influence this logarithmic relationship significantly. Calcium content was calculated from bone mineral content using the conversion equation from bone mineral content to calcium previously obtained in piglets ($Ca = 0.456BMC + 1.56$) and compared to reference values obtained chemically (2) or by neutron activation analysis (11) on stillbirths or dead newborn infants.

Centile values of bone mineral content were calculated using Altman's method, based on polynomial regression and modeling of the residual variation (12). All statistical tests were performed with statistical software for a personal computer, Statistica 5.0 for Windows 95 (Statsoft, Tulsa, Oklahoma, USA) at an adopted significance level of 0.05.

The DXA body weight was the major and only predictor of bone mineral status in infants, accounting for more than 90% of the variance of total bone mineral content and bone area (Fig. 2). The independent variables DXA weight, study weight, and birth weight are highly collinear and may be used interchangeably. Because the delay of a few days from birth to DXA analysis, even if it may influence total body water, does not significantly change bone mineral content or bone area, the data obtained may be considered an intrauterine reference.

A conversion equation for bone mineral content to calcium allowed the calcium contents to be compared with the data obtained from carcass analysis (2) or with neutron activation analysis (11) (Fig. 3). The perfect agreement between the *in vivo* calcium estimations and the reference values suggests that the translation equation calculated in newborn piglets may be applied in newborn infants scanned soon after birth with identical equipment. However, the validity of the equation for the conversion of bone mineral content to calcium content must be confirmed after the neonatal period in view of the major changes in bone growth and mineral deposition that occur after birth.

Normative data for preterm and term infants are extremely limited. Results are often difficult to compare because of the different equipment and software employed. Recently Koo *et al.* (13), using similar equipment in a similar population, reported a positive relationship between body weight and bone mineral content (BMC =

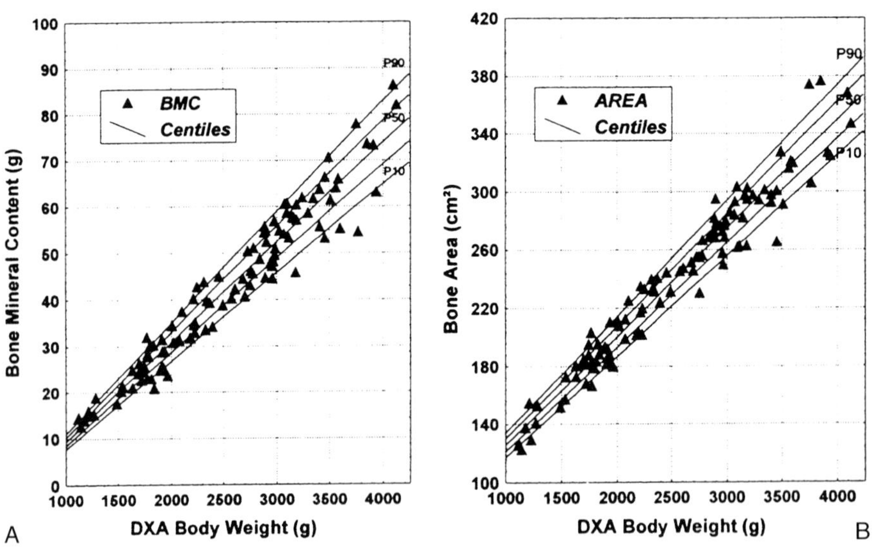

FIG. 2. Relationship between bone mineral content **(A)** and bone area **(B),** measured by DXA, and body mass at the time of study. Determination of centile reference values.

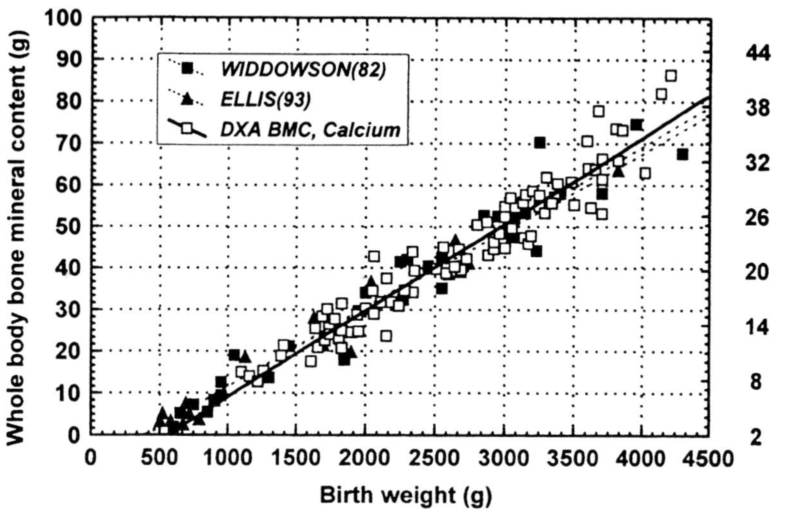

FIG. 3. Correlation between whole body calcium content estimated from bone mineral content, measured by DXA, and birth weight in 106 preterm and term newborn infants. Comparison with the reference values reported by Widdowson (2) and Ellis *et al.* (11).

0.0242BW − 11.1). From this study, bone mineral content represents 25.2 g at 1,500 g body weight and 73.0 g at 3,500 g instead of 20 g and 63 g in our study. The difference between these two studies could be related to the densitometer (QDR 1000 versus QDR 2000) or to a difference in the population studied. There is indeed evidence that in pregnant women, vitamin D status and dairy calcium supply may be different between the North America and the Belgian populations (14). Therefore, this study stresses the need for the development of an infant whole body phantom to compare equipments and populations.

In our study, DXA body weight was also the major predictor of bone mineral density, but gestational age was an additional significant independent variable (Table 2) in the final predictor equation. The proportional relationships (10) between bone mineral content and bone area, estimated from the logarithmic relationship, showed that a 1% increase in bone area was associated with a 1.71% increase in bone mineral content. The bone mineral density index, calculated as $BMDI = BMC/(BA)^{1.71}$, was not predictable by any of the independent variables. It remained stable despite changes in anthropometric variables, gestational age, or gender (Fig. 4). Its mean value was 3.41 ± 0.29, and this could be very helpful in comparing bone mineral density in various pathologic conditions (intrauterine growth retardation, infants of diabetic mothers, osteogenesis imperfecta, and so on) or during the follow-up of preterm infants (15,16). However, multivariate analysis showed that gestational age was an additional significant independent variable in the logarithmic relationship between bone mineral content and bone area. In multivariate analysis, a 1% increase in bone area was associated with a 1.5% increase in bone mineral content, and an

TABLE 2. *Best predictive equation of bone mineral content, bone area, and bone mineral density in preterm and term infants measured with DXA at birth*

Variable	Coefficient	SE	*t*-Ratio	*p*
BMC = C + DXA BW (r^2 = 0.94)				
Constant	−12.2	1.44	8.46	<0.00001
BW (10^{-3})	21.5	0.5	39.3	<0.00001
BA = C + DXA BW (r^2 = 0.95)				
C	51.3	4.5	11.5	<0.00001
BW (10^{-3})	74.6	1.7	43.7	<0.00001
BMD = C + DXA BW (r^2 = 0.82)				
C	71.7	4.6	15.7	<0.00001
BW (10^{-3})	38.5	1.7	22.1	<0.00001
BMD = C + DXA BW + GA (r^2 = 0.85)				
C	−8.3	19.2	−0.4	0.67(NS)
BW (10^{-3})	26.7	3.2	8.3	<0.00001
GA	3.0	0.7	4.3	=0.00004
log BMC = C + log BA (r^2 = 0.96)				
C	−5.7	0.17	32.6	<0.00001
ln BA	1.7	0.03	53.5	<0.00001
log BMC = C + log BA + GA (r^2 = 0.97)				
C	−5.1	0.2	−23.6	<0.00001
log BA	1.5	0.07	22.4	<0.00001
GA	0.02	0.005	3.8	=0.00023

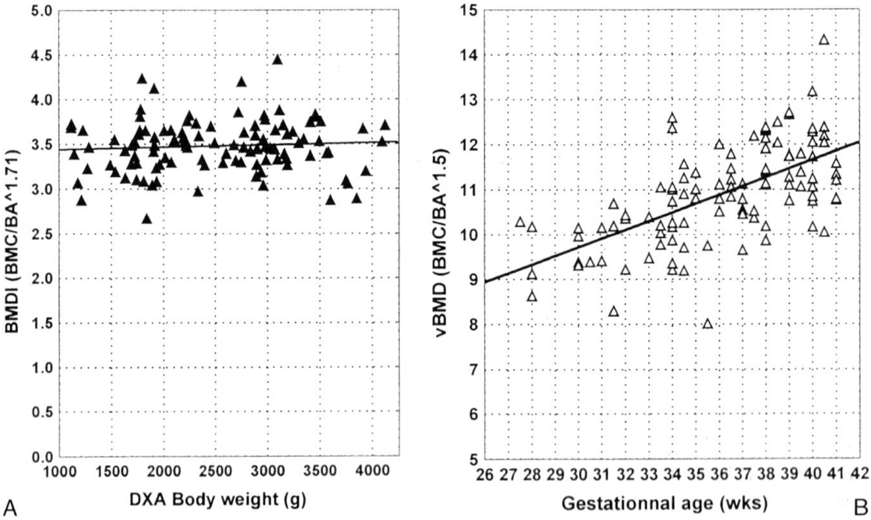

FIG. 4. Relationship between bone mineral density index and body mass **(A)** and between volumetric bone mineral density and gestational age **(B)** in preterm and term infants at birth.

additional increase resulted from gestational age (Table 2). These results indicate that during the last trimester of gestation, bone mineral content was related not only to bone growth but also to the exponential supply of calcium related to gestational age (4). The 1.5 coefficient of bone area observed in the multivariate relationship also suggests that bone area is an accurate index of bone growth or bone volume. Indeed, for a bone growing proportionally in length, width, and thickness, bone area at the power 1.5 ($BA^{1.5}$) represents a constant part of bone volume ($BA^{1.5} = kBV$). Therefore, volumetric bone mineral density was also estimated, as vBMD = BMC/$BA^{1.5}$, and was found to be significantly related to gestational age as well (Fig. 4).

BONE MINERALIZATION IN VERY-LOW-BIRTH-WEIGHT INFANTS ACCORDING TO FEEDING REGIMEN

For bone formation, an adequate supply of protein, energy, and minerals is necessary. Up to now, postnatal growth and mineral deposition in preterm infants have been estimated using metabolic and energy balance studies. Recently we observed a growth rate of 16 g/kg per day and a calcium retention of 90 mg/kg per day in VLBW infants fed fortified human milk (HMF) but a higher growth (20 g/kg per day) and a lower calcium retention (50 mg calcium/kg per day) in VLBW infants fed preterm formula (PTF). Because serial DXA measurements of bone mineral content and bone area permit estimation of bone growth and mineral accretion, DXA scans were performed twice, at about 3-week intervals, in VLBW infants fed HMF ($n = 10$) or PTF ($n = 24$) (Table 3). Weight gain, bone mineral, and bone area increases as well as various indices of bone mineralization were determined (Table 4).

TABLE 3. *Composition of diet and anthropometric parameters at birth and at the time of study in VLBW infants fed fortified human milk (HMF) or preterm formula (PTF)*

	HMF (n = 10)	PTF (n = 24)
Milk composition/dl		
Nitrogen (mg)	360	340
Fat (g)	3.3	4.1
Ca (mg)	110	78
P (mg)	56	50
Anthropometry at birth		
Birth weight (g)	1,387 ± 443	1,316 ± 302
Gestational age (weeks)	30.8 ± 3.4	30.1 ± 2.6
At DXA1		
Body weight (g)	1,540 ± 230	1,555 ± 228
Postnatal age (d)	22.8 ± 25	24.9 ± 16.5
BMDI[a]	3.4 ± 0.2	3.3 ± 0.4
At DXA2		
Body weight (g)	2,192 ± 149	2,483 ± 241*
Postnatal age (d)	46.0 ± 25.0	47.5 ± 17.6
BMDI	3.4 ± 0.4	3.0 ± 0.3*

[a] BMDI, bone mineral density index
* $p < 0.05$ vs HMF.

TABLE 4. *Various parameters of mineralization determined from the two DXA measurements in follow-up studies*

Bone mineral density index (BMDI)	$BMC/BA^{1.71}$
Volumetric bone mineral density (vBMD) (mg/kcm^3)	$BMC/BA^{1.5}$
BMC gain (%)/BA gain (%)	$(\log BMC_2 - \log BMC_1)/(\log BA_2 - \log BA_1)$
BMC gain (%)/volume gain (%)	$(\log BMC_2 - \log BMC_1)/[\log (BA_2)^{1.5} - \log (BA_1)^{1.5}]$

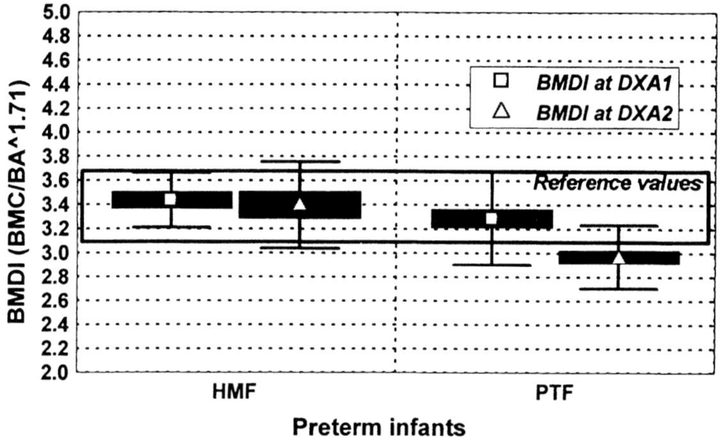

FIG. 5. Evaluation of bone mineral density index in very-low-birth-weight infants fed fortified human milk or preterm formula from two DXA measurements at 3-week intervals.

TABLE 5. *Composition and parameters of mineralization in VLBW infants fed HMF or preterm formula*[a]

	HMF (n = 10)	PTF (n = 24)
Interval between DXA$_2$ (days)	23 ± 8	23 ± 7
Mean vol. intake (ml/kg per day)	163 ± 13	144 ± 11*
Weight gain (g/kg per day)	15.5 ± 2.6	20.1 ± 2.9*
BMC gain (mg/kg per day)	290 ± 102	270 ± 72
Area gain (cm^2/day)	2.23 ± 0.77	2.92 ± 0.59*
BMDI gain	−0.04 ± 0.30	−0.32 ± 0.30*
vBMD gain	+0.46 ± 0.80	−0.27 ± 0.83*
BMC gain (%)/area gain (%)	1.74 ± 0.39	1.40 ± 0.25*
BMC gain (%)/area gain (%)	1.16 ± 0.26	0.94 ± 0.17*

[a] BMC, bone mineral content; BMD, bone mineral density; BMDI, bone mineral density index.
* $p < 0.05$ vs. HMF.

Weight gain and bone growth were significantly greater in the formula-fed infants, but bone mineral accretion was similar in the two groups (Table 5). All the various indices of bone mineralization were significantly greater in the HMF-fed infants. Thus, from the first to the second examination, no significant change in BMDI was observed in the HMF group, in contrast to a significant decrease measured in the PTF group (Fig. 5). Weight gain composition determining by DXA was similar to that previously obtained with metabolic and energy balance studies. Our data also suggest that the use of preterm formula may contribute to the development of osteopenia in VLBW infants by inducing greater bone growth in association with lower bone mineral deposition. Bone growth and bone mineral deposition appear to be two distinguishable phenomena that can be evaluated by DXA.

BONE MINERALIZATION IN VERY-LOW-BIRTH-WEIGHT INFANTS AFTER DISCHARGE

Bone growth and mineralization were also followed after discharge and during the subsequent 2 months in 16 very-low-birth-weight infants (Table 6). Those infants were divided into two groups according to their bone mineral density index at the time of discharge (<3,10; >3,10). Eight were considered osteopenic (BMDI = 2.99 ± 0.25), and eight were considered nonosteopenic (BMDI = 3.39 ± 0.10).

After 2 months, the increase of weight and bone area was similar in the two groups. However, the bone mineral accretion and the various indices of bone mineralization were significantly greater in the osteopenic group (Fig. 6). This preliminary study suggests that body growth as well as bone growth were similar in the two

TABLE 6. *Anthropometric variables at birth and at the time of study; weight gain composition and indices of mineralization in osteopenic and nonosteopenic very-low-birth-weight infants after birth*[a]

	Osteopenic (n = 8)	Nonosteopenic (n = 8)
Birth weight (g)	1,153 ± 274	1,400 ± 408
Gestational age (wks)	31.3 ± 1.6	30.9 ± 2.6
Postnatal age (d)	47.2 ± 19.9	32.9 ± 18.0
Body weight DXA1 (g)	2077 ± 252	2,012 ± 137
BMDI	2.99 ± 0.25	3.39 ± 0.10
Interval age (d)	62.9 ± 8.1	58.8 ± 4.2
Weight gain (g/d)	10.3 ± 1.0	10.3 ± 2.2
BMC gain (mg/kg/d)	206 ± 29	173 ± 40
BMC gain (mg/d)	625 ± 91	505 ± 132*
Area gain (cm^2/d)	2.32 ± 0.26	2.25 ± 0.64
BMDI gain	−0.03 ± 0.13	−0.42 ± 0.26*
vBMD gain	+1.00 ± 0.46	−0.28 ± 0.83*
BMC gain %/area gain % (%)	1.69 ± 0.09	1.41 ± 0.21*
BMC gain %/vol. gain % (%)	1.13 ± 0.06	0.94 ± 0.14*

[a] BW, birth weight; BMC, bone mineral content; BMD, bone mineral density; BMDI, bone mineral density index.

* $p < 0.05$ vs. osteopenic.

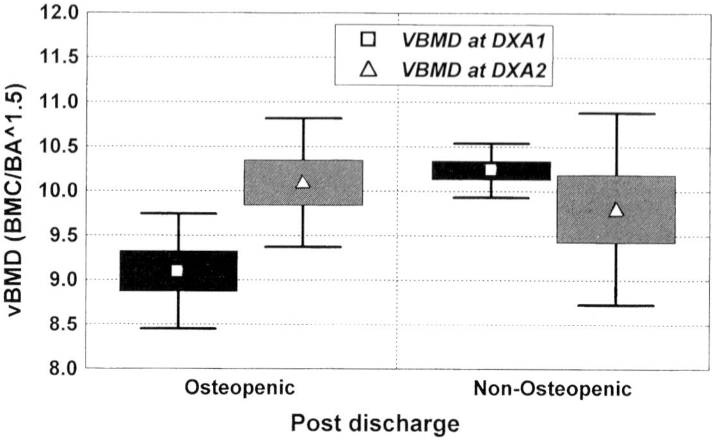

FIG. 6. Evolution of volumetric bone mineral density in very-low-birth-weight infants from discharge. Evidence of a catch-up mineralization in osteopenic preterm neonates.

groups, whereas mineral deposition was greater in the osteopenic preterm infants. This observation suggests that mineral status could be a trigger for bone mineral absorption and retention in preterm infants.

CONCLUSIONS

In summary, DXA appears as a new noninvasive, safe, and accurate method for evaluating bone mineral content. It can be used successfully for the determination of whole body mineral status even in small preterm infants. From the data obtained soon after birth in preterm and term infants, normative or intrauterine values were determined. These *in vivo* reference values were similar to previous reference values obtained from carcass analyses. A bone mineral density index was calculated and could be helpful in comparing bone mineral status in various clinical or pathologic conditions. Our data in preterm infants before and after discharge suggest that bone mineral content estimated from DXA does not represent a true measurement of hydroxyapatite content. Rather, the radiologic density measured by DXA appears to be the sum of the densities contributed by the bone matrix and by the bone mineral content. Therefore, bone growth and mineralization appear to be two distinguishable phenomena that can be evaluated with DXA. The relative osteopenia observed in preterm infants fed formula could be related to rapid bone growth in association with low mineral retention. After discharge this relatively low mineral density seems to trigger a catch up in mineral accretion independently of the diet.

In conclusion, the optimal nutritional strategy for bone mineralization needs to be determined. We do not at present know whether to promote bone growth or bone mineral deposition to obtain optimum development of bone mass during growth.

REFERENCES

1. American Academy of Pediatrics, Committee on Nutrition. Nutritional needs of low-birth-weight infants. *Pediatrics* 1977; 60: 519–530.
2. Widdowson EM. Importance of nutrition in development, with special reference to feeding low-birth infants. In: Sauls HS, Benson JD, eds. *Nutritional goals for low-birth-weight infants: Proceedings of the Second Ross Clinical Research Conference, Oct. 2–3, 1980.* Columbus, OH: Ross Laboratories, 1982: 4–11.
3. Garner SC, Anderson JJB, Ambrose WW. Skeletal tissues and mineralisation. In: Anderson JJB, Garner SC, eds. *Calcium and phosphorus in health and disease.* CRC Press: Boca Raton, 1995: 97–117.
4. Sparks JW. Human intrauterine growth and nutrient accretion. *Semin Perinatol* 1984; 8: 74–93.
5. Kahn B, Straub CP, Robbins PJ, Wellman HN, Seltzer RA, Telles NC. Intake and excretion of calcium and phosphorus by infants; calcium retention and model. *Pediatrics* 1969; Suppl 43, 4, part II: 668–686.
6. Dickerson JWT. Changes in the composition of the human femur during growth. *Biochem J* 1962; 82: 56–61.
7. Bronner F, Salle BL, Putet G, Rigo J, Senterre J. Net calcium absorption in premature. Results of 103 metabolic balance studies. *Am J Clin Nutr* 1992; 56: 1037–1044.
8. Koo WWK, Massom LR, Walters J. Validation of accuracy and precision of dual energy x-ray absorptiometry for infants. *J Bone Miner Res* 1995; 10: 1111–1115.
9. Picaud JC, Rigo J, Nyamugabo K, Milet J, Senterre J. Evaluation of dual energy x-ray absorptiometry (DXA) for body composition assessment in piglets and term human neonates. *Am J Clin Nutr* 1996; 63: 157–163.
10. Prentice A, Parsons TJ, Cole TJ. Uncritical use of bone mineral density in absorptiometry may lead to size-related artifacts in the identification of bone mineral determinants. *Am J Clin Nutr* 1994; 60: 837–842.
11. Ellis KJ, Shypailo RJ, Schanler RJ, Langston C. Body elemental composition of the neonate: new reference data. *Am J Hum Biol* 1993; 5: 323–330.
12. Altman DG. Construction of age-related reference centiles using absolute residuals. *Stat Med* 1993; 12: 917–924.
13. Koo WWK, Walthers J, Bush AJ, Chesney RW, Carlson SE. Dual-energy x-ray absorptiometry studies of bone mineral status in newborn infants. *J Bone Miner Res* 1996; 11: 997–1002.
14. Delvin EE, Salle BL, Glorieux FH, Adeline P, David LS. Vitamin D supplementation during pregnancy. Effect on neonatal calcium homeostasis. *J Pediatr* 1986; 109: 328–334.
15. Rigo J, De Curtis M, Pieltain C, Nyamugabo K, Senterre J. Bone mineral density index (BMDI) determined by whole body dual energy x-ray absorptiometry (DEXA) in IDM, IUGR and preterm infants. Comparison to intrauterine reference values. *Pediatr Res* 1996; 40(3): A548.
16. Rigo J, De Curtis M, Nyamugabo K, Pieltain C, Senterre J. Contribution of diet; human milk fortifier or preterm formula in the occurence of osteopenia in VLBW infants. *J Pediatr Gastroenterol Nutr* 1997; 24: A456.

DISCUSSION

Dr. Haschke: My question relates to your metabolic balance studies where you compared infants fed human milk with fortifier versus infants fed preterm formula. The data on your calcium and phosphorus retention in the first group fed human milk were 90 mg and 60 mg/kg per day, which is a ratio of 1.5 approximately, which one would expect. The retentions in your preterm-formula-fed infants were 56 mg calcium and 50 mg phosphorus, which is a ratio of 1.0. Isn't it possible that there was a problem with this infant formula and that the calcium was not absorbed very effectively for other reasons? The reason I ask is that it should not remain in use as a preterm formula if it gives poor calcium absorption. We did a study with you using another preterm formula where there was substantially better calcium retention.

Dr. Rigo: We carefully analyzed the phosphorus retention in our metabolic balance studies.

Phosphorus retention is related to calcium deposition, with a Ca/P ratio of 2/1, and to nitrogen retention, with a nitrogen/Ca ratio of 17/1. In our study, results of phosphorus retention can be accurately predicted by this equation. It means that the ratio between Ca and P retention is directly related to Ca retention and inversely related to nitrogen retention.

In the formula-fed group, fat absorption is high: 85% to 90%. Therefore, the relatively low Ca retention cannot be related to a poor fat absorption but is probably the result of the calcium salt used in the formula. As you mentioned in a more recent study, performed with a preterm formula from your company and containing a different calcium salt (Ca glycerophosphate), we obtained a higher Ca retention close to 90 mg/kg per day, which is similar to the values observed in the group fed the human milk fortifier. We are presently awaiting the results of bone mineral accretion in preterm infants fed this new preterm formula.

Dr. Klish: I'd like to ask about the interference with bone absorptiometry from the fat mantle overlying the bone. The DXA also can measure total body fat, so is it not possible to have an internal correction of the fat mantle from the DXA technique?

Dr. Rigo: Accurate measurement of whole body fat content in preterm infants is difficult to obtain, particularly in the smaller one. In fact, we observed that error of estimation was inversely related to fat mass (1).

Dr. Klish: But at least it measures the fat mantle that seems to be what causes the interference.

Dr. Rigo: When we include the fat content in a multivariate analysis, we don't get significant variables on the bone mineral content. So it is difficult at present to make any corrections. This is an important technical question: we need to undertake further studies to obtain data on interference between the fat and the bone mineral content.

Dr. Eisman: So, the problem with the fat mantle is not so much that it changes the value overall, it is that if the fat is not homogeneous, then you get very different results; that is what Dr. Gilsanz was referring to in terms of the big difference that can result from a 2-cm shift in fat from overlying the vertebrae to being on the side of the vertebrae. (See Discussion following Dr. Namgung's chapter.) It is lack of homogeneity that makes the big difference.

Dr. Gilsanz: When you do the whole body DXA, do you do it in a lateral or an AP position?

Dr. Rigo: It was done with the infant lying supine.

Dr. Gilsanz: I would like to see the correlation between the whole body mineral content in AP and lateral positions because, theoretically, the distribution of fat around the whole body is not a sphere, and the correlation would be far from 1. We need to measure the same bone in two different projections to see if the measurements they give us are the same.

Dr. Rigo: This study was performed partially by Koo and Coll (2). They did not find significant change in bone mineral content according to the position of the newborn infants, supine or lateral. In piglets, we also do not find any difference for bone mineral content according to prone or supine position. By contrast, bone area was modified. In the present study, the baby was carefully positioned on supine position in order to obtain reproducibility of area measurements. The interindividual variation of area measurement adjusted for body weight was small. In fact, reproducibility of area measurement, requiring three consecutive measurements in the same infants, was not performed for ethical reasons.

Dr. Eisman: I want clarification of a point that I did not fully understand. When you put all your data together initially, including both preterm and term infants, and did the mathematical analyses, you came out with a BMC log area of 1.71, yet when you split them up into the preterm and the term infants, you came up with a value of 1.5, with subtle differences in the constants that would have arisen depending on their age. I was wondering if you actually forced the 1.5 value, to approach some sort of volumetric concept, or whether that was the actual value that arose mathematically, and if so, can you explain why you got one value when you combined the two groups but a different value the same for both groups when you separated them.

Dr. Rigo: Thank you, this point needs to be clarified. In fact, in our first group, including preterm and term infants at birth, the "*in utero* reference group," we obtain a power coefficient of 1.71. The bone mineral density calculated as BMDI = $BMC/BA^{1.71}$ was independent of anthropometric parameters, i.e., body weight, length, gestational age. Therefore, contrary to BMC or BMD, this index does not need normalization for change in growth and is very useful for the study of infants of diabetic mothers, infants with intrauterine growth retardation, and preterm infants at the time of discharge (3,4).

However, using multivariate analysis, we showed that the power coefficient 1.71 was reduced to 1.5 when gestational age is taken into consideration as a dependent variable in the logarithmic relationship. This value of 1.5 was identical to that observed in our second group including healthy term infants measured during the first year of life. Considering that area at a power of 1.5 represents a volume, we suggested that $BMC/BA^{1.5}$ makes it possible to determine the change in volumetric bone mineral density at the perinatal period.

Dr. Prentice: One of the advantages of the approach you have been taking is that you actually look at the relationships within your data set, and you are not necessarily trying to come up with a predefined index. I think the discussion was moving to the question of whether or not the value of 1.5 represents something in physical terms. Often what happens is that bone area, either in a regression or on its own, gives information about other aspects in the child, and in this case it was gestational age, which reduces the power coefficient. If you put in other aspects as well, which you were not interested in, it would probably have reduced the coefficient still further. This is one of the advantages of not predefining indices before you have looked at the particular data set. This should then to some extent get away from the problems of overlying fat, because you are looking at the relationship within children, from low fat to high fat, that you are particularly interested in.

Dr. Eisman: But if you do that, you can't possibly use it to compare different groups, such as a diabetic group. You can only look within the group and look at the differences from that particular regression.

Dr. Prentice: It depends on the question you are asking yourself at the start. If you want to look at determinants for different effects, then it works very well. If you are trying to determine whether a particular child is different, then you have to take another approach.

Dr. Eisman: But differences are not defined within the group you are analyzing because diabetic children and so forth are not included within that group.

Dr. Prentice: You would put those in at the same time. If your hypothesis was to look at whether or not diabetic and nondiabetic children were different, that would be your data set.

Dr. Rigo: When we measured infants of diabetic mothers, we found that bone mineral content was slightly higher than our reference value and that bone area was also slightly higher. However, the bone mineral density index was in the range of the normal population at birth. Thus, in infants of diabetic mothers, bone mineral content appears to be appropriate for bone size. Bone volume increases in relation to body size, and mineralization is in the same range as *in utero*. This study demonstrates the role of this index for comparison of various groups of infants without the need of normalization for body size.

Dr. Seeman: With these pediatric programs, can't you measure the dimensions of the femur, the size and the width and the depth of either the vertebral column or one or two vertebrae, and then get your BMC and derive a volumetric density without having to resort to these equations that we all seem to be a little uncomfortable with?

Dr. Rigo: It is possible to obtain the projected area of one, but it is difficult with the whole body software to obtain accurate measurements and therefore to calculate the precise volume. We need to assess the shape of the femur precisly. By comparison with lumbar spine, we can assume that it is a cylinder or an ellipse, but all those mathematical models are dependent on the projected area measurements.

Dr Seeman: We always have to deal with the errors. But is the error greater with your formula than the error produced by assuming that the femur is a cylinder of a given length. Perhaps there is error in both, but the question is, which is the greater error? Maybe the alternative that I am suggesting has the smaller error.

Dr. Bonjour: In your conclusion you said that DXA allows one to measure bone matrix. Could you elaborate on that?

Dr. Rigo: In isolated femur obtained in fetuses and preterm infants, Salle *et al.* (in press) showed that calcified bone represents about 30% of whole volume. The DXA infant whole body software, using a low threshold level of bone detection, makes it possible to determine radiologic density of most of the whole bone and not only of the calcified one. So the BMC-to-calcium ratio may change according to bone growth and mineral deposition. It may be different from that obtained in adult.

Dr. Pettifor: I am confused because you showed a very good linear relationship between estimation of calcium mineral content by DXA and the estimations that were made by Widdowson and colleagues by ashing bone: she was measuring bone ash, you are measuring presumed mineral, and you have a very good correlation between the two for a very large weight range. So how can you say that hydroxyapatite or that matrix is actually interfering with your measurement?

Dr. Rigo: In our reference group *in utero,* our data suggest that the BMC-to-Ca ratio was constant. So we are able to calculate a calcium content that appears similar to that obtained by Widdowson on carcass analysis. It means that during gestation, bone growth and mineralization are proportionally constant. By contrast, after birth in a preterm infant, the ratio between growth and mineralization is modified. Growth is related to nitrogen and energy supply and is relatively high, whereas mineralization is related to calcium and phosphorus deposition and varies according to the diet: relatively high with the human milk fortifier and low with the preterm formula. Therefore, the challenge for neonatal nutrition is to make either a small amount of hard bone using the HMF or a large amount of soft bone using preterm formula?

Dr. Pettifor: I understand the issue that bone volume or bone growth does not necessarily parallel bone mineral content because you may get relative undermineralization of that bone, but that doesn't mean that you are measuring the matrix; perhaps all you are measuring is a thinner cortex, less trabeculae, or whatever happens to be in a bone that has grown in volume but has not been properly mineralized.

Dr. Rigo: I agree with you. In fact, technically the radiologic density measured with DXA is converted to hydroxyapatite equivalent using an internal standard. From the analysis of bone mineral content accretion and of bone area gain obtained in the two groups of preterm infants fed HMF or formula, we suggest that DXA takes into account matrix gain as well as calcium and phosphorus deposition. Indeed, Ca retention estimated from BMC gain was largely overestimated relative to metabolic balance studies.

REFERENCES

1. Picaud JC, Rigo J, Nyamugabo K, Milet J, Senterre J. Evaluation of dual energy x-ray absorptiometry (DXA) for body composition assessment in 1500 to 5500 g piglets and term human neonates. *Am J Clin Nutr* 1996; 63: 157–163.
2. Koo WWK, Massom LR, Walthers J. Validation of accuracy and precision of dual energy x-ray absorptiometry for infants. *J Bone Miner Res* 1995; 10: 1111–1115.
3. Rigo J, De Curtis M, Pieltain C, Nyamugabo K, Senterre J. Bone mineral density index (BMDI) determined by whole body dual energy x-ray absorptiometry (DEXA) in IDM, IUGR and preterm infants. Comparison to intrauterine reference values. *Pediatr Res* 1996; 40: A548.
4. Rigo J, De Curtis M, Nyamugabo K, Pieltain C, Senterre J. Contribution of diet; human milk fortifier or preterm formula in the occurance of osteopenia in VLBW infants. *J Pediatr Gastroenterol Nutr* 1997; 24: A456.

Nutrition and Bone Development, edited by
Jean-Philippe Bonjour and Reginald C. Tsang,
Nestlé Nutrition Workshop Series, Vol. 41, Nestec Ltd.,
Vevey/Lippincott–Raven Publishers,
Philadelphia © 1999.

Follow-Up Bone Development in Premature Infants

Richard J. Schanler

USDA/ARS Children's Nutrition Research Center and Section of Neonatology, Department of Pediatrics, Baylor College of Medicine, Houston, Texas 77030, USA

Much attention has been focused on increasing the survival of premature infants and improving their quality of survival by enhancing nutrition support regimens. To this end, during their time in hospital, premature infants receive specially designed commercial formulas containing more protein, energy, and minerals than formulas given to term infants. Because human milk has become a primary nutrient source for premature infants in many neonatal centers, various methods also are available to enhance the nutrient content of human milk to meet the greater nutritional needs of the preterm infant. Fortifiers are added to mothers milk to increase the content of protein and minerals, specifically calcium and phosphorus. Although postnatal intakes of calcium and phosphorus eventually meet estimates of intrauterine accretion, a cumulative deficit in mineral accumulation occurs by the time of hospital discharge. At the time of hospital discharge, which generally coincides with the attainment of term gestational age, premature infants have significantly lower bone mineral content than term infants. This difference in bone mineralization reflects the cumulative deficit in calcium and phosphorus accumulation. The consequences of inadequate mineral substrate during the period of rapid skeletal growth may be poor bone mineralization, reduced linear growth, rickets, or fractures (1–4).

The results of two prospective studies suggest that early nutrition affects later growth in premature infants. Koo *et al.* (1) demonstrated a relationship between radius bone mineral content and the subsequent development of rickets and fractures in later infancy. Lucas *et al.* (5) showed that abnormal biochemical indices of mineral status obtained during the neonatal period (for example, increased activity of serum alkaline phosphatase) were associated with reduced linear growth in follow-up at 9 and 18 months. Of note was the fact that the premature infants receiving the lowest calcium and phosphorus intake and having the greatest increase in alkaline phosphatase activity were those fed human milk.

Several questions arise from these comparisons. What is the significance of the differences in mineral accumulation between term and premature infants? Is the greater mineral deposition in term infants protective when breast feeding (for example, while feeding a low-mineral-containing milk)? Is subsequent growth affected by lower mineralization at the time of discharge? What are the effects and the long-term consequences of a mineral-enriched diet after hospital discharge?

BONE MINERALIZATION AFTER HOSPITAL DISCHARGE

Measurements of bone mineralization in the posthospital follow-up of premature infants were begun at The Children's Nutrition Research Center by evaluating the outcomes of infants fed fortified human milk (6,7). We evaluated bone mineral outcomes in premature infants who received fortified human milk during their hospital stay and who, at the time of discharge (10 weeks postnatal age), had attained term-equivalent age (Table 1). At discharge, nearly 50% of the infants were switched, by parental choice, from human milk to term infant formula. Two groups were followed: one continued to receive their mothers' milk and the other term formula. Both groups had similar measurements of growth and bone mineral content (using the distal third of the radius, as analyzed by single photon absorptiometry) at study entry, aged 10 weeks. In follow-up at 16, 25, and 52 weeks, however, infants who were breast-fed after discharge had lower bone mineral content than infants receiving term formula at home after discharge (Fig. 1). By 52 weeks, bone mineral content in those infants who received their mothers' milk after discharge remained significantly below that of infants receiving term formula (7). Those infants switched to term formula had a rapid increment in bone mineral content from 10 to 25 weeks compared with human-milk-fed infants. Premature infants who were breast-fed after hospital discharge also showed lower serum phosphorus and higher serum alkaline phosphatase activity throughout the 52 weeks compared with similar infants receiving term formula. The study population was small, and any differences in gender, race, or ethnicity could not be appreciated. The balance was such that, if differences in these variables were significant, bone mineral content in the human milk group would have been favored. No differences in body weight and length were noted between the two groups (Table 1). In both groups, however, the median weight and height were below the NCHS 50th centile (National Center for Health Statistics).

Even at term-equivalent age, both groups of premature infants had radius bone

TABLE 1. *After receiving fortified human milk in hospital, premature infants were breast-fed or switched to term formula after hospital discharge*

	Human milk (n = 10)	Term formula (n = 11)
Birth weight (kg)	1.1 ± 0.1[a]	1.1 ± 0.2
Gestational age (weeks)	28 ± 1	29 ± 1
Boys/girls (n)	9/1	5/6
White/Hispanic/black/Asian	5/1/3/1	10/0/1/0
Duration of human milk feeding (weeks; range)	31 ± 5 (20–72)	11 ± 3 (6–16)

[a] Mean ± SD.
From Abrams et al. (6,7).

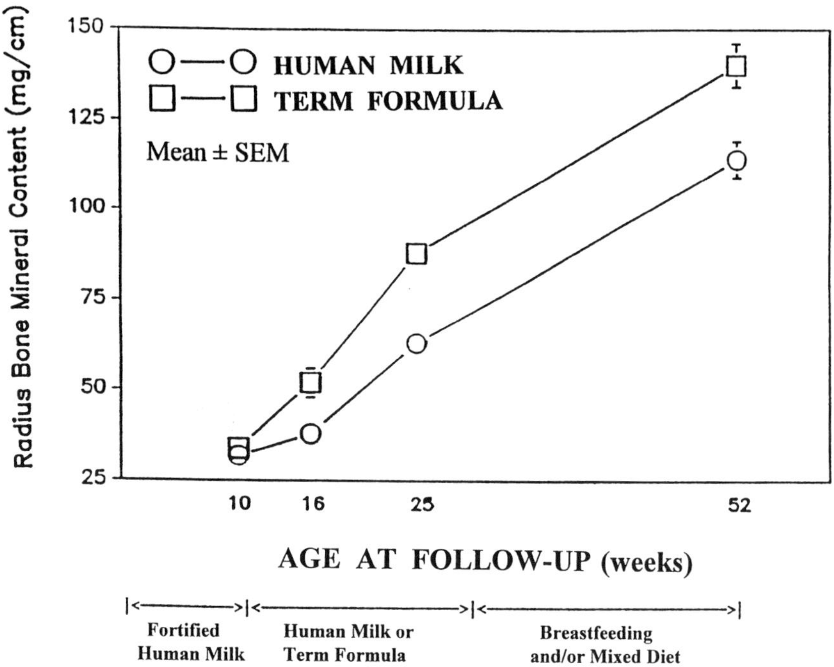

FIG. 1. Radius bone mineral content (BMC) in premature infants previously fed fortified human milk in hospital and either human milk or term formula after hospital discharge. The BMC in the human milk group is significantly lower than that in the term formula group at 16, 25, and 52 weeks. Adapted from Schanler *et al.* (8) and Schanler (28).

mineral content well below that of infants born at term (approximately 90 mg/cm). When they were switched to term formula after hospital discharge, the catch-up in bone mineralization was achieved between 6 and 12 months of corrected age. However, those infants who received human milk for more than 6 months after discharge failed to achieve catch-up bone mineralization until their second birthday (Fig. 2) (8). There is a striking difference in bone mineral content when human-milk-fed premature infants are compared with term infants receiving human milk, formula, or a mixed diet at 1 and 2 years of age or with premature infants fed formula (8). We believe catch-up mineralization might have occurred earlier if efforts at correcting the deficit in bone mineral mass had been made before discharge from hospital (8).

These data suggest that large deficits in bone mass arise before the infants are discharged from hospital. They further suggest that attempts should be focused on posthospital nutritional regimens that favor the accumulation of bone mineral mass. This focus might be appropriate because skeletal mass accumulates most rapidly in the first months after hospital discharge of a premature infant (9,10). Bone mineral measurements in premature infants fed term formula approximate measurements made in term babies by 6 months (11). Other investigators suggest that the mineral

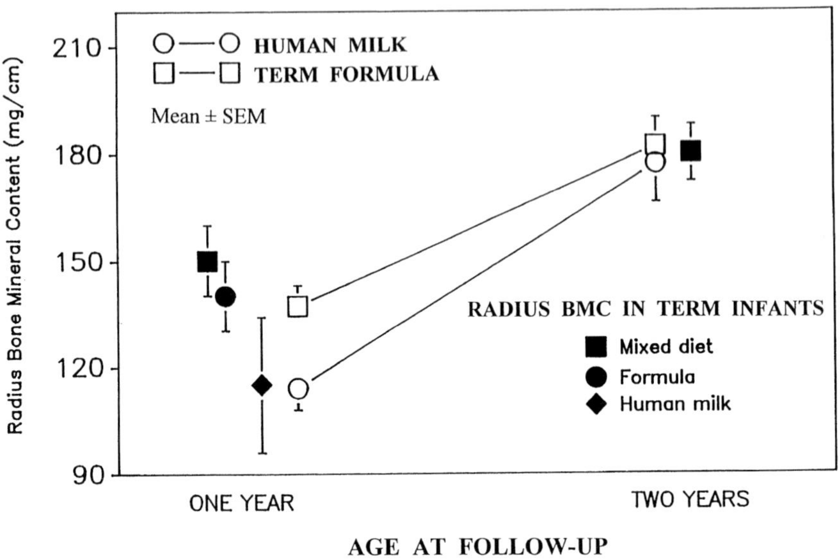

FIG. 2. Radius bone mineral content (BMC) at 1 and 2 years in premature infants previously fed fortified human milk in hospital compared with term infants fed human milk, formula, or mixed diets. HUMAN MILK, infants fed human milk after hospital discharge; TERM FORMULA: infants fed term formula after hospital discharge. Adapted from Schanler *et al.* (8) and Schanler (28).

accretion in premature infants catches up to the term infant as early as 8 to 16 weeks (9,12). There remains disagreement in this area (13).

ENRICHED DIETS AFTER DISCHARGE

Because it is not practicable to correct the mineral deficit before discharge from hospital, there have been several studies in premature infants evaluating the effects of a mineral-enriched diet on growth, serum biochemical indices, and bone mineral content after discharge home. The studies also differ in many aspects, the most significant difference being whether human milk or formula was used as the predominant mode of feeding.

Lucas *et al.* (14) investigated the growth of 32 premature infants fed an enriched formula (containing more energy, protein, and minerals) compared with a standard term infant formula. The study evaluated relatively large premature infants (32 weeks of gestation, 1.5 kg body weight at birth) who began the study diets at 37 weeks of postmenstrual age and were followed for 9 months corrected age. Infants receiving the enriched formula had greater gains in weight and increments in length throughout the study period than did infants fed standard formula. By 9 months corrected age, the infants in the enriched group had length increments at the 50th centile and weight gains at the 25th centile, while the standard group maintained their length growth at the 25th centile and weight gain at the third to tenth centile. Bishop *et al.* (15) provided data on bone mineral content of the distal third of the radius in this study population. There were no differences between groups at study entry, but by 3 and 9 months corrected age, the group receiving the enriched diet had significantly greater bone mineral content. No data were provided from either report to indicate whether growth centiles and bone mineral content were maintained once the study diet was terminated.

Friel *et al.* (16) studied 54 premature infants randomized to receive either an enriched or a standard formula. The enriched formula contained increased quantities of Ca (40%), P (21%), protein (10%), zinc (34%), vitamin D (38%), and vitamin C (100%) over the standard formula. In the 6-month follow-up there were no differences in growth as measured by NCHS *z* scores, corrected for age and gender. No data on bone mineralization were provided.

Wheeler and Hall (17) evaluated premature infants (birth weight 1.3 kg, gestational age 30 weeks) beginning at 36 weeks postmenstrual age, who were fed isoenergetic quantities of either preterm formula or standard formula. The preterm formula contained significantly more calcium (135%), phosphorus (54%), protein (22%), vitamin D (150%), and vitamin C (350%) than the standard formula. The group fed the enriched formula had a greater gain in length than the standard formula group. There were no differences in weight gain. The serum alkaline phosphatase activity was slightly greater in the standard group; there were no differences in serum calcium or phosphorus. Differences in length remained significant even at the 12-week visit (4 weeks after discontinuation of the enriched diet).

The study by Wheeler and Hall (17) also showed major differences in growth and serum biochemical indices between infants fed enriched formula or human milk in the 8 weeks after discharge from hospital. Premature infants fed human milk after discharge from hospital had slower gains in weight and length than infants fed enriched formula. Serum phosphorus was lower, and alkaline phosphatase activity was higher, in infants fed human milk than in those on enriched formula. No measures of bone density were reported.

Hall *et al.* (18) observed that a supplement of calcium and phosphorus in human-milk-fed premature infants did not affect growth but did affect biochemical indices after hospital discharge. A significantly lower incidence of hypophosphatemia was observed in the supplemented group. No length or bone density measures were reported.

Chan (19) evaluated growth, biochemical indices, and bone mineral content by single photon absorptiometry in an 8-week follow-up study of premature infants (birth weight 1.2 kg, gestational age 30 weeks) fed one of three formulas or human milk. After the follow-up study period, there was an 8-week washout period when formula-fed infants received standard formula. At 2, 8, and 16 weeks, body weight was significantly lower in the human milk than in the enriched formula group. All three formula groups had similar body weight at 8 and 16 weeks, and all were greater than the human milk group. The linear growth rate through 16 weeks was significantly greater in all the formula groups compared with the human milk group.

Serum calcium and 25-hydroxyvitamin D were similar among the four study groups. Serum phosphorus was lower and alkaline phosphatase higher in human milk than in formula groups. There were no differences among formula groups for any biochemical index.

Bone mineral content measured at 2 weeks was similar among the four groups. At 8 weeks there were marked differences among the groups. Bone mineral content was significantly greater in the group receiving the most nutrient-enriched formula and was the lowest in the human milk group. At 16 weeks, all formula groups had similar bone mineral content; all were significantly greater than in the human milk group.

Thus, Chan and his colleagues (19,20) suggested that mineral-enriched formulas were indicated in the posthospital nutritional management of premature infants. However, it is noteworthy that although infants receiving the enriched formula diet had a greater bone mineral content while on that diet, after an additional 8 weeks on standard formula there were no significant differences in bone mineral content among the formula groups. Furthermore, differences among formula groups were not observed for growth measures or serum indices. From analyses of these data it is difficult, therefore, to make firm recommendations. It is unclear why greater mineral intakes were associated with only transient increases in bone mineralization and no increases in growth. Few studies have provided follow-up beyond the period of enriched formula feeding. The long-term consequences of such practices are unknown.

LONG-TERM STUDIES

Furthermore, the data are a concern for the separate group of premature infants fed human milk. Most post-hospital follow-up studies have focused on growth and mineral status of formula fed premature infants. Those studies that included human milk fed infants found that they had slower rates of growth and bone mineralization than formula fed infants. No study has evaluated a practical method for providing an enriched diet to the breast-fed premature infant after hospital discharge. The implications of this practice are a concern.

However, data published by Bishop *et al.* (21) suggest paradoxic effects in long-term studies of bone mineralization. Premature infants fed human milk during their hospital stay were evaluated at 5 years. Bone mineral content, measured by single photon absorptiometry, was directly proportional to the quantity of human milk they received while in hospital, especially when the data were adjusted for differences in body weight. These data are distinct from other observations of long-term bone mineralization, which suggest that premature infants at 4 to 16 years have similar bone mineralization to term infants and that early diet does not appear to be a significant determinant of later bone mineralization (22,23).

Newer methodologies using dual-energy x-ray absorptiometry are now in use to investigate bone mineral development in premature infants (24–26). Several factors should be included in subsequent large-scale studies, with sufficient statistical power

TABLE 2. *Follow-up studies in premature infants: standard versus enriched diet*

		Standard diet		Enriched diet	
Reference	Duration	Calcium[a]	Phosphorus[a]	Calcium[a]	Phosphorus[a]
Lucas et al. (14)	9 months	350	290	200	350
Bishop et al. (15)	9 months	350	290	700	350
Wheeler and Hall (17)	2 months	510	390	1,200	600
Friel et al. (16)	6 months	490	345	680	416
Chan (19); Chan	2 months	535–539	392–462	624–686	361–392
et al. (20)	2 months	535–539	392–462	1208–1364	616–703

[a] Expressed in milligrams per liter.

to identify important covariates so as to provide a best estimate of bone development. Current and previous diet, gender, race and ethnicity, season, body weight, and age are all considered to be potential confounders in the analyses (13,25–27). Studies of enriched diets have employed a variety of nutrient adjustments, making it impossible to identify specific nutrient combinations directly affecting bone growth and development. For example, Table 2 shows the range of calcium and phosphorus concentrations found in the various enriched diets that have been investigated.

NUTRITIONAL RECOMMENDATIONS AFTER DISCHARGE

The postdischarge studies have many interpretations. Not all premature infants may be at nutritional risk at hospital discharge. Specific criteria may be needed to indicate which, if any, infant needs an enriched diet after discharge. The infant who is unable to consume sufficient volumes of milk *ad libitum* to satisfy growth needs is at greatest risk. The infant who, before discharge, is noted to have biochemical indicators of nutritional risk (low serum albumin and phosphorus concentrations and increased serum alkaline phosphatase activity) may also benefit from an enriched diet after discharge. The infant with residual cardiopulmonary or gastrointestinal disease may be at particular risk. These studies raise many questions regarding the recommendations for appropriate nutrition of premature infants after hospital discharge. If the goal is to match the rate of growth and bone mineral deposition of the term infant soon after discharge, then it may be prudent to use enriched formulas. It is unclear, however, how this approach can be adapted for the exclusively breast-fed premature infant at home. Further studies on the consequences of an enriched diet during the posthospital phase of rapid bone development are warranted.

CONCLUSIONS

At the time of hospital discharge, which generally coincides with the attainment of term gestational age, premature infants have significantly lower bone mineral content than term infants. The consequences of inadequate mineral substrate deposition during the period of rapid skeletal growth may be manifested as poor bone mineralization, reduced linear growth, rickets, or fractures. The results of prospective studies suggest that early nutrition affects later growth, specifically linear growth, in premature infants. Follow-up studies of premature infants after discharge from hospital suggest that bone mineralization is affected negatively by feeding unfortified human milk and positively by feeding enriched formula diets. The long-term consequences of these studies indicate that catch-up bone mineralization is possible. The bone development of the premature infant is complex, and further studies delineating the major confounding factors and using newer methodologies are warranted to address the potential consequences.

ACKNOWLEDGMENTS

These studies were supported in part by the General Clinical Research Center, Baylor College of Medicine/Texas Children's Hospital Clinical Research Center, Grant No. MO1-RR-00188, National Institutes of Health. This work is a publication of the USDA/ARS Children's Nutrition Research Center, Department of Pediatrics, Baylor College of Medicine and Texas Children's Hospital, Houston, Texas, USA. Funding has been provided from the USDA/ARS under Cooperative Agreement No. 58-6250-1-003. The contents of this publication do not necessarily reflect the views or policies of the USDA, nor does mention of trade names, commercial products, or organizations imply endorsement by the US Government.

REFERENCES

1. Koo WWK, Sherman R, Succop P, *et al.* Sequential bone mineral content in small preterm infants with and without fractures and rickets. *J Bone Miner Res* 1988; 3: 193–197.
2. Dahlenburg SL, Bishop NJ, Lucas A. Are preterm infants at risk for subsequent fractures? *Arch Dis Child* 1989; 64: 1384–1393.
3. Bishop NJ. Long-term effects of early diet on bone mineralisation in children born prematurely. In: Schonau E, ed. *Paediatric Osteology: New Developments in Diagnostics and Therapy.* Amsterdam: Elsevier Science, 1996: 115–120.
4. Ryan S. Bone mineralization and growth. *Eur J Clin Nutr* 1992; 46: S41–S44.
5. Lucas A, Brooke OG, Baker BA, Bishop N, Morley R. High alkaline phosphatase activity and growth in preterm neonates. *Arch Dis Child* 1989; 64: 902–909.
6. Abrams SA, Schanler RJ, Garza C. Bone mineralization in former very low birth weight infants fed either human milk or commercial formula. *J Pediatr* 1988; 112: 956–962.
7. Abrams SA, Schanler RJ, Tsang RC, Garza C. Bone mineralization in former very low birth weight infants fed either human milk or commercial formula: one year follow-up observation. *J Pediatr* 1989; 114: 1041–1044.
8. Schanler RJ, Burns PA, Abrams SA, Garza C. Bone mineralization outcomes in human milk-fed preterm infants. *Pediatr Res* 1992; 31: 583–586.
9. Congdon PJ, Horsman A, Ryan SW, Truscott JG, Durward H. Spontaneous resolution of bone mineral depletion in preterm infants. *Arch Dis Child* 1990; 65: 1038–1042.
10. Horsman A, Ryan SW, Congdon PJ, Truscott JG, Simpson M. Bone mineral content and body size 65 to 100 weeks postconception in preterm and full term infants. *Arch Dis Child* 1989; 64: 1579–1586.
11. Lapillonne AA, Glorieux FH, Salle BL, *et al.* Mineral balance and whole body bone mineral content in very low-birth-weight infants. *Acta Paediatr Suppl* 1994; 405: 117–122.

12. Pittard WB, Geddes KM, Sutherland SE, Miller MC, Hollis BW. Longitudinal changes in the bone mineral content of term and premature infants. *Am J Dis Child* 1990; 144: 36–40.
13. Hori C, Tsukahara H, Fujii Y, *et al.* Bone mineral status in preterm-born children: assessment by dual-energy x-ray absorptiometry. *Biol Neonate* 1995; 68: 254–258.
14. Lucas A, Bishop NJ, King FJ, Cole TJ. Randomized trial of nutrition for preterm infants after discharge. *Arch Dis Child* 1992; 67: 324–327.
15. Bishop NJ, King FJ, Lucas A. Increased bone mineral content of preterm infants fed with a nutrient enriched formula after discharge from hospital. *Arch Dis Child* 1993; 68: 573–578.
16. Friel JK, Andrews WL, Matthew JD, McKim E, French S, Long DR. Improved growth of very low birthweight infants. *Nutr Res* 1993; 13: 611–620.
17. Wheeler RE, Hall RT. Feeding of premature infant formula after hospital discharge of infants weighing less than 1800 grams at birth. *J Perinatol* 1996; 16: 111–116.
18. Hall RT, Wheeler RE, Rippetoe LE. Calcium and phosphorus supplementation after initial hospital discharge in breast-fed infants of less than 1800 grams birth weight. *J Perinatol* 1993; 13: 272–278.
19. Chan GM. Growth and bone mineral status of discharged very low birth weight infants fed different formulas or human milk. *J Pediatr* 1993; 123: 439–443.
20. Chan GM, Borschel MW, Jacobs JJ. Effects of human milk or formula feeding on the growth, behavior, and protein status of preterm infants discharged from the newborn intensive care unit. *Am J Clin Nutr* 1994; 60: 710–716.
21. Bishop NJ, Dahlenburg SL, Fewtrell MS, Morley R, Lucas A. Early diet of preterm infants and bone mineralization at age five years. *Acta Paediatr* 1996; 85: 230–236.
22. Helin I, Landin LA, Nilsson BE. Bone mineral content in preterm infants at age 4 to 16. *Acta Paediatr Scand* 1985; 74: 264–267.
23. Rubinacci A, Sirtori P, Moro G, Galli L, Minoli I, Tessari L. Is there an impact of birth weight and early life nutrition on bone mineral content in preterm born infants and children? *Acta Paediatr* 1993; 82: 711–713.
24. Braillon PM, Salle BL, Brunet J, Glorieux FH, Delmas PD, Meunier PJ. Dual energy x-ray absorptiometry measurement of bone mineral content in newborns: validation of the technique. *Pediatr Res* 1992; 32: 77–80.
25. Koo WWK, Walters J, Bush AJ, Chesney RW, Carlson SE. Dual-energy x-ray absorptiometry studies of bone mineral status in newborn infants. *J Bone Miner Res* 1996; 11: 997–1002.
26. Salle BL, Glorieux FH. Assessment of bone mineral content in infants: the new age. *Acta Paediatr* 1993; 82: 709–710.
27. Rubinacci A, Moro GE, Resmini G, *et al.* Sex-related differences of bone mineral content in low birthweight infants fed cow's milk formula. *Acta Paediatr Scand* 1990; 79: 866–868.
28. Schanler RJ. Body outcomes: bone mineral in preterm infants post discharge. In: Hay WW, Lucas A, eds. *Posthospital Nutrition in the Preterm Infant.* Columbus: Ross Products Division, Abbott Laboratories, 1996: 104–109.

DISCUSSION

Dr. Eisman: In those last data you presented, were the children of comparable stature irrespective of what they had been fed?

Dr. Schanler: There was a range of stature, and they corrected for that. There were all about the same age.

Dr. Eisman: From what we were saying before, one of the problems might be that if you feed a higher protein intake, the babies will grow faster but may not mineralize. If you correct for that, which is what you said they did, it might look as though they do better with less formula.

Dr. Schanler: The differences in the diets were only during the hospitalization, that is, for the first 3 months, and here we are talking about 5 years later.

Dr. Eisman: But it would be nice to know whether there was an inverse relation of stature or weight with the percentage of mother's own milk.

Dr. Tsang: I share the same concerns. Those babies were actually shorter, so one wonders if there was another interaction there.

Dr. Schanler: At 5 years?

Dr. Tsang: At least at 18 months. Then there is the issue of the proportion of breast milk: if there was more breast milk, does that mean that the mother was more motivated? What are the driving factors that are associated with this variation? In some way could that be what is causing the higher bone mineral content later? Human milk feeding is such an emotional issue.

Dr. Schanler: Certainly more holding of the baby, more stimulation perhaps.

Dr. Haschke: The data on bone fractures in the premature infants were not particularly alarming: only 1% in your cohort had fractures, less than the expected rate of 5% approximately. Are we doing any harm to infants if we just let them gradually make up their bone mineral by the time they are 2 years old? Should we be so careful? What are your concerns?

Dr. Schanler: We don't know if there is a concern. Our own data were on a very small sample size, and one of our concerns was that we couldn't adjust for factors that we thought might be affecting the outcome, at least by 2 years that is: gender and ethnicity. The only data that would cause me concern at present were the linear growth deficits in the infants fed the human milk, who were as much as 2 cm shorter when they were measured at 18 months.

Dr. Pettifor: If you used your data and, correcting for body size, produced centiles, is there any evidence of tracking of bone mineral measurement over age?

Dr. Schanler: We did that a while ago. The babies who were lower early on seem to be the ones who remain lower.

Dr. Pettifor: After correcting for body size at each of the age groups, so that you do not have an influence of body size?

Dr. Schanler: There was never a difference in body size at the times that we measured our infants.

Dr. Pettifor: But what happens is that the child who is, say, 2 SD below the norm for body weight tends to remain 2 SD below the norm at 3, 6, 9, 10 months, etc., and therefore, one would expect that if you just measured BMC, the smaller babies would have a lower BMC. But if you correct for their differences in body size at each of those ages, is there still tracking of bone mineral content?

Dr. Schanler: I need to look at that.

Dr. Prentice: The studies that Nick Bishop and Alan Lucas performed at our nutrition unit (1) showed that children who received human milk were shorter and had smaller bone areas at 5 years, even when corrected for body size. I know that Nick Bishop himself interprets this as showing evidence of some form of programming that the children who had human milk earlier on had smaller, denser bones. These data were obtained with single-photon absorptiometry, so there are perhaps concerns about them. I am now cosupervisor with Alan Lucas of a research fellow who has brought those children back yet again at 10 to 15 years of age, and we are doing DXA measurements on them. We have no results yet, but they will be out fairly soon.

Dr. Seeman: Let me reinforce this; the question is so important. We know in longitudinal studies that height does track, and as far as I am aware there is no crossing of height centiles. But the real question is, do you cross centiles for bone mass, and if you do, why do you? That is fundamental to the problem of fractures later in life. If you don't cross centiles, that means that the risk of osteoporosis is established at birth, if not before.

Dr. Haschke: Height does cross centiles, if not during the first 2 years than certainly later on at adolescence. It depends on how height is considered. If height for age is the reference, then tracking certainly does not occur, because height for age takes no account of early or late sexual development. So the question is, what is the right reference?

Dr. Gilsanz: You mean that children who are short can be tall after puberty?

Dr. Haschke: Yes, if puberty is delayed.

Dr. Prentice: But in general, there is tracking. Height at 1 year will predict adult stature very well. Cyrus Cooper at the Southampton Epidemiology Unit has looked at bone as well, and it does seem to track, but it is related to the height phenomenon, that is, the size of the skeleton (2).

Dr. Tsang: Cyrus Cooper's data were birth weight or 1-year weight relative to bone mineral content later, so it really wasn't bone mass tracking.

Dr. Pohlandt: Some babies develop severe skeletal deformation as a result of bone demineralization postnatally, and I wonder if these deformations are still recognizable 2 years after birth, when the bone mineral content has normalized.

Dr. Schanler: It would be interesting to follow that up.

REFERENCES

1. Bishop NJ, Dahlenburg SL, Fewtrell MS, Morley R, Lucas A. Early diet of preterm infants and bone mineralization at age five years. *Acta Paediatr* 1996; 85: 230–236.
2. Cooper C, Cawley M, Bhalla A, Egger P, Rung F, Morton L, Barker D. Childhood growth, physical activity and peak bone mass in women. *J Bone Miner Res* 1995; 10: 940–947.

Nutrition and Bone Development, edited by
Jean-Philippe Bonjour and Reginald C. Tsang,
Nestlé Nutrition Workshop Series, Vol. 41, Nestec Ltd.,
Vevey/Lippincott–Raven Publishers,
Philadelphia © 1999.

Factors Affecting Bone Mass in Infants and Toddlers

Bonny L. Specker

Ethel Austin Martin Endowed Program in Human Nutrition, South Dakota State University, Brookings, South Dakota 57007, USA

DEVELOPMENT OF METHODS FOR ASSESSING BONE MASS

Over the last two decades, many pediatric studies have been completed that have used various methods of bone densitometry to determine factors that affect bone mineralization during growth and to ascertain whether different interventions affect bone mass accretion. With each new method, greater insight into the complexities of skeletal growth has been gained.

In the 1960s several methods were used to assess bone mass in infants. Trotter and co-workers established normative data in 16-week-old fetuses to a 100-year-old subject in skeletal weight, density, and percentage ash weight, by weighing the skeletons and determining the volume by displacement of millet seed (1). Garn *et al.* used radiographs of the hand to assess skeletal maturity and mass (2). This method has been abandoned in studies of neonatal bone metabolism and studies in infants because radiographic changes are notoriously imprecise, as major shifts in bone mineral content are required before significant alterations in the image become apparent.

Also in the 1960s, photon absorptiometry was introduced by Cameron and Sorenson (3). By the early 1970s, single-beam photon absorptiometry (SPA) methods were used in pediatric populations to measure the bone mineral content of the distal radius. The infant is placed in a supine position, and the arm is held in place as it is scanned. A monoenergetic photon source, usually iodine-125 (^{125}I), is used in conjunction with a detector. The beam intensity in single-beam photon absorptiometry is proportional to the bone mineral density and the soft tissue thickness. The variability introduced by the soft tissue thickness is overcome by holding the arm in place with a bag containing deionized and demineralized water, which has absorption properties for ^{125}I similar to that of soft tissue. The amount of bone mineral content in the 1-cm width of the beam path and the bone width are determined. From these two measurements, bone mineral density is calculated in grams per square centimeter.

Single-beam photon absorptiometry has been used in many pediatric studies on bone mineralization. However, it measures primarily cortical bone, and the turnover rate of cortical bone is significantly less than that of trabecular bone. Therefore, cortical bone measurements are a less sensitive indicator of changes in density resulting from metabolic stimuli than is trabecular bone. Despite this limitation, the use of this technique has led to an understanding of many aspects of bone mineralization (see below).

In the early 1980s, dual-photon absorptiometry (DPA) was fast replacing single-beam photon absorptiometry for the measurement of bone mineral density in adults. The use of photons at two different energy levels eliminated the need for a constant soft tissue thickness across the scan path, allowing for the measurement of more peripheral bone sites. The primary use of dual-photon absorptiometry was in the measurement of the lumbar spine, which is primarily trabecular bone and is also the site of compression fractures in elderly people. Dual-photon absorptiometry was never used extensively in pediatric populations, perhaps because of the lack of pediatric software, long scanning times, and relatively high radiation exposures. Other methods for determining bone mineral density, such as computed tomography and neutron activation, have not been used in pediatric populations for similar reasons.

In the late 1980s, dual-energy x-ray absorptiometry (DXA) became available for use in pediatric populations, although algorithms for the software continue to be developed. The radiation dose for the pediatric total body scan is very low, equivalent to approximately 2 days of background radiation. The DXA technique is similar to DPA in that two different energy levels are used to measure the bone mineral content of the body. It differs, however, in that x-rays are used as the energy source rather than radioactive isotopes. The increased output of energy with an x-ray tube compared with an isotope source has led to increased resolution, improved precision, and reduced scanning time. Both DPA and DXA measure the density of the skeleton. In addition, the bone area can be determined from the image by identifying each pixel as either bone, fat, or lean tissue, thus allowing a calculation of bone mass in grams. Because the scan is obtained in two dimensions, certain assumptions regarding bone geometry are made within the computer software. The total body scans provide not only measurements of total body bone mineral content, bone area, and therefore bone mineral density but measurements of fat and lean mass as well. In addition to total body scans, other regional scans are available, as well as regional analyses from the total body scans (Fig. 1). The use of DXA to measure bone mass in small infants and toddlers has been validated by several investigators (4,5), and DXA total body bone mineral content measurements correlate significantly with total body calcium measured in the same subjects *in vivo* by neutron activation analysis (6).

Because peripheral quantitative computed tomography provides a cross-sectional analysis of bone, the density and thickness of cortical bone can be determined as well as the density of the trabecular bone. This method has been used in older children and adolescents and provides a true density measurement of the different

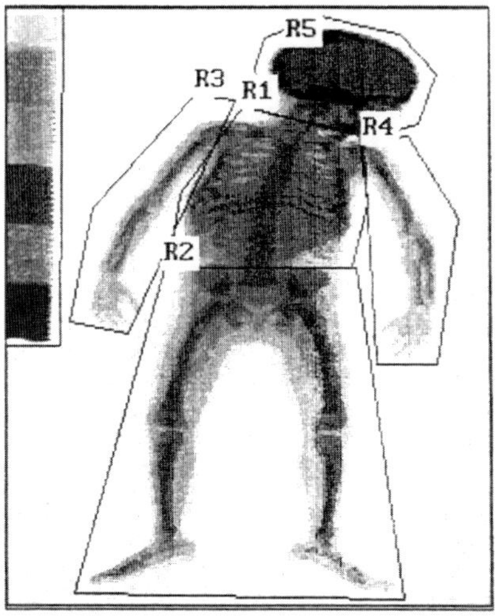

Region	BMC (grams)	Fat (grams)	Lean (grams)	Lean+BMC (grams)	Total (grams)	% Fat (%)
GLOBAL	230.5	2326.8	8562.6	8793.1	11119.9	20.9
R1	41.5	351.0	3333.5	3375.0	3726.0	9.4
R2	79.7	1534.3	2636.8	2716.5	4250.8	36.1
R3	14.0	164.7	383.2	397.2	561.8	29.3
R4	12.5	172.2	359.6	372.1	544.3	31.6
R5	83.2	116.8	1906.7	1989.9	2106.7	5.5

FIG. 1. Total body scans provide measurements of total body bone mineral content and bone area. Regional analyses from the total body scans are also possible.

types of bone (7). However, the method, although helpful in studies of older children, has not been validated in the infant and small child.

Unfortunately, bone mineral density cannot always be equated with bone strength. Ultrasound methods for estimating bone strength may prove valuable in this regard because it is thought that ultrasound not only measures bone quantity but also estimates bone quality (8). This technique makes measurements of the attenuation of ultrasound by bony structures over a wide frequency range (broadband). Although this technique is worth evaluation because the transmission of a sound wave through a limb is painless, noninvasive, and radiation-free, reliable methods have not been developed for the small infant and young child.

In summary, there have been recent advances in the development of new methods for assessing bone mass during infancy and early childhood. The use of these methods is allowing investigators to determine factors that influence bone growth early in life and to determine whether bone growth can be altered during this period of rapid growth. The development of new techniques for this age group may allow investigators in the future to determine whether environmental or genetic factors affect specific types of bone as well as the quality of the bone.

EFFECT OF ANTHROPOMETRIC, DEMOGRAPHIC, AND GENETIC FACTORS ON BONE MASS

Bone mineral content is consistently found to increase with increasing body weight and length in infants and children (9,10). Whether gender differences in bone mass or density exist in early life is not clear. Inconsistent findings have been reported and may reflect differences in the bone sites measured, use of different absorptiometers, or sample sizes insufficient to detect gender differences (9,11,12). A higher total body bone mass has been observed in male infants than in female infants 1 to 18 months of age, even after controlling for age, weight, length, and race (10).

Black adults have a greater bone mass and density than white adults (13), and a higher radius bone mineral density is observed in black children 1 to 7 years of age than in white children (9). No race differences in bone mineral density are observed in term infants at birth (14,15). The age at which race differences occur has not been determined, and the reason for these differences is not clear (10). Both decreased urinary calcium excretion and increased intestinal absorption have been found in older black children compared to white children (16); similar studies have not been done in infants.

Genes that may play a role in determining bone mass may be involved in race differences in bone mass. Restriction fragment length polymorphisms in the gene encoding the vitamin D receptor (VDR) have been shown to influence bone mass (17), although it is likely that more than one gene is involved. It was recently suggested that although racial differences in the vitamin D endocrine system may contribute to the racial differences in bone density, it is also possible that the VDR alleles may explain some of the racial differences that are observed. Racial differences in allele frequencies have been reported by some, but not all, investigators (18,19). Responsiveness to 1,25-dihydroxyvitamin D appears to differ depending on VDR alleles, although the mechanism for these differences is still unclear (20). Preliminary results indicate no relationship between variations in the VDR allele and bone mass accretion during infancy (21). If a genetic component of bone mass accretion during infancy is identified, it may be possible to determine whether certain interventions are more effective in increasing bone mass early in life in certain genotypes.

DIETARY FACTORS

Vitamin D and calcium may affect bone mass accretion during infancy and early childhood. However, it is not clear whether vitamin D levels within the normal range

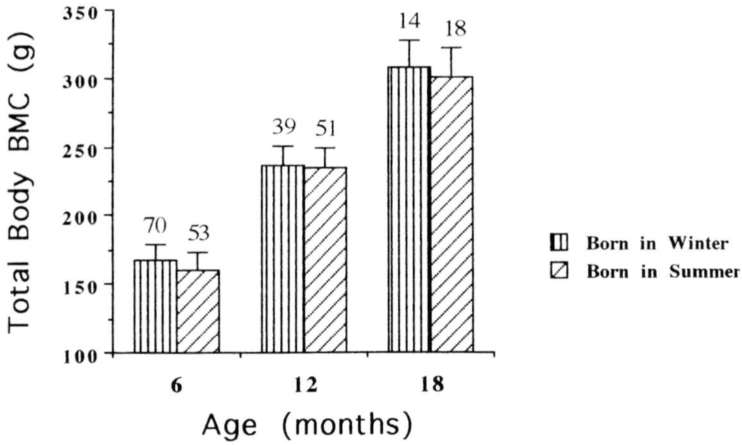

FIG. 2. Mean (± SD) total body bone mineral content by age and season of birth in formula-fed infants. Numbers of infants are given above each *bar.*

are associated with bone mass. Figure 2 illustrates mean total body bone mineral content, adjusted for weight and bone area, in infants born in winter or summer by age. Data from several studies were combined for this comparison (B.L. Specker, *unpublished observations*). There is no consistent trend of higher bone mineral content in summer compared to winter. However, all infants were formula-fed and were likely to have sufficient vitamin D stores.

Many studies on the effect of different diet regimens on infant bone metabolism have been completed using single-beam photon absorptiometry. In these studies, bone mineral content was measured either at the distal one-third or the distal one-tenth of the left radius or at the midpoint of the left humerus. Investigators have studied either the effect of human milk fortified with vitamin D versus human milk alone (22–24) or human milk versus formula (either soy based or cow milk based) (25–28). Some studies have found no differences in bone mineral content in infants fed human milk with or without vitamin D supplements (22,23), although others found a significantly lower bone mineral content in infants fed human milk alone than in infants fed human milk plus vitamin D (29). Older studies comparing soy-based formula with human milk or with formulas based on cow's milk found that bone mineral content in infants fed soy formulas was lower than that in infants fed human milk or cow's milk-based formula (25,28). Other studies found no difference (11,26). Findings from these early infant feeding studies have led to recommendations concerning vitamin D supplementation among human-milk-fed infants living in northern latitudes and to improvements in infant formula composition for the term infant.

Although rickets is usually associated with vitamin D deficiency, there is evidence that inadequate calcium intake also may be important (30–32). In addition to vitamin

D and calcium intake, sodium intake may theoretically influence bone mass accretion. Increased sodium intake significantly increases urinary calcium excretion in older children (33) and may lead to reduced calcium retention and bone mineral accretion. No data are available in infants and young children on the role of sodium intake on bone mass accretion.

The use of DXA now enables investigators to assess total body bone mass accretion in infants and young children and will allow better estimates of mineral accretion during infancy. Past estimates of mineral accretion have been based primarily on cadaver data (34). A recent randomized trial of formulas with varying mineral content found that total body bone mass accretion was greater during the first 6 months of life in infants fed a formula containing a moderate amount of mineral than in infants fed either a low-mineral-containing formula or human milk (35) (Fig. 3). At 6 months of age, all infants were rerandomized to either moderate- or high-mineral formulas. During the second 6 months of life, infants previously fed the moderate-mineral formula had less gain in bone mass than infants fed low-mineral formula or human milk. These results are consistent with randomized trials of calcium supplementation in prepubertal children older than 6 years, which showed that the beneficial effect of calcium supplementation does not persist beyond the supplementation period (36,37).

In 1984, the Consensus Development Conference on Osteoporosis suggested that increased calcium intake might help prevent osteoporosis by maximizing peak bone mass (38), and in 1994, the NIH Consensus Development Panel on Optimal Calcium Intake recommended 800 mg/day for children 1 to 5 years of age, despite a lack of data for this age group (39). As described above, calcium supplementation trials in

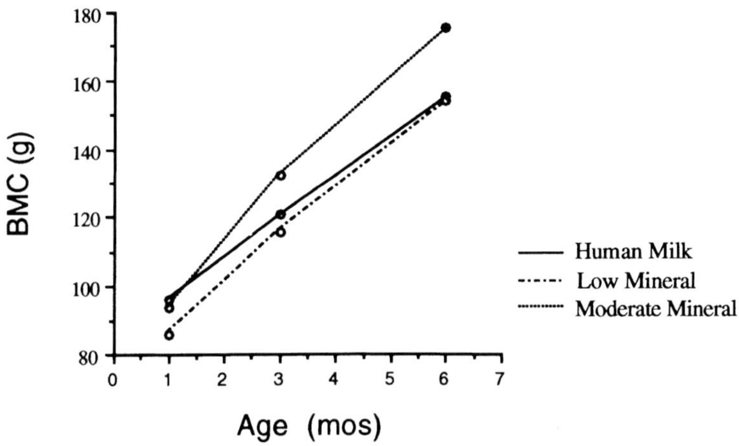

FIG. 3. Total body bone mineral accretion during the first 6 months of life is significantly affected by the mineral content of the infant's diet. Infants fed moderate mineral formula had a significantly greater bone mass at 3 and 6 months of age than infants fed human milk or low-mineral formula ($p < 0.001$ at both ages). From Specker *et al.* (35).

prepubertal children older than 6 years have found a beneficial effect of calcium supplementation that did not persist beyond the supplementation period (36,37). Very few studies have been conducted in young children between 1 and 6 years of age. In one small cross-sectional study of children aged 2 to 16 years, those children who received at least 1,000 mg calcium/day had a greater bone mass than children receiving less than this amount (40). In addition, bone mass at 5 years of age is associated with cumulative calcium intake from birth (41). There are no trials on the effect of calcium supplementation on bone mass in young children.

PHYSICAL ACTIVITY

The effect of weight-bearing activity and muscle contraction on bone growth is evident early in development. Infants with intrinsic fetal akinesia resulting from congenital neuromuscular diseases have significant osteopenia at birth (42). These findings have been supported by animal studies showing that the main mechanical factor related to fetal bone modeling is muscular strength (43). During growth, bone modeling results from both increased osteoclast activity and osteoblast proliferation. During weight bearing and muscle contraction, bones are slightly deformed, and during periods of relaxed pressure they tend to return to their normal form (44). This deformation and recoil stimulates osteoblastic activity. Intermittently loaded bone has been shown to increase in cross-sectional area, and this should theoretically allow a greater number of mineralization sites, thereby providing the framework for a larger bone mass (44). Physical activity in young growing rats is associated with an initial increase in bone resorption and formation, followed by a decrease in resorption and a sustained increase in bone formation. Overall, an increase in calcium retention is observed among young animals randomized to a regimen of increased physical activity (45).

There are no randomized trials in humans showing that activity during growth can affect bone mass accretion. However, recommendations are being made that physical activity be increased early in life to maximize peak bone mass (46–48). There are a few cross-sectional studies showing greater bone mineral density among active older children (>6 years of age) compared to sedentary children (49,50), and children participating in competitive sports with significant bone loading have a greater bone mineral density than control children (51). It has been speculated that more active children may emerge from adolescence with 5% to 10% greater bone mass (50).

Bone mass of postmenopausal women and young adults has been found to be positively related to the assessment of past childhood activity levels (52,53). Recent results of longitudinal studies indicate that weight-bearing activity during childhood is more important in determining bone mineral density of young adults (54,55). These studies support the hypothesis that weight-bearing activity during childhood is associated with a higher peak bone mass.

Although exercise has been shown to have a positive influence on bone mineralization in children aged 6 to 14 years (49), preliminary reports on the effect of physical

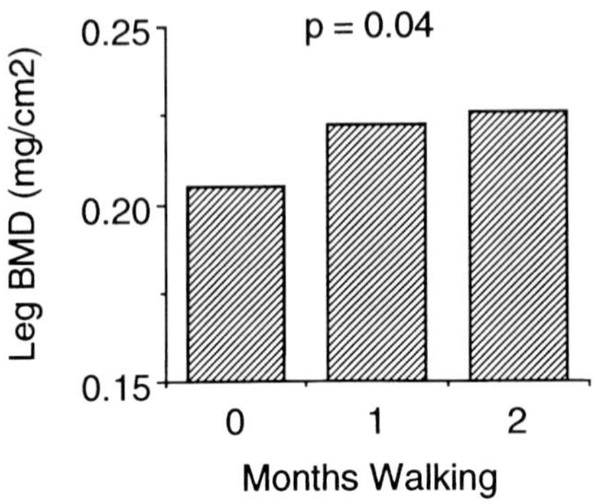

FIG. 4. Leg and arm bone mineral density in 1-year-old infants is greater the longer they have been walking.

activity on bone mass accretion in infants and young children have only recently been published. In an ongoing study designed to determine whether infants randomized to a 1-year gross motor activity program have a greater increase in bone mass accretion than infants randomized to a fine motor activity program, we found that leg and arm bone density at 1 year of age was correlated with the number of months the infant had been walking: infants who had been walking for 2 months had greater density than infants who had been walking for 1 month, which in turn was greater than infants who were not yet walking (56) (Fig. 4). Total body bone measurements were similar, indicating that the effects of bone loading on increasing density at this age are local rather than systemic. These results are consistent with a recent preliminary report showing that the most important predictor of total body bone mineral content in children 3 to 5.5 years of age, after controlling for age, weight, and height, was not previous calcium or phosphorus intake but the age at which the child began walking (57).

DISORDERS AFFECTING BONE MASS IN INFANTS AND YOUNG CHILDREN

There are several diseases that may lead to significant osteopenia in infants and young children. These conditions were recently reviewed by Gertner (58) and include genetic defects of bone matrix such as osteogenesis imperfecta, homocystinuria, and Menke's syndrome; hormonal conditions such as glucocorticoid excess and hyperparathyroidism; nutritional and metabolic conditions such as liver disease, vitamin D or C deficiency, and calcium or copper deficiency.

DOES MORE MEAN BETTER?

Although studies are just now beginning to appear on factors affecting total body bone mass accretion in infants and young children, they illustrate the types of questions that can be asked. Why should we want to increase the bone mass accretion in infants and young children? Decreased bone mineral content is associated with increased fracture risk in adults (47). Whether a similar relationship exists in childhood is not known, but if it does hold, interventions for preventing childhood fractures could begin early in life.

Increasing bone mineral content at a young age also may have long-term implications. Both peak bone mass and the rate at which bone is lost later in life are the two strongest predictors for subsequent risk of fractures and osteoporosis (47,59). For many years, osteoporosis research has focused on ways of minimizing bone loss in older individuals, and little attention has been paid to ways of maximizing bone gain. Some investigators now support the view that optimizing peak bone mass in childhood by providing an adequate calcium intake and moderate weight-bearing activity might serve as a means of preventing or delaying osteoporotic fracture (46). It will be important to determine whether these interventions, as well as others, early in life can affect bone mass accretion. Equally important is the need to clarify the role of early bone mass accretion on subsequent peak bone mass. It is likely that the prevention of osteoporosis must begin early in life, and as recently stated "... the prevention of osteoporosis, often deemed a geriatric disorder, may now be considered the legitimate domain of pediatricians" (60).

SUMMARY

Over the last two decades many pediatric studies of bone mineral density have been completed. Although these studies used various methods for assessing bone changes, much knowledge has been gained concerning skeletal growth. With the recent development of dual-energy x-ray absorptiometry, knowledge regarding genetic and environmental factors that affect total body bone mass accretion throughout infancy and early childhood is being gained. The ultimate goal of research in this area is to provide insight into possible interventions that may maximize the bone mass an individual achieves early in life.

REFERENCES

1. Trotter M, Broman GE, Peterson RR. Densities of bones of white and Negro skeletons. *J Bone Joint Surg* 1960; 42: 50–58.
2. Garn SM, Sundusky ST, Nagy JM, McCann MB. Advanced skeletal development in low-income Negro children. *J Pediatr* 1972; 80: 965–969.
3. Cameron JR, Sorenson JA. Measurement of bone mineral *in vivo:* an improved method. *Science* 1963; 142: 230.
4. Koo WWK, Massom LR, Walters J. Validation of accuracy and precision of dual energy x-ray absorptiometry for infants. *J Bone Miner Res* 1995; 10: 1111–1115.
5. Brunton JA, Bayler HS, Atkinson SA. Validation and application of dual-energy x-ray absorptiometry to measure bone mass and body composition in small infants. *Am J Clin Nutr* 1993; 58: 839–845.
6. Ellis KJ, Shypailo RJ, Hergenroeder A, Perez M, Abrams S. Total body calcium and bone mineral content: comparison of dual-energy x-ray absorptiometry with neutron activation analysis. *J Bone Miner Res* 1996; 11: 843–848.
7. Gilsanz V, Roe TF, Mora S, Costin G, Goodman WG. Changes in vertebral bone density in black girls and white girls during childhood and puberty. *N Engl J Med* 1991; 325: 1597–1600.

8. Kaufman JJ, Einhorn TA. Perspectives: ultrasound assessment of bone. *J Bone Miner Res* 1993; 8: 517–525.
9. Li JY, Specker BL, Ho ML, Tsang RC. Bone mineral content in black and white children 1 to 6 years of age. *Am J Dis Child* 1989; 143: 1346–1349.
10. Rupich RC, Specker BL, Lieuw-A-Fam N, Ho M. Gender and race differences in bone mass during infancy. *Calcif Tissue Int* 1996; 58: 395–397.
11. Chan GM, Robert CC, Folland D, Jackson R. Growth and bone mineralization of normal breast-fed infants and the effects of lactation on maternal bone mineral status. *Am J Clin Nutr* 1982; 36: 438–443.
12. Specker BL, Brazerol W, Tsang RC, Levin R, Searcy J, Steichen J. Bone mineral content in children 1 to 6 years of age: detectable sex differences after 4 years of age. *Am J Dis Child* 1987; 141: 343–344.
13. Mangaroo J, Glasser JH, Roht LH, Kapadia AS. Prevalence of bone demineralization in the United States. *Bone* 1985; 6: 135–139.
14. Steichen JJ, Kaplan B, Edwards N, Tsang RC. Bone mineral content in full-term infants measured by direct photon absorptiometry. *Am J Roentgenol* 1976; 126: 1283–1285.
15. Namgung R, Mimouni F, Campaigne BN, Ho ML, Tsang RC. Low bone mineral content in summer compared with winter-born infants. *J Pediatr Gastroenterol Nutr* 1993; 15: 285–288.
16. Abrams SA, O'Brien KO, Liang LK, Stuff JE. Differences in calcium absorption and kinetics between black and white girls aged 5–16 years. *J Bone Miner Res* 1995; 10: 829–833.
17. Morrison NA, Qui JC, Tokita A, *et al.* Prediction of bone density from vitamin D receptor alleles. *Nature* 1994; 367: 284–287.
18. Hustmyer FG, DeLuca HF, Peacock M. ApaI, BsmI, EcoRV and TaqI polymorphisms at the human vitamin D receptor gene locus in Caucasians, blacks and Asians. *Hum Mol Genet* 1993; 2: 487.
19. Fleet JC, Harris SS, Wood RJ, Dawson-Hughes B. The BsmI vitamin D receptor restriction fragment length polymorphism (BB) predicts low bone density in premenopausal black and white women. *J Bone Metab Res* 1995; 10: 985–990.
20. Howard G, Kelly PJ, Morrison NA, *et al.* Functional significance of vitamin D receptor alleles: response of bone turnover indices to calcitriol stimulation. *J Clin Encdocrinol Metab* 1996; 80: 2800–2805.
21. Specker BL, Williams LA, Kalkwarf H, *et al.* Vitamin D receptor genotype and its relation to bone growth and bone mineralization in infants 3 to 12 months of age (abstract). *J Bone Metab Res* 1995; 10: S188.
22. Greer F, Marshall S. Bone mineral content, serum vitamin D metabolite concentrations, and ultraviolet B light exposure in infants fed human milk with and without vitamin D_2 supplements. *J Pediatr* 1989; 114: 204–212.
23. Roberts CC, Chan GM, Folland D, Rayburn C, Jackson R. Adequate bone mineralization in breast fed infants. *J Pediatr* 1981; 99: 192–196.
24. Greer FR, Searcy JE, Levin RS, Steichen JJ, Steichen-Asche PS, Tsang RC. Bone mineral content and serum 25-hydroxyvitamin D concentrations in breast-fed infants with and without supplemental vitamin D: one-year follow-up. *J Pediatr* 1982; 100: 919–922.
25. Steichen JJ, Tsang RC. Bone mineralization and growth in term infants fed soy-based or cow milk-based formula. *J Pediatr* 1987; 110: 687–692.
26. Hillman LS. Bone mineral content in term infants fed human milk, cow milk-based formula, or soy-based formula. *J Pediatr* 1988; 113: 208–212.
27. Bainbridge RR, Mimouni F, Tsang RC. Bone mineral content of infants fed soy based formula. *J Pediatr* 1988; 113: 205–207.
28. Chan GM, Leeper L, Book LS. Effects of soy formulas on mineral metabolism in term infants. *Am J Dis Child* 1987; 141: 527–530.
29. Greer FR, Searcy JF, Levin RS, Steichen JJ, Steichen-Asch P, Tsang RC. Bone mineral content and serum 25-hydroxyvitamin D concentration in breast-fed infants with and without supplemental vitamin D. *J Pediatr* 1981; 98: 696–701.
30. Legius E, Proesmans W, Eggermont E, Vandamme-Lombaerts R, Bouillon R, Smet M. Rickets due to dietary calcium deficiency. *Eur J Pediatr* 1989; 148: 784–785.
31. Dagnelie PC, Vergote FJ, van Staveren WA, van den Berg H, Dingjan PG, Hautvast JGAJ. High prevalence of rickets in infants on macrobiotic diets. *Am J Clin Nutr* 1990; 51: 202–208.
32. Pettifor JM, Ross FP, Moodley G, Wang J, Margo G, Skjolde C. Serum calcium, magnesium, phos-

phorus, alkaline phosphatase and 25-hydroxyvitamin D concentrations in children. *S Afr Med J* 1978; 53: 751–754.
33. O'Brien KO, Abrams SA, Stuff JE, Liang LK, Welch TR. Variables related to urinary calcium excretion in young girls. *J Pediatr Gastrenterol Nutr* 1996; 23: 8–12.
34. Widdowson EM, McCance RA, Spray CM. The chemical composition of the human body. *Clin Sci* 1951; 10: 113–125.
35. Specker BL, Beck A, Kalkwarf H, Ho M. Randomized trial of varying mineral intake on total body bone mineral accretion over the first year of life. *Pediatrics* 1997; 99: e12.
36. Lee WTK, Leung SSF, Leung DMY, Cheng JCY. A follow-up study on the effects of calcium-supplement withdrawal and puberty on bone acquisition of children. *Am J Clin Nutr* 1996; 64: 71–77.
37. Slemenda CW, Reister TK, Peacock M, Johnston CC. Bone growth in children following cessation of calcium supplementation (abstract). *J Bone Miner Res* 1993; 8: S154.
38. Consensus Conference: Osteoporosis. *JAMA* 1984; 252: 799–802.
39. Food and Nutrition Board NRC. *Recommended Dietary Allowances, 10th ed.* Washington DC: National Academy Press, 1989.
40. Chan GM. Dietary calcium and bone mineral status of children and adolescents. *Am J Dis Child* 1991; 145: 631–634.
41. Lee WTK, Leung SSF, Lui SSH. Relationship between long-term calcium intake and bone mineral content of children from birth to 5 years. *Br J Nutr* 1993; 70: 235–248.
42. Rodriguez JI, Garcia-Alix A, Palacios J, Paniagua R. Changes in the long bones due to fetal immobility caused by neuromuscular disease. *J Bone Joint Surg [Am]* 1988; 70A: 1052–1060.
43. Palacios J, Rodriguez JI, Ruiz A, Sanchez M, Alvarez I, DeMiguel E. Long bone development in extrinsic fetal akinesia: An experimental study in rat fetuses subjected to oligohydramnios. *Teratology* 1992; 46: 79–84.
44. Lanyon LE, Rubin CT. Static vs dynamic loads as an influence on bone remodelling. *J Biomech* 1984; 17: 897–905.
45. Yeh JK, Liu CC, Aloia JF. Effects of exercise and immobilization on bone formation and resorption in young rats. *Am J Physiol* 1993; 264: E182–E189.
46. Anderson JJB, Metz JA. Contributions of dietary calcium and physical activity to primary prevention of osteoporosis in females. *J Am Coll Nutr* 1993; 12: 378–383.
47. Seeman E, Allen T. Risk factors for osteoporosis. *Aust NZ J Med* 1989; 19: 69–75.
48. USDHHS. *Healthy People 2000: National Health Promotion and Disease Prevention Objectives.* Washington DC: US Government Printing Office, 1991.
49. Slemenda CW, Reister TK, Hui SL, Miller JZ, Christian JC, Johnston CC. Influences of skeletal mineralization in children and adolescents: Evidence for varying effects of sexual maturation and physical activity. *J Pediatr* 1994; 125: 201–207.
50. Slemenda CW, Miller JZ, Hui SL, Resiter TK, Johnston CC. Role of physical activity in the development of skeletal mass in children. *J Bone Miner Res* 1991; 6: 1227–1233.
51. Cassell C, Benedict M, Specker B. Bone mineral density in elite 7–9 year old female gymnasts and swimmers. *Med Sci Sports Exerc* 1996; 28: 1243–1246.
52. Metz JA, Anderson JJB, Gallagher PN. Intakes of calcium, phosphorus, and protein, and physical activity level are related to radial bone mass in young adult women. *Am J Clin Nutr* 1993; 58: 537–542.
53. McCulloch RG, Bailey DA, Houston CS, Dodd BL. Effects of physical activity, dietary calcium intake and selected lifestyle factors on bone density in young women. *Can Med Assoc J* 1990; 142: 221–227.
54. Welten DC, Kemper HCG, Post GB, *et al.* Weight-bearing activity during youth is a more important factor for peak bone mass than calcium intake. *J Bone Miner Res* 1994; 9: 1089–1096.
55. Valimaki MJ, Karkkainen M, Lamberg-Allardt C, *et al.* Exercise, smoking, and calcium intake during adolescence and early adulthood as determinants of peak bone mass. *Br Med J* 1994; 309: 230–231.
56. O'Connor L, Buckley D, Ho M, Uetrecht G, Kalkwarf H, Specker B. Walking and bone mineral density at one year of age (abstract). *J Bone Miner Res* 1993; 8: S249.
57. Lasekan J, Specker B, Neylan M, Uetrecht G, Jones W, Tsang R. Early age of walking, calcium intake during infancy and bone mineralization at 3–5.5 years of age (abstract). *Pediatr Res* 1996; 39: 122A.
58. Gertner JM. Osteoporotic syndromes in children. *Growth Genet Horm* 1996; 12: 17–22.
59. Cummings SR, Kelsey JL, Neitt MD, O'Dowd KJ. Epidemiology of osteoporosis and osteoporotic fractures. *Epidemiol Rev* 1985; 7: 178–208.
60. Kreipe RE. Bones of today, bones of tomorrow. *Am J Dis Child* 1992; 146: 22–25.

DISCUSSION

Dr. Seeman: Could you just remind me how many people were in the physical activity trial and how many dropped out?

Dr. Specker: We enrolled about 70 infants, and about 60 completed. We looked at the reasons for dropping out. The usual one was that the infant was withdrawn from that particular day care center and moved to another where we weren't conducting a study. Those infants were no different from the ones who remained in the study up until the time that they withdrew.

Dr. Bachrach: How did you control for the background activity of these children? Twenty minutes a day is a fraction of what they were doing the rest of the time, and how do you know you didn't have slugs in the intervention group and more active infants in the nonintervention group?

Dr. Specker: We measured that in two different ways. One way is that we had 48-hour sensor readings every month on all infants; we did both the arm and the leg, so we have actual sensor counts. Those counts are comparable between the two groups. We also have 6 hours of direct observation of activity every 3 months. We did that because you can have very active children at this age who lie on their backs shaking their arms but not bearing weight at all, so to try to get information on weight bearing, we actually recorded whether or not they were bearing weight and on what extremities.

Dr. Pettifor: A walking toddler or toddler who is crawling is fairly active. I am interested in what sort of exercise you got them to do that was more physically active than either walking or crawling for a 20-minute period.

Dr. Specker: One thing I have learned from looking at the literature on activity in this age group is how inactive young children are. Adults have the conception that a toddler or an infant is a very active, but from our sensor counts over 24-hour periods we found that peak activity in toddlers is between 6:00 and 7:30 at night, which is the time that parents usually see most of them, but for the rest of the day it is very low and has small sporadic surges of activity. To get a 3- or 4-year-old to do, say, 30 minutes of sustained activity is very difficult, and to get them to do 20 minutes is not easy. For the really young ones in the gross motor group, we had four different exercises, each being either bending, tension, torsion, or compression, and we had a physical therapist working with us who came up with developmentally appropriate activities that were changed every 3 months. For fine motor activity, we did things like reading to them or just holding them because we wanted the physical contact to be the same in case that was affecting growth. Examples of activities in the younger ones are placing them on their hands and knees and rocking them back and forth and pulling them to a standing position. In the older ones (12 to 15 months), one of the activities was simply crawling around on the floor, but it is extremely difficult to get a 12-month-old who has just learned to walk to go back to crawling!

Dr. Pettifor: In relation to the difference in bone mass at the arm and the leg in the exercise groups, did you look at bone age? It is possible that those who were walking earlier may have had a more advanced bone age than those who didn't.

Dr. Specker: We didn't look at bone age *per se,* but what you are implying is important: that maybe you don't walk until your bones are strong enough to support you. The way I tried to address that problem was to look at the bone density at 9 months of age, because we had a scan at 9 months, and we found there was no difference between the two groups at 9 months, though there was at 12 months. We couldn't measure bone age because we only did the total body DXA.

Dr. Seeman: Karlberg divides growth into an infancy childhood pattern (1) and an apparent acceleration of growth at 12 months of age that appears to correspond to the appearance of growth hormone receptors in chondrocytes. This acceleration is of leg growth, not of trunk growth, whereas at puberty the main acceleration is in trunk growth, and leg growth ceases. I wonder whether exercising children at 1 year of age might be enhancing or impairing that phenomenon. I think it is important to look at the regions very carefully. I agree with you that it is very hard to define the regions on DXA.

Dr. Specker: That is interesting because of its relevance to studies on gymnasts who have shown reduced height (2). You can actually see from our data what appears to be a very large increase in the leg bone mass at around 11 months of age, which might be what you are talking about.

Dr. Seeman: We have done some work on international gymnasts. We find that in prepubertal female international gymnasts, the bone density is about two to three standard deviations above the predicted mean, and they are slightly short. We have also looked at a group who have been retired for 8 years, and despite their retirement, their bone mass is maintained. There are other data by Karlsson *et al.* (3) that support the idea that the effects of exercise in the prepubertal years, because it affects the modeling of bone, may be maintained into adulthood, and I think that this is an important window of opportunity for exercise. John Walk's group in Melbourne have done an intervention trial, not yet published, showing quite remarkable effects of physical activity in 8- to 9-year-olds compared to a control group. So I think that is a very important time of life. Whether 12 months is as important I don't know.

Dr. Specker: I think 12 months is probably a bad time to be doing this. In relation to the long-term effects of loading on bone, there was a study presented last year at Society for Pediatric Research that we were involved with (2) that had to do with bone density at 3 to 5 years of age in children who had previously been fed different mineral intakes during the first year of life. The only significant predictor of bone density that they found was the age when they began walking. There was no effect at all of mineral intake at any time of life. So physical activity may be the one thing that can have a long-term impact. And if you get the children active early in life, they may maintain a higher activity level beyond the intervention period.

Dr. Mughal: Afro-Caribbeans tend to have accelerated motor development in the first 2 years of life. They walk sooner and generally achieve the motor development sooner than white Caucasians. Do you think that might explain their increased bone density?

Dr. Specker: The rationale for our study was to try to explain those differences. The study was designed to have equal numbers of whites and blacks. Black infants in the United States do walk on average at about a month earlier than white infants, so they are loading their skeletons at a younger age. The problem we had was that black infants are enrolled at a much older age than white infants in our day care centers, and because we had to enroll them by 6 months of age, we ended up with too few black infants to address the question.

Dr. Pettifor: There is an important issue of which comes first: is it that early walking produces an increase in bone mass, or is it in fact a genetic factor? We know that most major motor development appears to be genetic. Perhaps children who walk early tend to have a higher bone mass not because of their early walking but because of a hereditary attribute that increases their bone mass.

Dr. Specker: Randomized trials will give the answer to that, because the age at walking is no longer of importance if children are randomized to different treatment groups. That is why it is so necessary to have a trial looking at the effect of physical activity on bone mass in this age.

Dr. Eisman: We have done some studies on physical activity in older people, and I have been impressed by our inability to really change the exercise patterns that the people choose. We did some studies in twins, and the twins were meant to be randomized to exercise or not, but we found that both twins exercised or neither exercised, even though they tried to be very cooperative. I just wonder how much these built-in characteristics may override any interventions you might apply.

Dr. Specker: I think that when trying to get young children to exercise, you cannot target the young children alone: you have to get the entire family to do it, or it is not going to be effective.

Dr. Eisman: Can you estimate what sort of relative change there would have been in the children who were randomized to additional gross motor activity compared to the underlying loading activity. Was it a 5% difference over what they were already doing? 50%? 100%? What sort of percentage change were you looking at?

Dr. Specker: In the 3- to 5-year-olds, the increase was about 15%. Whether that is true in the infants I am not sure. I would think that in the infants it is even higher, because children at 6 to 18 months are not that mobile: they sleep a lot at that age.

Dr. Gilsanz: Did you see any gender difference in physical activity in the age groups you studied?

Dr. Specker: Yes, there are differences in physical activity by gender. The boys had higher sensor counts than the girls on the leg, but the girls had higher arm counts.

Dr. Prentice: What was the level of calcium intake in the lower quartile?

Dr. Specker: It was less than about 550 to 600 mg.

Dr. Prentice: To what extent did it reflect the food intake of the children at that age? Were they the ones who were eating less food and therefore perhaps the ones who were growing more slowly?

Dr. Specker: In the data I presented, body weight was allowed for in the model.

Dr. Prentice: But energy intake, if it was measured adequately, would give you an indication of activity patterns as well, and if low calcium intake was related to other low intakes in the diet, one couldn't necessarily conclude that there was calcium insufficiency. It could be protein deficiency, for example. You did not look at this?

Dr. Specker: No, I only looked at calcium.

Dr. Tsang: I still think this is rather confusing. The low is normal actually!

Dr. Specker: It was low to moderate, the lowest quartile.

Dr. Tsang: But the low intake is actually a normal intake, only low in terms of the study. The high intake was actually high.

Dr. Prentice: What foods were the children in the high quartile of calcium intake consuming?

Dr. Specker: Most of the increased calcium came from cow's milk at that age.

Dr. Frenk: What about the passive mobilization? I am thinking especially of Mexico, where babies are carried around a lot. Has this ever been examined?

Dr. Specker: There are studies showing that just touching and holding an infant may affect growth. That is why we felt it was important to have a fine motor group—if this is an issue, we wanted to include it. But we didn't really look at how the infants were being held outside of the intervention program.

Dr. Bachrach: What are you intending to do with the blood and urine that you collected in the study?

Dr. Specker: We have already looked at quite a few things. Our numbers are not large enough to look at gross versus fine motor groups, and we have not been able to get sufficient numbers to analyze the effect of calcium intake, but the gross motor group has lower urinary calcium excretion and a slight but not statistically significant trend to a higher PTH.

REFERENCES

1. Karlberg J. A biologically-oriented mathematical model (ICP) for human growth. *Acta Paediatr Suppl* 1989; 350: 70–94.
2. Theintz GE, Howald H, Weiss U, Sizeonenko PC. Evidence for a reduction of growth potential in adolescent female gymnasts. *J Pediatr* 1993; 122: 306–313.
3. Karlsson MK, Johnell O, Obrant KJ. Bone mineral density in weight lifters. *Calcif Tissue Int* 1993; 52: 212–215.
4. Lasekan J, Specker B, Neylan M, Uetrecht G, Jones W, Tsang RC. Early age of walking, calcium intake during infancy and bone mineralization at 3–5.5 years of age. *Pediatr Res* 1996; 39: 122A.

Nutrition and Bone Development, edited by
Jean-Philippe Bonjour and Reginald C. Tsang,
Nestlé Nutrition Workshop Series, Vol. 41, Nestec Ltd.,
Vevey/Lippincott–Raven Publishers,
Philadelphia © 1999.

Lactation and Bone Development: Implications for the Calcium Requirements of Infants and Lactating Mothers

Ann Prentice, M. Ann Laskey, and Landing M. A. Jarjou

Medical Research Council Dunn Nutrition Unit, Cambridge, United Kingdom and Keneba, The Gambia

Full breastfeeding is associated with the transfer of approximately 200 mg/day of calcium from mother to infant. This amount is close to the theoretical calcium accretion rate required for optimal skeletal growth in early infancy (1). It also represents a sizable proportion of the mother's dietary calcium intake, placing her calcium economy under strain at a time when peak bone mineral mass should be achieved (2). Potentially, therefore, breastfeeding could have profound effects on the bone development of the infant and the bone health of the mother. These issues are important because current recommendations on infant feeding encourage exclusive breastfeeding for 3 to 6 months, followed by a period of partial breastfeeding (3,4).

Several studies have demonstrated that infants who are breast-fed for 3 to 6 months or longer have a different pattern of growth from babies who are formula-fed or weaned early from the breast (5–7). In particular, breast-fed children tend to be shorter and lighter in the second half of infancy, irrespective of the timing of the introduction of weaning foods, and remain so after weaning. Feeding mode has also been reported to influence the bone mineral content and bone mineral density of babies born at term in some studies but not others (8,9). This is discussed in more detail elsewhere in this volume. However, interpretation of these studies is problematic because these measures of bone mineral status, obtained by absorptiometry, are a function of bone and body size and are unable to distinguish between effects of feeding mode on growth and on bone mineralization unless adequate corrections are made (9–11).

There are similar difficulties in the interpretation of studies relating bone mineral density and fracture incidence of postmenopausal women to previous lactation history. There are conflicting reports suggesting that lactation increases the risk, decreases the risk, or has no influence on the incidence of osteoporosis (2,12). One reason may be related to the problem of confounding factors such as social class differentials in breastfeeding incidence and in body size. Another is the difficulty of defining lactation adequately, especially in retrospect. The term "lactation" encompasses a spectrum of breastfeeding behaviors that differ in the duration of exclusive and partial breastfeeding, the number of breastfeedings given per day, the time at which weaning foods are introduced, the extent to which they are used, and the lactational performance of the mother.

Lactational performance, in terms of the quality and quantity of breast milk produced, varies considerably among individual mother–infant pairs. These differences provide a useful model for exploring the impact of lactation on the bone development of the infant and on the bone mineral status of the mother. We have been conducting a series of prospective investigations to examine this issue. These are based in two very disparate groups of breastfeeding mothers living in Cambridge, England, and in Keneba, The Gambia. Cambridge is an affluent university city where breastfeeding for more than 3 months is more common among educated women of middle to high socioeconomic status. Many of these women have their first baby in their late 20s and generally have a total of one to four children. Typically, the calcium intake of lactating women in Cambridge is moderate to high at around 1,250 mg/day, the main sources being cow's milk, dairy products, and calcium-fortified white flour (13). Keneba, on the other hand, is a poor farming village in sub-Sahelian West Africa. In this region, all mothers breastfeed their children on demand for at least 2 years, introducing solid foods at around 3 to 4 months. The calcium intake of lactating mothers in this part of The Gambia is very low, at only 300 to 400 mg/day, and comes primarily from leaves, fish, groundnuts, and cereals (12,14,15). In addition, unlike Cambridge, women in Keneba have their first pregnancy shortly after menarche, which occurs at a median age of 16 years, and they continue with regular cycles of pregnancy and lactation throughout their reproductive lives, many ultimately having 10 or more children.

This chapter briefly summarizes our current understanding of variations in the amount of calcium transferred during breastfeeding and the likely impact of lactation on the bone mineral status of the mother and infant, drawing largely on our studies in Keneba and Cambridge as examples. The implications of the findings for the definition of calcium requirements are discussed.

BREAST MILK CALCIUM

The concentration of calcium in mature breast milk during the first 6 to 12 weeks of lactation is similar to that in early and transitional milk but declines progressively in later lactation (Fig. 1) (16,17). Variations in calcium concentration over the short term, for example during a single breastfeed or during the course of 24 hours, are small, and no special collection protocol is required to obtain representative samples of breast milk for calcium analysis (17). There are, however, substantial differences in the calcium concentration of mature breast milk between mothers, which are maintained throughout the lactation period (15,17,18). This is illustrated in Fig. 1 for two Gambian mothers followed through 18 months of lactation, one with a calcium concentration above the average for women in Keneba, the other with a

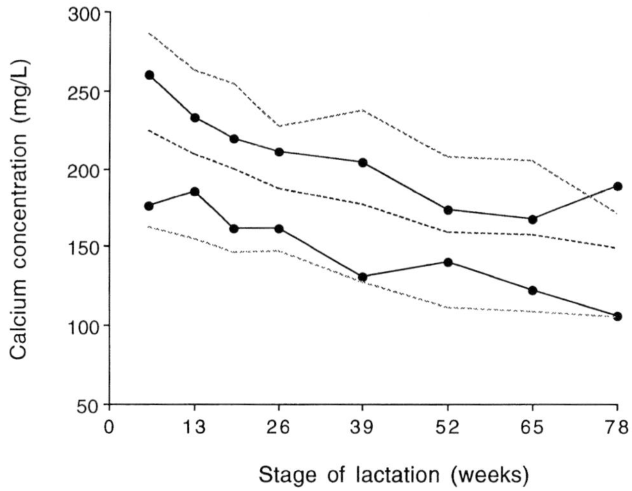

FIG. 1. Effect of stage of lactation on breast milk calcium concentration for two Gambian women. The *dotted lines* represent the mean ± 2 SD for 60 Gambian women collected from 1990 to 1992 (15). The *solid lines* are values from two individuals collected in the same period.

content below the average. Typically, the coefficient of variation of breast milk calcium concentration, after adjustment for lactation duration, is 20% to 30% (Table 1), implying a greater than twofold range of values between mothers at the same stage of lactation in the same community. No obvious reason has been identified for these differences between individuals. For example, most studies find no associations with either maternal age or parity (17,19–22). One Californian study has suggested that teenagers may have a lower breast milk calcium concentration than adult mothers (Table 1) (23), although this has not been observed in our Gambian studies (17).

In addition, there are substantial regional variations in the calcium concentration of mature breast milk (17,24). Table 1 gives a selection of published values from different areas for the concentration of calcium in breast milk at around 3 months of lactation. Mean values range from around 200 mg/l in some regions of West Africa, India, and Papua New Guinea to approximately 300 mg/l in parts of the United States and Europe. Although methodologic differences may be partly responsible for these effects, comparisons between more recent studies are valid because of the use of standardized methodology and accuracy control materials. For our cross-cultural studies in Cambridge and Keneba, for example, samples were collected and stored using the same protocol and identical equipment and were analyzed concurrently in the same laboratory (Table 1). The observed differences in breast milk calcium concentrations were highly significant at all stages of lactation (15,17,31).

TABLE 1. *Regional variations in mature breast milk calcium concentration*[a]

State	City	Group	*n*	Lactation month	Ca conc (mg/liter) Mean	SD	CV	Reference
United States								
California	Davis	UL	52	3	235	58	25	(25)
California	Davis	UL,T	13	3	215	79	37	(23)
California	Davis	UX	18	3	270	59	22	(23)
Georgia	Athens	UH	159	1–2	262	63	24	(20)
Illinois	Champaign-Urbana	UX	26	3	286	50	17	(21)
Indiana	West Lafayette	UH	45	3	265	60	23	(22)
Nebraska	Lincoln	UX	28	1–3	257	153	60	(16)
Ohio	Cincinnati	UX	18	3	270	34	13	(26)
Texas	Houston	UX	45	3	292	35	12	(19)
Europe, Australasia								
Australia	Canberra	UX	40	3	296	—	—	(27)
Australia	Melbourne	UX	18	3	338	—	—	(28)
Netherlands	Wageningen	UX,M	9	2–3	266	40	15	(29)
Netherlands	Wageningen	UX,O	10	2–3	298	39	13	(29)
UK	London	UX	12	1.5	276	55	20	(30)
UK	Cambridge	UH	29	0.5–3	301	54	18	(31)
Africa								
Egypt	Kalama	RL	53	3	258	54	21	(24)
Kenya	Nairobi	UM	21	1–6	245	40	16	(24)
Nigeria	Lagos	UX	14	3	197	46	23	(24)
Nigeria	Ibadan	UL	10	1–6	195	56	29	(24)
The Gambia	Keneba (1985–8)	RL	22	0.5–3	260	42	16	(31)
The Gambia	Keneba (1989)	RL	14	0.5–3	269	45	17	(31)
The Gambia	Keneba (1990–2)	RL	40	0.5–3	217	25	12	(31)
The Gambia	Manduar/K-Kunda	RL	31	0.5–3	218	28	13	(31)
Zaire	Yasa-Bongo	RL	12	2.5	260	59	23	(24)
Asia and South America								
Brazil	São Paulo	UH	6	3	236	67	28	(24)
Brazil	São Paulo	UL	8	3	273	58	21	(24)
India	Baroda	UX	59	3–4	208	52	25	(24)
India	Coonoor	UL	43	2–6	363	129	36	(24)
Korea	Seoul	UH	13	3	272	—	—	(24)
Nepal	Katmandu Valley	RL	26	2–6	264	143	54	(24)
Pakistan	Karachi	UL	9	1.5–6	284	74	26	(24)
PNG	Biak Island	RL	3	2–5	186	—	—	(24)
Taiwan	Taipei	UX	—	3	275	—	—	(24)
Vanatu	Port Vila	RL	18	2–5	274	42	15	(24)

[a] Data are those presented in the original reference for samples collected at the time closest to 3 months postpartum. Groups: R, rural; U, urban; L, low to middle income; H, middle to high income; X, mixed income or not stated; T, teen-aged mothers; M, macrobiotic diet; O, omnivorous diet.

MATERNAL CALCIUM INTAKE AND BREAST MILK CALCIUM

One plausible explanation for variations in calcium concentration is that breast milk calcium content is influenced by maternal diet. In The Netherlands, for example, women consuming a macrobiotic diet were found to have significantly lower calcium concentrations than omnivorous mothers (Table 1, $p < 0.04$) (29). The possibility that the calcium intake of the mother may influence her breast milk calcium concentration has been suggested by the fact that low milk calcium concentrations tend to occur in regions of the world where maternal calcium intakes are particularly low (Table 1), by a few observational studies that have reported significant associations between maternal calcium intake and breast milk concentration (26), and by early uncontrolled intervention studies on small numbers of women (27). However, moderate to high calcium concentrations have been recorded in some regions where the maternal diet is low in calcium, such as Egypt, Nepal, and Pakistan (Table 1) (22,32,33), and most observational studies in Western countries have not found relationships between maternal calcium intake or the use of mineral supplements and the content of calcium in breast milk (13,16,22,25,34). In a recent study in Cambridge, for example, we found no evidence of any association between breast milk calcium concentration and maternal calcium intake in the range 640 to 2,280 mg calcium/day (Fig. 2) (13).

The discrepancies between studies may be explained if there is a threshold calcium intake below which breast milk calcium concentrations are reduced. In order to test whether the calcium intake of lactating mothers accustomed to a very low calcium

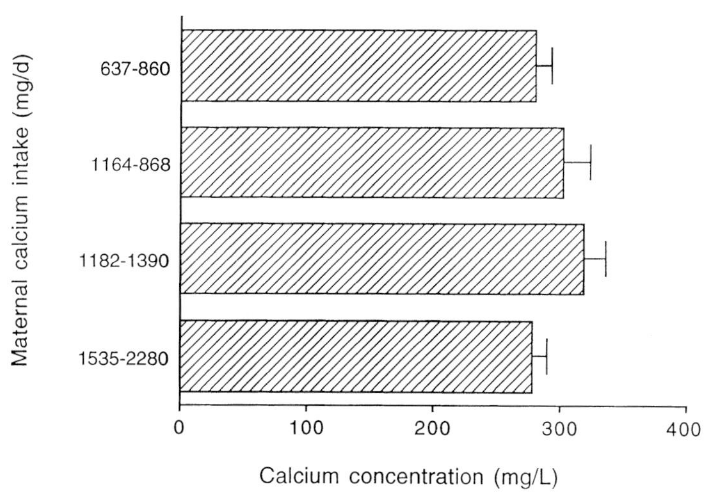

FIG. 2. Lack of a relationship between maternal calcium intake and breast milk calcium concentration in British women. Data are from Laskey *et al.* (13) and represent mean + SE. Results are from 40 women at 2 months postpartum, divided into four equal groups according to their calcium intake. There was no significant effect of maternal calcium intake on breast milk calcium concentration, as demonstrated by analysis of variance or regression analysis.

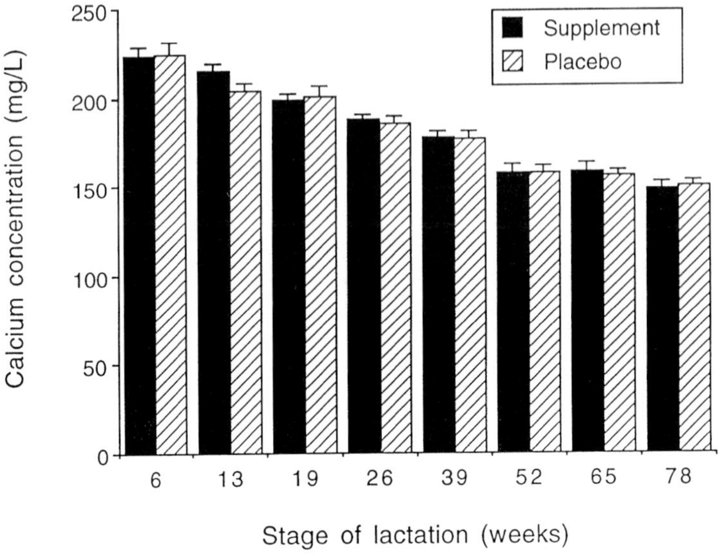

FIG. 3. Effect of a calcium supplement on the breast milk calcium concentration of Gambian women. Data are from Prentice *et al.* (15) and represent mean + SE. *Solid bars,* women supplemented with 714 mg calcium/day for first 12 months of lactation ($n = 30$); *hatched bars,* women receiving placebo for the same period ($n = 30$). There were no statistically significant differences between the groups at any stage of lactation, as demonstrated by analysis of variance.

intake influences breast milk calcium concentration, we conducted a randomized, double-blind, placebo-controlled supplementation study in Keneba (15). Sixty women were recruited to receive either a calcium supplement (1,000 mg/day calcium as the carbonate, 5 days per week) or a placebo (dextrose) for the first 12 months of lactation, starting 10 days after delivery. Breast milk samples were collected regularly during the supplementation period and during the succeeding 6 months. The tablets were delivered to the subjects on a daily basis and were consumed in front of research staff. Compliance with the regimen was 100%, and the expected increase in 24-hour urinary calcium output of 7% of the ingested dose was observed in the supplemented women (15). The calcium supplement effectively tripled the calcium intake of the mothers in the supplemented group and brought the intake close to internationally recommended levels for lactating women. Despite this, there were no significant differences in breast milk calcium concentration between the supplemented and placebo groups at any stage of lactation between 6 and 78 weeks (Fig. 3) (15). This result, coupled with the observational studies in mothers on a higher plane of calcium nutrition, indicates that breast milk calcium content is not responsive to maternal calcium intake during the lactation period.

Evidence emerged during the Gambian study that maternal calcium intake during the previous pregnancy may have some influence on breast milk concentration (31). Breast milk calcium concentrations measured in Keneba during the supplementation trial were significantly lower than those obtained during earlier studies in the same population using identical methods (Table 1, $p < 0.001$) (31). In the period between the previous studies (1985 to 1988 and 1989) and the supplementation trial, conducted in 1990 to 1992, a food supplement, routinely supplied to pregnant Gambian mothers in this village, had been modified to maintain the macronutrient content but to remove the dried skim milk component, thereby reducing the calcium intake of the women. We are currently testing the possibility that breast milk calcium concentration is influenced by calcium intake during the preceding pregnancy by a detailed supplementation study of pregnant women in Keneba. The first results from this investigation should be available in 1998.

BREAST MILK CALCIUM INTAKE

The amount of calcium transferred from the mother to the breast-fed infant depends on both the calcium concentration of the breast milk and the volume of breast milk ingested by the baby. These two variables are independent of one another, even during exclusive breastfeeding (17). As a consequence, the calcium intake of breast-fed infants varies widely. We have recently explored the extent of this variation in data from a subset of British and Gambian mothers who were participating in our detailed longitudinal studies of calcium and bone metabolism during lactation. The women who were included in this analysis—38 in Cambridge and 22 in Keneba—were selected because they had breast-fed their babies exclusively for at least 2 to 3 months and continued to breastfeed well beyond 3 months. The breast milk calcium concentration and the breast milk intake of the infant had been quantified for each individual toward the end of the period of exclusive breastfeeding (Table 2) (13,15,17,35). The results showed a range of measured breast milk calcium intake that was more than threefold in each community and was significantly lower in The Gambia. Overall there was a fivefold range of measured calcium intake. This finding of a wide range of calcium intakes by exclusively breast-fed infants supports our

TABLE 2. *Breast milk calcium intake of exclusively breast-fed infants at 2 to 3 months postpartum in Britain and The Gambia*[a]

		Breast-milk calcium intake (mg/day)			
Country	*n*	Mean	SD	Min	Max
Britain	38	263	78	130	450
The Gambia	22	187	48	79	293

[a] Data obtained by combining measurements of breast milk calcium concentration and breast milk intake for each individual mother–child pair. The subjects, selected because the infants were exclusively breast-fed for at least 2 to 3 months, were a subset of larger cohorts (13,15). Breast milk calcium analysis was performed by spectrophotometry on whole-milk samples that had been ashed and digested (17). Breast milk intake was measured over 14 days by deuterium oxide dilution, using the dose-to-mother method (35). The difference in means between the British and Gambian data is highly significant ($p < 0.0001$).

earlier observations on smaller numbers (17) and those of other researchers in the United States (19).

GROWTH AND BONE DEVELOPMENT IN BREAST-FED INFANTS

Despite such large differences in calcium intake, analysis of anthropometric data from these 60 exclusively breast-fed British and Gambian infants provided little evidence to suggest that the differences are reflected in variations in growth rate or bone development in the first months of life. The Gambian infants (G), 11 boys and 11 girls, were somewhat lighter and shorter than the British children (B), 16 boys and 22 girls, at both 0.5 and 3 months of age ($p < 0.0001$). Their mean (SD) weight at 0.5 months was G = 3.2 (0.6) kg, B = 3.9 (0.4) kg; and at 3 months, G = 5.8 (0.8) kg, B = 6.2 (0.6) kg. Their length at 0.5 months was G = 49.4 (1.3) cm, B = 52.6 (2.3) cm; and at 3 months, G = 58.9 (2.2) cm, B = 61.7 (2.0) cm. However, weight and length gains between 0.5 and 3 months were satisfactory in both cohorts, close to international reference median values, and were not significantly different between the two groups ($p > 0.3$, NS). Their weight gain was G = 2.6 (0.9) kg, B = 2.3 (0.6) kg; and their length gain was G = 9.5 (2.2) cm, B = 9.0 (1.9) cm. With multiple regression analysis in which initial value, sex, and country were also included, no relationships were found between infant gain in length and breast milk volume, breast milk calcium concentration, or breast milk calcium intake. Gain in weight, however, was positively related to breast milk volume ($p < 0.0001$; total $R^2 = 69\%$). This is in line with other studies, including our own, that suggest that human milk production is not limited by the secretory capacity of the breast but is controlled by infant demand (36,37). However, breast milk calcium concentration was not a significant predictor of weight gain when entered as an independent variable in the regression model ($p = 0.85$, NS; total $R^2 = 68\%$). Substituting breast milk calcium intake for breast milk volume and calcium concentration resulted in a significant correlation with weight gain, but the proportion of the variance that could be accounted for by the model was reduced ($p < 0.0001$; total $R^2 = 62\%$). These results indicate that weight gain in the first months of infancy, but not linear growth, is related to the total amount of breast milk ingested but that variations in breast milk calcium *per se* have little influence.

In the Gambian cohort, bone mineral measurements at the radius shaft using single-photon absorptiometry were also available at 3 months. No significant relationships were observed between breast milk volume, breast milk calcium concentration, or breast milk calcium intake and the infant's bone mineral content at 3 months, with or without adjustment for bone and body size.

In a previous, more detailed comparative study of growth and bone mineral status in Gambian and British children aged 0 to 36 months, we showed that the Gambians fall behind their British counterparts during infancy in terms of weight, height, and size-adjusted bone mineral content of the radius (38). Whether growth and bone development in these children is limited by their low calcium intake during later infancy, which averages about 200 mg/day because of a combination of the low breast milk calcium concentration and poor quality weaning foods, needs further exploration (1,12). However, it is unlikely that calcium intake is the main factor involved; a calcium-rich weaning food supplement provided to all infants aged 3 to 12 months in Keneba over a period of several years did not improve growth or bone mineral status relative to infants in neighboring villages (38,39).

LACTATION AND BONE MINERAL STATUS OF THE MOTHER

Because the amount of calcium secreted into breast milk represents a substantial proportion of the daily calcium intake of the mother, it is possible that calcium is mobilized from bone to support lactation. Potentially, this could compromise the optimal development of peak bone mineral mass, especially in women with inadequate dietary calcium intake.

It is now well recognized that breastfeeding is accompanied by reductions in bone mineral content, which reverse toward the end of lactation and after weaning (2,12,40–42). The effects are most pronounced in axial regions of the skeleton,

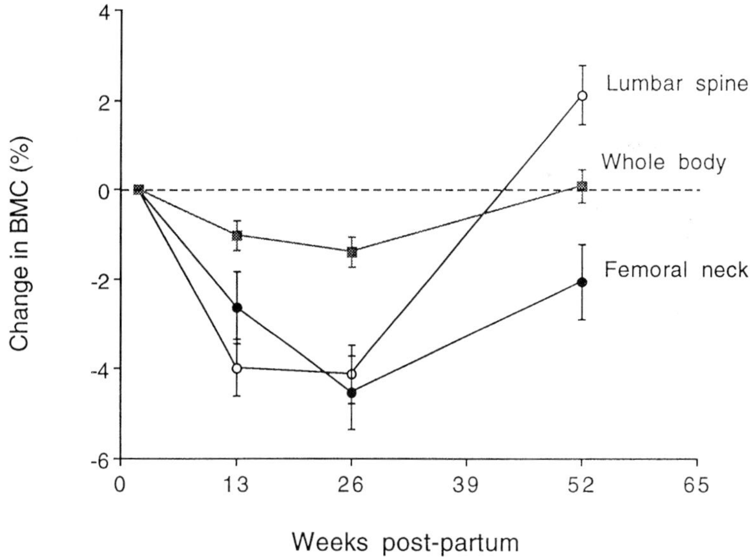

FIG. 4. Effect of lactation on change in maternal bone mineral content in British women. Data represent the percentage change in bone mineral content from 0.5 months postpartum (mean ± SE) at 3, 6, and 12 months postpartum for 38 women who breast-fed exclusively for at least 2 months. These women are a subset of a larger cohort, as detailed by Laskey *et al.* (42). Scanning was performed using a Hologic 1000/w dual x-ray absorptiometer with a long-term imprecision <1%. The patterns of change across time were significantly different from zero at each site illustrated (analysis of variance, $p < 0.0001$). No significant changes were observed over time in mothers who chose not to breast-feed or in a group of nonpregnant, nonlactating controls.

especially those rich in trabecular bone such as the spine. For example, in the 38 exclusively breastfeeding British mothers described above, highly significant changes ($p < 0.0001$) were observed over 12 months in the bone mineral content at the lumbar spine and femoral neck (Fig. 4), which were reflected in changes in whole body bone mineral content, but there were no significant changes in forearm bone mineral content. No such effects were observed in 11 mothers who had chosen not to breastfeed their infants (non-BF) or in 22 nonpregnant, nonlactating women of similar age (NPNL).

The skeletal response to lactation is very variable between women. For example, the mean (SD) change in spinal bone mineral content after 3 months in the 38 British mothers was −4.0 (3.1)% and ranged from −9.4% to 2.4%. This is similar to the result obtained with larger numbers in the Cambridge study when lactating mothers who had introduced small quantities of weaning foods before 2 to 3 months were also included (43). The bone changes observed in breastfeeding mothers contrasts with the small, nonsignificant changes seen in the two groups of control women over the same period [non-BF = −1.0 (3.7)%, NPNL = 0.4 (2.1)%]. The variation in response during lactation is illustrated in Fig. 5, which gives the spinal bone mineral content values for two of the mothers, one of whom experienced no reduction, the other of whom showed a marked but temporary decrease. Breast milk volume at 2 to 3 months, but not breast milk calcium concentration, was found to be a major determinant of the decrease in spinal bone mineral content between 0.5 and 3 months in the Cambridge women, suggesting that the skeletal effect is a

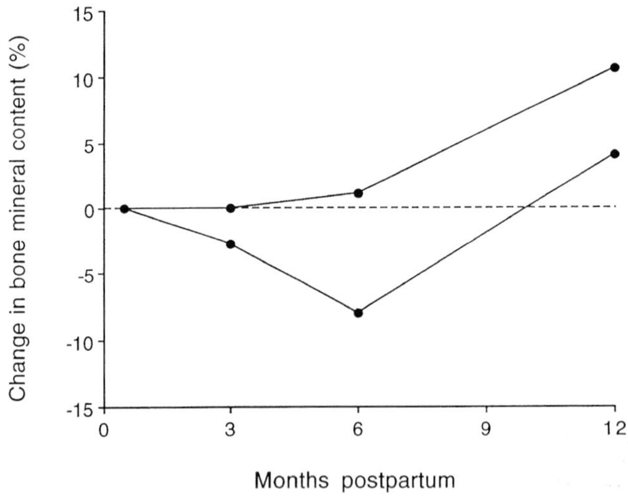

FIG. 5. The change in bone mineral content of the lumbar spine in two individuals during lactation. Data represent the percentage change in bone mineral content from 0.5 months at 3, 6, and 12 months postpartum in two Cambridge mothers. Both women breast-fed exclusively for at least 3 months and did not terminate breastfeeding until after 9 months.

TABLE 3. *Longitudinal studies that investigated a possible link between maternal calcium intake and bone changes in lactation*[a]

Location	Numbers			Baseline	Mean Ca intake at 1–3 months lactation	Scan sites	Effect of calcium intake	Reference
	BF	Non-BF	NPNL					
Observational studies								
Chile	30	—	26	1 month	1,480	Sp Hp	0	44
England	47	11	22	2 weeks	1,250	WB SP HP RS RD	0	43
United States	12	7	—	2 days	1,790	Sp RS RD	0	45
United States	90	20	—	2 weeks	1,300	Sp Hp	0	40
United States	35	25	—	Delivery	1,100, 1,500, 1,900	Sp RX	+	46
Supplementation studies								
Australia	79	—	—	1 week	1,050 (+1,000)	Sp HP FS FD	0	47
The Gambia	60	—	—	1.5 weeks	280, (+700)	RS RD	0	15
United States	79, 57	69, 60	—	2 weeks, 4–6 months	<800 (+1,000)	Sp	0[b]	48
United States	15	—	—	<2 weeks	1,300 (+1,000)	WB Sp RS RD US UD	0	49

[a] All studies demonstrated significant changes in bone mineral at one or more skeletal site in lactating women that were not seen in the controls.
Numbers: BF, breastfeeding mothers; FF, mothers not breastfeeding; NPNL, nonpregnant, nonlactating premenopausal women.
Baseline, days, weeks, or months postpartum when first measurement was made.
Scanned sites: WB, whole body; Sp, lumbar spine; Hp, hip sites; RS, radius shaft; RD, distal radius; US, ulna shaft; UD, distal ulna; FS, forearm (radius + ulna) shaft; FD, distal forearm. Calcium effect: 0, no correlation between bone change and Ca intake; +, smaller decrease in bone mineral associated with higher calcium intake.
[b] Calcium supplementation increased BMD in both lactating and nonlactating women but had no effect on the patterns of change postpartum.

response to suckling, possibly mediated by mammary parathyroid hormone related protein (PTHrP) (43).

Evidence is accumulating that the skeletal response to lactation is independent of maternal calcium intake. In the Cambridge study, maternal calcium intake was not an independent predictor of change in bone mineral at any skeletal site (43). Scrutiny of published reports indicates that bone mineral changes of similar magnitude have been observed in different groups of lactating women irrespective of their mean calcium intake, ranging from low (<800 mg/day) to high (>1,600 mg/day). In those prospective longitudinal studies that have explored a possible link with maternal diet, most have been unable to show any relationship between current calcium intake and bone mineral changes in lactation (Table 3) (15,40,43–49). Recent randomized placebo-controlled supplementation trials support this conclusion (Table 3). Our calcium supplementation study of lactating Gambian women showed bone and biochemical effects in the first months of lactation, including renal calcium conservation, decreases in bone mineral content, and raised circulating osteocalcin levels, but these were not affected by calcium supplementation (15). Results from the three other supplementation studies that are currently available (two only in preliminary communications) (47,48) paint a similar picture (Table 3). An exception comes from an early uncontrolled intervention study in the United States where changes in forearm bone mineral were observed in adolescent mothers consuming an average of 900 mg calcium/day but not in a similar group advised to consume 1,850 mg calcium/day (50).

CONCLUSIONS

There are wide variations in the amount of calcium ingested by breast-fed infants of the same age. These result from differences in the volume of milk drawn from the breast by the baby and from the characteristic concentration of calcium in the breast milk produced by the mother. Despite this, there is no evidence that differences in breast milk calcium intake influence linear growth or bone mineral status in early infancy. Infant weight gain is correlated with breast milk volume, as would be expected if breast milk intake is controlled by infant appetite, but not with breast milk calcium concentration. Breastfeeding is accompanied by a decrease in the bone mineral content of some women, but prospective studies indicate that this is transitory and unlikely to compromise long-term bone health. There is no evidence that either the mother's skeletal response to lactation or her breast milk calcium concentration are affected by current maternal calcium intake in the range commonly found in human diets.

The results of this overview imply that normal growth, bone development, and lactation in the human can occur in the face of substantial differences in dietary calcium intake. This raises a number of questions such as how the human body copes with differences in calcium supply and at what cost, what determines the skeletal response to lactation and the incorporation of calcium into breast milk, whether exposure at an early age to a particular calcium intake has any long-term effects on the individual's calcium metabolism, and what we should be recommending as an optimum calcium intake at a population level. The challenge for the future is to define the limits of the adaptive response to different calcium intakes. In order to do this, we need to place more emphasis on the biological mechanisms that underpin adaptation and calcium homeostasis, including genetic effects. We also need to intensify the search for sensitive indicators of optimum calcium handling and of bone health. Only in this way will we be better able to define the calcium requirements of infants and reproductive women.

ACKNOWLEDGMENTS

We are grateful to our many colleagues in Cambridge and The Gambia who have helped us in this research and to all the women and children who have taken part in our investigations. The longitudinal study of lactating women in Cambridge was partly funded by the Sainsbury Charitable Fund; the calcium supplementation study of lactating Gambian women was partly funded by the European Commission under the Science and Technology for Development Programme, TS2*.0028.UK(JR).

REFERENCES

1. Prentice A, Bates CJ. An appraisal of the adequacy of dietary mineral intakes in developing countries for bone growth and development in children. *Nutr Res Rev* 1993; 6: 51–59.
2. Prentice A. Maternal calcium requirements during pregnancy and lactation. *Am J Clin Nutr* 1994; 59S: 477–483.
3. Department of Health. *Weaning and the Weaning Diet. Report on Health and Social Subjects No 45.* London: HMSO, 1994.
4. National Academy of Sciences. *Nutrition During Lactation.* Washington, DC: National Academy Press, 1991.
5. Prentice A. Breastfeeding and the older infant. *Acta Paediatr Scand* 1991; Suppl 374: 78–88.
6. Whitehead RG, Paul AA, Ahmed EA. Weaning practices in the United Kingdom and variations in anthropometric development. *Acta Paediatr Scand* 1986; Suppl 323: 14–23.
7. Hitchcock NE, Gracey M, Gilmour AI. The growth of breast fed and artificially fed infants from birth to twelve months. *Acta Paediatr Scand* 1985; 74: 240–245.
8. Bainbridge RR, Mimouni F, Tsang RC. Bone mineral content of infants fed soy-based formula. *J Pediatr* 1988; 113: 205–207.
9. Hillman LS. Bone mineral content in term infants fed human milk, cow milk-based formula, or soy-based formula. *J Pediatr* 1988; 113: 208–212.
10. Prentice A, Parsons TJ, Cole TJ. Uncritical use of bone mineral density in absorptiometry may lead to size-related artifacts in the identification of bone mineral determinants. *Am J Clin Nutr* 1994; 60: 837–842.
11. Mimouni F, Tsang RC. Bone mineral content: data analysis. *J Pediatr* 1988; 113: 178–180.
12. Prentice A. Calcium intakes and bone densities of lactating women and breast-fed infants in The Gambia. *Adv Exp Med Biol* 1994; 352: 243–255.
13. Laskey MA, Jarjou L, Dibba B, Prentice A. Does maternal calcium intake influence the calcium nutrition of the breast-fed baby? *Proc Nutr Soc* 1997; 56: 6A.
14. Prentice A, Laskey MA, Shaw J, *et al.* The calcium and phosphorus intakes of rural Gambian women during pregnancy and lactation. *Br J Nutr* 1993; 69: 885–896.
15. Prentice A, Jarjou LMA, Cole TJ, Stirling DM, Dibba B, Fairweather-Tait S. Calcium requirements of lactating Gambian mothers: effects of a calcium supplement on breast-milk calcium concentration, maternal bone mineral content and urinary calcium excretion. *Am J Clin Nutr* 1995; 62: 58–67.

16. Vaughan LA, Weber CW, Kemberling SR. Longitudinal changes in the mineral content of human milk. *Am J Clin Nutr* 1979; 32: 2301–2306.
17. Laskey MA, Prentice A, Shaw J, Zachou T, Ceesay SM. Breast-milk calcium concentrations during prolonged lactation in British and rural Gambian mothers. *Acta Paediatr Scand* 1990; 79: 507–512.
18. Prentice A, Barclay DV. Breast-milk calcium and phosphorus concentrations of mothers in rural Zaire. *Eur J Clin Nutr* 1991; 45: 611–617.
19. Butte NF, Garza C, O'Brian Smith E, Wills C, Nichols BL. Macro- and trace-mineral intakes of exclusively breast-fed infants. *Am J Clin Nutr* 1987; 45: 42–48.
20. Feeley RM, Eitenmiller RR, Jones JB, Barnhart H. Calcium, phosphorus and magnesium contents of human milk during early lactation. *J Pediatr Gastroenterol Nutr* 1983; 2: 262–267.
21. Picciano MF, Calkins EJ, Garrick JR, Deering RH. Milk and mineral intakes of breastfed infants. *Acta Paediatr Scand* 1981; 70: 189–194.
22. Karra MV, Kirksey A, Galal O, Bassily NS, Harrison GG, Jerome NW. Zinc, calcium and magnesium concentrations in milk from American and Egyptian women throughout the first 6 months of lactation. *Am J Clin Nutr* 1988; 47: 642–648.
23. Lipsman S, Dewey KG, Lonnerdal B. Breastfeeding among teenage girls: milk composition, infant growth and maternal dietary intake. *J Pediatr Gastroenterol Nutr* 1985; 4: 426–434.
24. Prentice A. Regional variations in the composition of human milk. In: Jensen RG, ed. *Handbook of Milk Composition.* San Diego: Academic Press, 1995: 115–221.
25. Finley DA, Lonnerdal B, Dewey KC, Grivetti LE. Inorganic constituents of breast milk from vegetarian and nonvegetarian women: relationships with each other and with organic constituents. *J Nutr* 1985; 115: 772–781.
26. Greer FR, Tsang RC, Levin RS, Searcy JE, Wu R, Steichen JJ. Increasing serum calcium and magnesium concentrations in breast-fed infants: longitudinal studies of minerals in human milk and in sera of nursing mothers and their infants. *J Pediatr* 1982; 100: 59–64.
27. Ritchie BV. The calcium and phosphorus content of milk from Australian women. *Med J Aust* 1942; i: 331–336.
28. Winikoff D. Calcium, magnesium and phosphorus in the milk of Australian women. *Med J Aust* 1944; ii: 660–665.
29. Dagnelie PC, van Staveren WA, Roos AH, Tuinstra LGMT, Burema J. Nutrients and contaminants in human milk from mothers on macrobiotic and omnivorous diets. *Eur J Clin Nutr* 1992; 46: 355–366.
30. Barltrop D, Hillier R. Calcium and phosphorus content of transitional and mature human milk. *Acta Paediatr Scand* 1974; 63: 347–350.
31. Prentice A, Dibba B, Jarjou LMA, Laskey MA, Paul AA. Is breast-milk calcium concentration influenced by calcium intake during pregnancy? *Lancet* 1994; 344: 411–412.
32. Lindblad BS, Rahimtoola RJ. A pilot study of the quality of human milk in a low socioeconomic group in Karachi, Pakistan. *Acta Paediatr Scand* 1974; 63: 125–128.
33. Moser PB, Reynolds RD, Acharya S, Howard MP, Andon MB. Calcium and magnesium dietary intakes and plasma and milk concentrations of Nepalese lactating women. *Am J Clin Nutr* 1988; 47: 735–739.
34. Kirksey A, Ernst JA, Roepke JL, Tsai T-L. Influence of mineral intake and use of oral contraceptives before pregnancy on the mineral content of human colostrum and of more mature milk. *Am J Clin Nutr* 1979; 32: 30–39.
35. Coward WA, Cole TJ, Sawyer MB, Prentice AM, Orr-Ewing AK. Breast-milk intake measurement in mixed-fed infants by administration of deuterium oxide to their mothers. *Hum Nutr Clin Nutr* 1982; 36C: 141–148.
36. Prentice AM, Paul AA, Prentice A, Black AE, Cole TJ, Whitehead RG. Cross-cultural differences in lactational performance. In: Hamosh M, Goldman AS, eds. *Human Lactation 2: Maternal and Environmental Factors.* New York: Plenum Press, 1986: 13–44.
37. Dewey KG, Heinig MJ, Nommsen LA, Lonnerdal B. Maternal versus infant factors related to breast milk intake and residual milk volume: The DARLING study. *Pediatrics* 1991; 87: 829–837.
38. Prentice A, Laskey MA, Shaw J, Cole TJ, Fraser DR. Bone mineral content of Gambian and British children aged 0–36 months. *Bone Miner* 1990; 10: 211–224.
39. Prentice A. Nutrient requirements for growth, pregnancy and lactation: the Keneba experience. *S Afr J Clin Nutr* 1993; 6: 33–38.
40. Sowers MF, Corton G, Shapiro B, *et al.* Changes in bone density with lactation. *JAMA* 1993; 269: 3130–3135.

41. Kalkwarf HJ, Specker BL. Bone mineral loss during lactation and recovery after weaning. *Obstet Gynecol* 1995; 86: 26–32.
42. Laskey MA, Prentice A, Cole TJ. Bone mineral changes at different skeletal sites in mothers breastfeeding for 6 months. *Bone* 1994; 15: 729.
43. Laskey MA, Prentice A, Jarjou LMA, Beavan S. Lactational changes in bone mineral of the lumbar spine are influenced by breast-milk output but not calcium intake, breast-milk calcium concentration or vitamin D receptor genotype (abstract). *J Bone Miner Res* 1996; 11: 1815.
44. Lopez JM, Gonzalez G, Reyes V, Campino C, Diaz S. Bone turnover and density in healthy women during breastfeeding and after weaning. *Osteoporosis Int* 1996; 6: 153–159.
45. Hayslip CC, Klein TA, Wray HL, Duncan WE. The effects of lactation on bone mineral content in healthy postpartum women. *Obstet Gynecol* 1989; 73: 588–592.
46. Morales A, Tud-Tud Hans L, Herber M, Taylor AK, Baylink DJ. Lactation is associated with an increase in spinal bone density (abstract). *J Bone Miner Res* 1995; 8: S156.
47. Kent GN, Price RI, Gutteridge DH, *et al.* Site-specific reduction in bone loss by calcium supplements in normal lactation. *Osteoporosis Int* 1995; 5: 315.
48. Kalkwarf HJ, Specker BL, Bianchi DC, Ranz J. Calcium supplementation: does it prevent bone loss during lactation and augment gain after weaning? *J Bone Miner Res* 1995; 10: S259.
49. Cross NA, Hillman LS, Allen SH, Krause GF. Changes in bone mineral density and markers of bone remodeling during lactation and postweaning in women consuming high amounts of calcium. *J Bone Miner Res* 1995; 10: 1312–1320.
50. Chan GM, McMurry M, Westover K, Engelbert-Fenton K, Thomas MR. Effects of increased dietary calcium intake upon the calcium and bone mineral status of lactating adolescent and adult women. *Am J Clin Nutr* 1987; 46: 319–323.

DISCUSSION

Dr. Tsang: I am interested in the issue of the low calcium intake and size. The issue seems to be whether the calcium intake in these Gambian children is appropriate for their size. I suppose the ultimate question is whether adult Gambians have reduced or increased prevalence of fractures or osteoporosis. Do you have any idea? Life-style differences make this a complicated issue, I know.

Dr. Prentice: The most difficult thing, of course, is getting accurate health statistics in a country that has one hospital. People with femoral neck fracture don't tend to walk 200 miles to present themselves! We have been trying to investigate this for several years now, and we are convinced that the rate of fractures is very low in older people. The people just don't know what we mean when we talk about osteoporotic fractures. They don't see them at all in the hospitals. The women are ramrod straight when they are older, so spinal osteoporosis doesn't seem to be a problem. Our opinions from The Gambia tend to be reflected by much larger studies in Nigeria, Ghana, South Africa, and so on, which also indicate low rates of osteoporotic fractures in African black people. The curious thing is that from our work in the older people in The Gambia, we know that they have low bone mineral status however you want to define it, and they lose bone at the menopause in just the same way as Europeans, so clearly bone mineral density is not a useful marker for osteoporosis in that community. The other interesting thing is the way these children grow. Their growth is very slow, and men will still be growing at the age of 25 or so in Keneba. However, there are many factors that are likely to affect growth in that population.

Dr. Haschke: Have you ever looked at women who give birth to a child and who do not breastfeed? What happens to their bone mineral content during the month after delivery? You showed changes in lactating mothers and interpreted the data as being an effect of lactation, but there could be other contributing factors such as the hormonal changes after pregnancy, which could substantially influence bone mineral content.

Dr. Prentice: Thank you very much for that question. We did have a group of non-breastfeeding women in our studies, and my initial hypothesis was that the change in bone mineral content was a response to the pregnancy rather than to the breastfeeding. In fact, that was not the case, and we did not see these changes in formula-feeding women or in nonlactating controls nor in women who initiated breastfeeding and then stopped feeding quite soon afterward. The changes seem to be those of a dose–response relationship, and we saw an earlier return of bone mineral content in mothers who weaned earlier than in those who weaned later. It really seems to be quite exquisitely related to the suckling response of the infant.

Dr. Specker: We found that the return of menses was one of the biggest predictors of change in bone, at least the upswing between 3 and 6 months. Have you looked at this in The Gambia?

Dr. Prentice: Like you I felt that that the return of menses was likely to be the driving factor. In the Cambridge study we are still a little uncertain, and we do have some women there who are showing the upswing before their menses return. But of course the further you go into lactation, the more likely it is that menstruation will return, so those two things are going to be correlated anyway. In The Gambia women are amenorrheic for well over the first year, and they tend to come back into fertility in the second year of lactation. In those women we have found that osteocalcin levels and bone mineral content return to normal by 12 months.

Dr. Specker: You looked at milk output and also the calcium concentration in milk. If you look at total calcium output what do you find?

Dr. Prentice: For total calcium output, you will get exactly the same result as if you use breast milk volume on its own, so in other words, there is an association among a decrease in bone mineral and the amount of milk that the mother is producing and the total amount of calcium that is being secreted. But if you separate out the two components into volume and calcium concentration, it is the volume that is the important predictor. Certainly, women who produce the most breast milk tend to be the ones who transfer the most calcium, but we could just as easily talk in terms of phosphorus, protein, or anything else. At the moment I find the most plausible way to explain it is that there is a suckling reflex in the breast that produces a signal that acts on the mother's skeleton, directly or indirectly, as a physiological response of lactation to allow the mother to produce breast milk irrespective of the dietary supply.

Dr. Guesry: You hypothesize that the calcium homeostasis could be under the influence of early calcium intake, but I think that your supplement study in Keneba goes against this. It seems to me that there is evidence of very fine day-to-day regulation. Have you done calcium balances, which would tell you if mothers receiving calcium supplements were able to retain the calcium and build up calcium stock in their bones, or whether they eliminate all the extra calcium that you provide?

Dr. Prentice: We didn't undertake detailed balance studies, but we did look at 24-hour urinary calcium excretion and showed that women in the supplemented group excreted 7% of the dose they were given. That is in line with every other calcium supplementation or depletion study, where urinary calcium output represents about 7% of the intake, so we feel quite confident that the calcium supplement was being utilized by the mother. We looked at calcium absorption efficiency using stable isotope methodology and showed that the Gambian women had very high calcium absorption efficiencies on a loading dose of 100 mg of calcium. This was not affected by the supplement, so that the women who were receiving the supplement also had high calcium absorption efficiency.

Dr. Marini: You said that in The Gambia in 1989 you had a calcium supplementation program for pregnant women. At what time of gestation did this start?

Dr. Prentice: That was actually a public health supplementation program. It was a food supplement for pregnant women to try and improve the birth weight of the babies. It started off as a scientific experiment back in the early 1980s and was shown to be successful. Once it was shown to work, it became a public health measure and remained in Keneba. Those women were entitled to receive their food supplement as soon as they presented at the antenatal clinic, so that was their own choice, but generally this was around 12 to 16 weeks of gestation.

Dr. Marini: Do you have data on blood pressure in these pregnant women?

Dr. Prentice: We are doing that at the moment. The main reason for the calcium supplementation study is to answer that particular question whether increasing the calcium intake of women in The Gambia could benefit them by reducing the incidence of pregnancy-induced hypertension. One in 600 women in The Gambia die in childbirth as a result of eclampsia; it is one of the major obstetric problems.

Dr. Bonjour: You mentioned a study in which you gave calcium supplements to children in The Gambia and didn't observe any effect on bone growth. This is very important information. Could you tell us what was the population, what was the basic diet, what was the calcium salt that you used? Your conclusion was that calcium was not a limiting factor for bone growth, so I would like to know on what basis you concluded that.

Dr. Prentice: I am not sure I concluded that for the older infants. I said that of the various factors affecting bone growth, we have little evidence at the moment to suggest that in the Gambian situation calcium is one of them. That information did not come from a controlled calcium supplementation study. It was a weaning food supplement study for all children in Keneba between the ages of 3 and 12 months. It was designed to try to prevent growth retardation in the second half of infancy. The supplement itself consisted mostly of high-energy sources—oil, sugar, protein—and included milk, so the milk component was providing the calcium and phosphate. The study was conducted over 14 years in Keneba, with the neighboring villages for controls, and we found no differences in length, growth, weight, or bone mineral status measured by single-photon absorptiometry at the forearm between the villages over that time period. But it was not a controlled study.

Dr. Pettifor: How do you think Keneba women are able to improve their bone mass with continued increases in loss of calcium during lactation? And what do you believe is the biochemical drive for the increase in bone loss that occurs during lactation?

Dr. Prentice: We are still in the middle of the biochemical measurements in Cambridge, but on what we have at the moment, I speculate that we are seeing an increase in bone turnover switched on by some signal from the breast—PTHrP, prolactin perhaps, I don't know—so that you get an increase in the number of activation sites on the surface of the bone, which for a short time, 3 or 6 months, allows for an increase in the amount of calcium that could be available for breast milk production, phosphate, protein, whatever is needed, and is then shut off again as the other aspects of calcium metabolism are able to catch up. In The Gambia we see marked renal conservation of calcium during lactation, where their calcium outputs halve from very low down to almost unmeasurable, from 50 mg a day in the urine down to 25 mg. In both communities we see a rise in osteocalcin levels at about 3 months with a steady decline afterward, while parathyroid hormone levels tend to be slightly lower in early lactation, becoming higher than normal in the postweaning period. So there are some very marked changes in the biochemistry of lactating mothers, but they do not appear to be responsive to or affected by the mother's calcium supply.

Dr. Eisman: I would strongly recommend that we stop thinking about the skeleton as "the skeleton.'' The skeleton is heterogeneous. When we talk about growth or the effects of exercise or calcium, we have to think about the region that is growing, axial versus appendicular, cortical versus trabecular; a proximal limb segment grows differently from a more distal limb segment, and so presumably if there is a calcium source or a calcium effect, it may be affecting the region that is growing rather than another region that is growing more slowly.

Dr. Prentice: I absolutely agree. One of the fascinating things with these lactating women is that you can find women who have marked effects at the femoral neck and you don't see anything in the spine, and *vice versa.* Why do some women respond to lactation and other women don't, and why is it that some respond in some parts of the skeleton and others don't? I think that holds important clues for us as to why some women lose more bone at the menopause than others in different parts of the skeleton.

Dr. Jüppner: When you said that the PTH levels increase in lactating women in The Gambia, how high do they rise? And secondly, do you also see a rise in PTH-related peptide?

Dr. Prentice: We haven't measured PTH-related peptide. The PTH levels in Cambridge and The Gambia are somewhat lower than those of nonlactating women in early lactation and increase slightly above them later. In The Gambia, PTH levels are much higher than in Cambridge, toward the top end of the normal range in both lactating and nonlactating women.

Dr. Eisman: I was very interested in your comment about some of the predictors of the change in bone. I am surprised that changing bone area was a predictor. It is of concern that it might relate to changes in abdominal fat in women after pregnancy. Are there comparable changes in bone area in the women who are not lactating?

Dr. Prentice: There are two aspects of that. You are going to get a change in bone area if you take measurements separated by 3 months, even if the bone is not changing. That is what I meant by movement artifact or short-term biological variation. If we take the data further out into lactation, 6 months or so, and look at the pattern, we do see a small but significant decrease in bone area in those women who have large decreases in bone mineral content and a rise again, and this suggests that probably we are seeing differences in the way that the machine can detect the bone edges.

Dr. Alliet: Most black Africans become lactase-deficient as adults. Could the apparent low calcium need in Gambians be a genetic adaptation related to the development of the adult type of lactase deficiency with a lower dietary calcium intake later in life?

Dr. Prentice: It is difficult to say that their low calcium intake is an adaptation to the fact that they can't digest milk, but you are right of course that many black Africans do have lactase insufficiency, although in this group of individuals very few cannot tolerate a 100-ml dose of milk, so they are lactase insufficient rather than deficient. Whether it is an adaptation or not I don't know.

Dr. Eisman: It is an important point that the people in The Gambia have been there for a very long time, and their diet has presumably not changed materially over that time in terms of calcium and protein sources. So there is a sense in which they really have to have adapted to those diets or they would be dead. They have adjusted somehow, most likely by genetic selection, to allow them to survive under those circumstances. But where it is important is that it may be very difficult on any rational basis to compare what you see in Gambian women and children and Cambridge women and children, where they really are genetically different and would have been selected very differently, in the same way as it would be difficult to compare a study that was comparing a rabbit with a guinea pig. You have to look at the same circumstances.

Dr. Prentice: Of course I agree, and we don't know at what stage the ability to adjust is initiated. It may be in infancy, it may be genetic effects, it may be a mixture of both, we just don't know. But I think it is still too soon to assume that people who live as the Gambians do are somehow different from people in other parts of the world and therefore have different sets of requirements.

Dr. Klish: I would like to remind you that we probably all lived like the Gambians just a few centuries ago, so the adaptive processes that have taken place in Gambians have also taken place in us. I think a good demonstration of that is the obesity genes that are being described. At least five now have been identified, and they are obviously survival genes, genes that were mutated to allow us to use energy more efficiently. We have them just as frequently in the United States as in other parts of the world, so I am not sure that is a very good argument.

Dr. Prentice: And if we believed the evolutionists, all human beings started off having incredibly high calcium intakes. This is half of the rationale for the push to increase calcium intakes in all of us to levels that for many of us who work in Africa would regard as pharmacologic.

Nutrition and Bone Development, edited by
Jean-Philippe Bonjour and Reginald C. Tsang,
Nestlé Nutrition Workshop Series, Vol. 41, Nestec Ltd.,
Vevey/Lippincott–Raven Publishers,
Philadelphia © 1999.

Assessment of Bone Mass Development During Childhood and Adolescence by Quantitative Imaging Techniques

Vicente Gilsanz

Radiology Department, Children's Hospital Los Angeles, Los Angeles, California 90027, USA

Bone is a composite material of approximately one-third organic (mostly collagen) and two-thirds inorganic components. The inorganic component consists of crystals of basic carbonate that contain a form of calcium phosphate called hydroxyapatite (1). Because of its higher attenuation coefficient, the mineral fraction accounts for the radiographic depiction of bone (2). The subjective evaluation of bone mineral in the skeleton by conventional radiography is relatively insensitive, as bone mass may have already decreased by 30% to 40% by the time osteoporosis is appreciated (2). Thus, the recent development of more accurate methods for measuring bone mineral content has improved our ability to assess changes in bone mass significantly.

There are two main reasons for measuring bone mineral content in children: first, to diagnose and quantify the loss of bone mineral associated with the various disorders that cause osteopenia in children (3); and second, to improve our understanding of the childhood antecedents of a condition that happens to manifest itself in elderly subjects: osteoporosis. Although most research on osteoporosis has focused on the bone loss that occurs with aging, studies are needed to assess the amount of bone that is gained during growth and its determinants (4).

Several techniques are available for bone mass measurements for both research and clinical purposes in pediatrics. Ideally, the technique employed should have the following properties:

1. It should be easy to perform without the need for sedation in young children.
2. It should be noninvasive and harmless.
3. It should be accurate and reproducible.
4. It should allow assessment of both the axial and appendicular skeletons.
5. It should allow assessment of both cancellous and cortical bone.
6. It should allow assessment of skeletal size.
7. It should allow separate assessment of the two components of bone mass: bone volume and bone density.

8. Measurements should not be influenced by the size of the bones.
9. Measurements should not be influenced by body size or soft tissues.
10. It should be inexpensive.

Unfortunately, none of the methods currently available fulfills all the above criteria. Single-photon absorptiometry (SPA) and dual-photon absorptiometry (DPA) have been used extensively in the past but have been superseded. Magnetic resonance imaging is a promising technique for the analysis of cancellous bone, but it is still under investigation. In this chapter, the advantages and disadvantages of the three methods most commonly employed in pediatrics—dual-energy x-ray absorptiometry (DXA), quantitative computed tomography (QCT), and quantitative ultrasound (QUS)—are described. Comparison among these techniques, which are totally dissimilar in the way they acquire data, is difficult, and more often than not judgment regarding their value has been at least partially subjective.

DUAL-ENERGY X-RAY ABSORPTIOMETRY

Since its introduction in 1987, DXA has become the most commonly employed technique for the assessment of bone mineral content. It represents an evolution of another projection method, DPA, which used a radionuclide source (gadolinium-153) (5). With DXA, an x-ray tube is the source of photons, resulting in a 1,000-fold higher photon flux, better edge detection, and, therefore, better precision. Bone mineral measurements by DXA rely on the attenuation (absorption) of energy that occurs as the beam of x-ray photons scans across the region of interest. Two different energy photons are used: the low-energy photons penetrate only the soft tissue surrounding bone, whereas the high-energy photons penetrate both the soft tissue and the bone. A detector measures the exiting photons from the region of interest, and a computer subtracts the low-energy values from the high-energy measurements. The attenuation values are converted into measurements of mass of mineral with the use of calibration materials, and the results are expressed as bone mineral content (BMC, in grams). Frequently, BMC values are divided by the projected area of the bone analyzed, and the resulting measurements are conventionally referred to as bone mineral density (BMD, in grams per square centimeter). Because these measurements are not representative of the true density of bone, they are commonly referred to as area density.

The preferred anatomic sites for DXA measurements of bone mineral include the lumbar spine, the proximal femur, and the whole body, but peripheral sites, such as the forearm and the hand, can also be scanned. With the initial DXA devices, the examination procedure took 6 to 15 minutes, but newly developed devices using enhanced generators or a fan beam instead of a pencil beam x-ray source have shortened the examination time to 2 minutes.

The *in vivo* precision of the posteroanterior DXA measurements has been calculated as ranging from 0.8% to 2.3% in children (6–8) and from 1.55% to 2.5% in infants (9–11). It should, however, be noted that bone measurements with DXA "densitometers" from different manufacturers display substantial variation in BMD values of the same bone. This variation arises from differences in bone standards, edge detection algorithms, and regions of interest that are incorporated into the different devices. Recently, leading manufacturers of DXA equipment have proposed a standardization of BMD for measurements in the lumbar spine (Fig. 1) (12). To provide similar standardization at other sites, such as the femoral neck, changes of the analysis software may be required because of substantial differences in the regions of interest that the various manufacturers have incorporated into the design of their devices.

Radiation exposure involved in DXA examinations is extremely low. The subject effective dose has been estimated to be about 1 μSv for lumbar spine measurements (13) and about 4 μSv for whole skeleton scans (Table 1) (14). Low radiation dose, ability to measure most skeletal sites, availability, and ease of use have made DXA the most widely used technique for bone measurements worldwide. However, several limitations—especially with reference to bone measurements during growth, when major changes in body composition, body size, and skeletal mass occur—need to be addressed.

The DXA is a projectional technique, and its measurements are based on the two-dimensional projection of a three-dimensional structure. Thus, DXA values are a function of three skeletal variables: the size of the bone being examined, the volume of the bone, and its mineral density (15). These values are frequently expressed as measurements of the bone content per surface area (grams per square centimeter), as determined by scan radiographs. However, scan radiographs provide only an approximation of the size of the bone, and any correction based on these radiographs is only a very rough estimate of the "density." Attempts to overcome this disadvantage with the use of correction factors—for example, the square root of the projected area, the height of the subject, or the width of the bone, assuming the cross-sectional area of the vertebra is a square, a circle, or an ellipse, or that the femur can be modeled as a cylinder, etc. (7,16–19)—are subject to error, as there is no closed formula that defines the size of the vertebrae or the femur. Although the inability of DXA to account for bone size is not of great concern in studying the mature skeleton, in growing children, longitudinal DXA values are subject to considerable error, as they reflect the changes in both skeletal size and bone mass.

The DXA values are also influenced by the unknown composition of soft tissues in the beam path of the region of interest. Because corrections for the soft tissues are based on a homogeneous distribution of fat around the bone, changes in DXA measurements are observed if fat is distributed inhomogeneously around the bone measured. It has been determined that an inhomogeneous fat distribution in soft tissues, resulting in a difference of 2 cm of fat layer between soft tissue area and bone area, will influence DXA measurements by 10% (20). Although this is not a limitation in studying subjects whose weight and body size remain constant, longitudinal DXA values in children are subject to considerable error, as the measurements may reflect the changes in body size and composition that occur with growth more

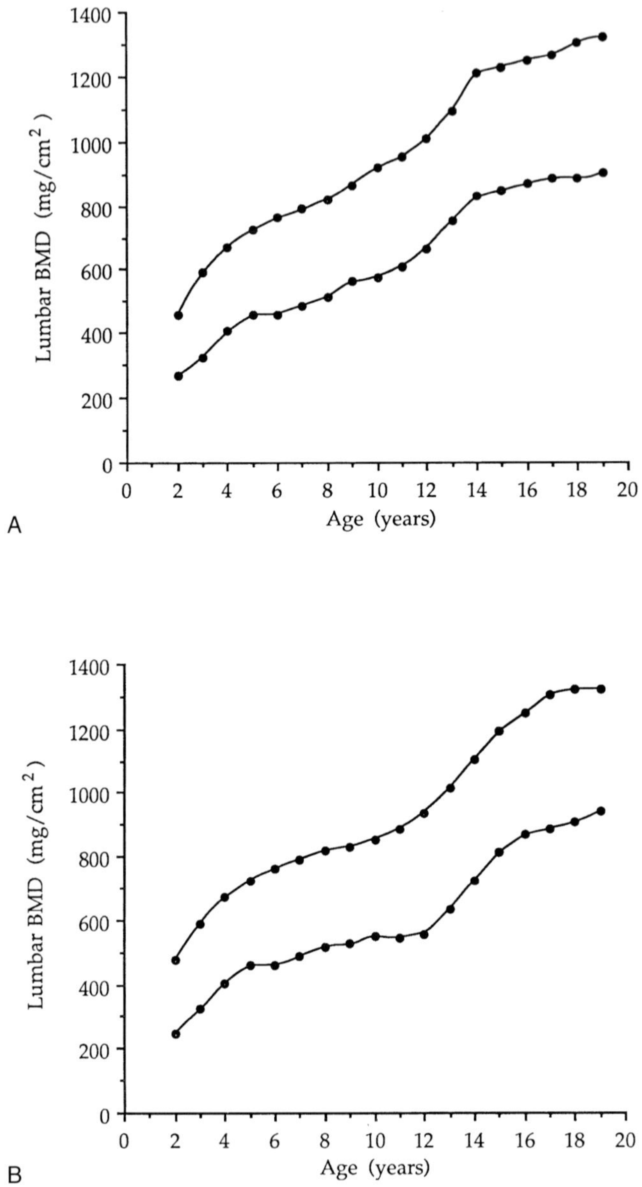

FIG. 1. Dual-energy x-ray absorptiometry values for the lumbar spine in relation to age in healthy Caucasian girls **(A)** and boys **(B).** Measurements were obtained with a Lunar DPX-L absorptiometer (Lunar Corp., Madison, Wisconsin, USA) (6) and have been standardized according to the method of Genant (12). Values represent 95% confidence limits and are expressed in milligrams per square centimeter.

TABLE 1. *Whole-body equivalent doses in microsievierts (μSv) for children at different ages*

Exam	Age (years) 5	10	20
Chest x-ray	44	39	32
Lumbar spine			
Anteroposterior	21	20	18
Lateral	131	121	112
DXA			
PA spine	~1	~1	~1
Lat spine	~3	~3	~3
Proximal femur	~1	~1	~1
Whole body	~4	~4	~4
QCT spine			
Scout view	48	45	41
Axial scan	9	9	8
Natural background (per month)	224	181	107
Transcontinental flight	37	30	18

Adapted from Kalender (13), Lewis et al. (14), and Cann (43).

than true changes in bone mineral content. This disadvantage especially limits studies in children with eating disorders, such as obesity or anorexia nervosa.

Other limitations of DXA studies in very young children include their lack of cooperation, resulting in motion and the presence of artifacts in the scan. Recent studies have shown that motion artifacts may increase the values of the projected bone area by 9%, of BMC by 13%, and of BMD by 4% (21). In an attempt to overcome these errors, children have been restrained (6,10), sedated (9,22), or studied while asleep (23). It should also be noted that the standard software from most DXA manufacturers was designed for adults. Although several manufacturers have developed special software to be used in pediatrics, this software requires longer scanning time, which makes cooperation from children more difficult. Correct positioning is also of the utmost importance in studies of children. Lumbar studies may be inaccurate with even the mildest bending of the trunk, and exact positioning of the foot is required for proper assessment of the proximal femur. Last, it should be stressed that DXA measurements in children, like those in adults, reflect a composite of cancellous and cortical bone and that these two compartments cannot be independently assessed with this technique, in either the axial or the appendicular skeleton.

Normative data for DXA values in pediatrics are available in published reports and are included in most DXA software packages (Table 2). However, caution is advised before using published normative data for clinical use, and institutional and device-specific norms are preferable to published references. Marked differences have been described in normal DXA values, mainly attributable to variations between devices, scanning protocols, and body size of the subjects studied.

Bone determinations in children with DXA have been done at all ages, including newborns (9,11,22) and infants (10,23,24). In general, values measured at different skeletal sites increase from infancy to adulthood (6,8,16,18,25–32). The relationship

TABLE 2. *DXA measurements of healthy Caucasian children[a]*

Age (years)	Boys			Girls		
	Femoral neck	Trochanter	Total body	Femoral neck	Trochanter	Total body
2	0.22–0.82	0.29–0.61	0.59–0.78	0.42–0.50	0.28–0.48	0.66–0.81
3	0.34–0.74	0.16–0.80	0.62–0.87	0.38–0.62	0.20–0.64	0.60–0.90
4	0.41–0.73	0.26–0.74	0.64–0.94	0.27–0.79	0.22–0.70	0.65–0.84
5	0.41–0.89	0.28–0.84	0.71–0.90	0.18–0.98	0.13–0.85	0.63–0.94
6	0.4–1.0	0.29–0.85	0.62–0.98	0.28–0.96	0.25–0.77	0.70–0.85
7	0.41–1.01	0.33–0.89	0.72–0.91	0.35–0.91	0.29–0.77	0.70–0.89
8	0.43–1.03	0.30–0.98	0.74–0.91	0.32–0.96	0.20–0.88	0.68–0.90
9	0.41–1.09	0.32–0.92	0.72–0.94	0.37–0.93	0.23–0.87	0.70–0.91
10	0.45–1.09	0.26–1.02	0.10–0.70	0.53–0.85	0.39–0.75	0.68–0.90
11	0.44–1.12	0.32–0.96	0.83–0.87	0.38–1.06	0.45–0.77	0.70–0.91
12	0.48–1.12	0.35–0.99	0.74–1.01	0.35–1.19	0.51–0.83	0.65–1.01
13	0.42–1.30	0.54–1.02	0.91–0.96	0.43–1.31	0.55–0.91	0.74–0.96
14	1.42–1.38	0.33–1.29	0.93–1.01	0.46–1.46	0.56–0.96	0.68–1.05
15	0.57–1.45	0.48–1.32	0.83–1.16	0.41–1.45	0.52–1.00	0.76–1.17
16	0.55–1.63	0.42–1.50	0.94–1.26	0.40–1.48	0.56–0.96	0.82–1.19
17	0.47–1.83	0.46–1.46	0.93–1.34	0.46–1.38	0.38–1.14	0.85–1.24
18–20	0.46–1.86	0.32–1.56	0.95–1.38	0.29–1.61	0.26–1.26	0.92–1.23

[a] Values represent the 95% confidence intervals for BMD measurements, are expressed as g/cm^2, and were obtained from Zanchetta et al. (8) with a Norland XR-26 absorptiometer (Norland Corp., Fort Atkinson, WI, USA).

between age and bone mineral content in the lumbar spine appears to be represented by a segmented polynomial curve (6,8,26,28,29); a rapid increase during childhood is followed by an even greater increase during puberty that ends in the third decade of life (6–8,17,18,25,28,29,33). Similar relationships may be seen in the femoral neck (8,25,26,29) and for the entire skeleton (8,26,27,29). However, radial DXA values in children have not been found to be influenced by puberty (8).

The majority of the studies on gender differences using DXA indicate that by the age of 12 or 13 years girls have greater BMD than boys in the lumbar spine (6,16,25,28,30). Most (8,16,25,26), but not all (19,29), of the studies in the femoral neck have found greater BMC in boys than in girls at 14 to 16 years of age. Measurements in the radius have yielded discrepant results: one study found no gender differences (8), but boys had greater values than girls in another study (30).

Studies examining racial differences in bone mass in children have yielded conflicting results. Some investigators have found no differences in bone measurements between African-American girls and Caucasian girls (18,31), but others report higher values for African-American girls at all ages (34). A recent study found that Asian-American children have lower spine, femur, and whole body DXA values than Caucasian children, and it was suggested that the difference is size related (35).

In summary, the relatively low cost, availability, and ease of use are the main advantages of DXA. This technique provides an accurate and precise quantitation of bone mass in the mature skeleton. Unfortunately, the inability of DXA to account for the large changes in body and skeletal size that occur during growth limits its use in longitudinal studies in children.

QUANTITATIVE COMPUTED TOMOGRAPHY

Computed tomography introduced the technique of digital imaging to diagnostic radiology. The transverse anatomic sections afforded by this digital technique provide a three-dimensional image unobscured by overlying structures. The data displayed as the CT image are actually a representation of attenuation values or CT numbers of the object scanned. These numerical values are stored in digital form and are accessible for future study, as needed. The use of this digital information to provide quantitative information has been labeled quantitative computed tomography (QCT).

With QCT, bone measurements can be obtained at any skeletal site with a standard clinical CT scanner using an external bone mineral reference phantom for calibration and specially developed software. Unfortunately, CT scanners are large, expensive, nonportable machines that require costly maintenance and considerable technological expertise for proper function. Moreover, this equipment is usually located in a radiology department and is under constant clinical demand, creating a lack of accessibility. These disadvantages have partially been overcome by the recent development of smaller, mobile, less expensive peripheral QCT scanners designed exclusively for bone measurements. These scanners, however, can only assess the bones of the appendicular skeleton.

In the past, QCT has principally been employed to determine cancellous bone density (milligrams per cubic centimeter) in the vertebral bodies. Cancellous bone exists as a three-dimensional lattice of plates and columns (trabeculae). The trabeculae divide the interior volume of the bone into intercommunicating pores, which are filled with a variable mixture of red and yellow marrow (36). Because of the relatively small size of the trabeculae when compared to the pixel (the CT unit of measurement), QCT values for cancellous bone density reflect not only the amount of mineralized bone and osteoid but also the amount of marrow per pixel (37). Similar limitations apply to *in vitro* determinations of the volumetric density of trabecular bone, which are obtained by washing the marrow from the pores of a specimen of cancellous bone, weighing it, and dividing the weight by the volume of the specimen, including the pores (36). Both QCT and *in vitro* bone density determinations of cancellous bone are therefore directly proportional to the bone volume fraction and inversely proportional to the porosity of the bone. The relatively large coefficient of variation for values of cancellous bone density reflect the considerable variations in the dimensions of the pores throughout the vertebral body. It should be noted that the precision and accuracy of QCT cancellous bone density determinations depend on the percentage of fat in the marrow, and, as the marrow of children contains little fat, the precision of cancellous measurements by QCT in children is considerably better than that reported for adults: approximately 1% to 2% (38).

In addition to measurements of cancellous bone density, the dimensions of the vertebrae can be obtained from the same QCT scans. Coefficients of variation for determinations of vertebral body heights and vertebral cross-sectional area have been calculated as 1.3% and 0.8%, respectively (39).

The recent application of QCT to assess the appendicular skeleton has significantly improved the ability to measure cortical bone. Three bone parameters can be measured by QCT in the appendicular skeleton: the cross-sectional area of the bone, the cortical bone area, and the cortical bone density (3,40). To do this, the outer and inner boundaries of the cortex are identified by specially developed software at the place of the maximum slope of the profile through the bone; the area within the outer cortical shell represents the cross-sectional area, whereas the area between the outer and inner shells represents the cortical bone area; the mean CT numbers of the pixels within the inner and outer cortical shells provide the average density of bone. The coefficients of variation for repeated QCT measurements of cortical bone density, cortical bone area, and cross-sectional area of the femur range between 0.6% and 1.5% (41).

Quantitative CT measurements of the density of cortical bone reflect, because of its relative lack of porosity, the material density of the bone (the amount of collagen and mineral in a given volume of bone) if the cortex is sufficiently thick to circumvent volume averaging errors (40). The minimum thickness necessary for an accurate density evaluation of cortical bone by QCT is 2 to 2.5 mm; below this threshold QCT values fall in a linear way relative to width. Above this thickness, the measured pixel represents the combination of the attenuation coefficients defined by the densities and concentrations of osteoid and mineral. Although the nonmineral fraction may contribute to minor fluctuations in measurements of cortical bone density, QCT numbers are primarily based on the calcified bone fraction, which has a high attenuation coefficient (40). These measurements are analogous to *in vitro* determinations of the intrinsic mineral density of bone, which are commonly expressed as the ash weight per unit volume of bone (42). In children, the material density of cortical bone in the appendicular skeleton when measured by QCT remains fairly constant, at 2.00 ± 0.065 g/cm^3 (Fig. 2) (40).

The radiation exposure from QCT measurements is related to the technique employed and can be as low as 150 mrem (1.5 mSv) localized to the region of interest in the appendicular or axial skeleton. The total body equivalent dose of radiation is approximately 4 to 9 mrem (40 to 90 μSv), and this figure includes the radiation associated with screening digital radiographs used to localize the site of measurement (13,43). This amount of radiation is far lower than that associated with other CT imaging procedures, accounting for the wide range of published figures for the radiation dose associated with CT measurements. It is also less than many other commonly used radiographic diagnostic tests. By comparison, a round-trip transcontinental flight in North America exposes a child to roughly 6 to 8 mrem (60 to 80 μSv) of ionizing radiation (Table 1) (13,43). Therefore, bone measurement determinations using QCT, like those using DXA, do not expose children to amounts of ionizing

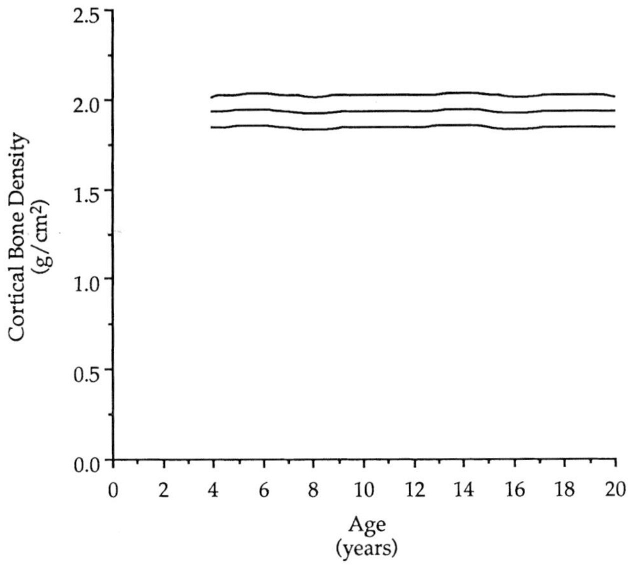

FIG. 2. Quantitative computed tomography values for cortical bone density at the midshaft of the femur in healthy children. Values represent the mean ± 1 SD, are expressed in grams per square centimeter, and were obtained from Hangartner and Gilsanz (40).

radiation that deviate from the amount that constitutes part of their normal life experience.

Studies in healthy children using QCT have shown that events during puberty are the major determinants of the increases in cancellous bone density during growth (44) and that the density of cancellous bone reaches its peak around the time of cessation of longitudinal growth and epiphyseal closure (40,45). Quantitative CT studies have also shown a greater increase in vertebral cancellous bone density in African-American girls than in Caucasian girls during the later stages of puberty (Fig. 3) (46,47). Other studies have analyzed the influence of gender on the amount of bone that is gained during childhood and adolescence (39,48). Quantitative CT has helped establish that the lower vertebral bone mass of girls, when compared to that in boys, results from early gender differences in the size of the bones rather than differences in cancellous bone density (39,48). Even after accounting for differences in body size, the cross-sectional area of the vertebral body is approximately 20% smaller in girls than in boys (Fig. 4) (39).

In contrast to these findings, the cross-sectional area at the midshaft of the femur does not differ between boys and girls matched for age and anthropometric variables (41). Quantitative CT values for the size and the amount of bone in the appendicular skeleton do, however, correlate strongly with all anthropometric indices, suggesting that weight bearing and mechanical stresses are the major determinants of the increases in the size and the volume of cortical bone during growth (Fig. 5) (44).

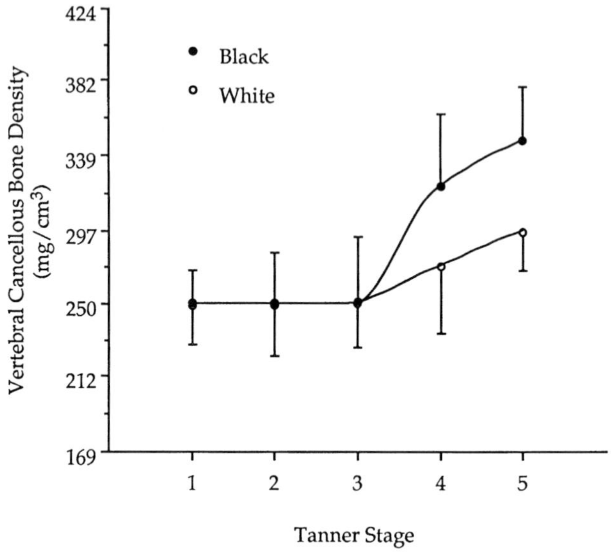

FIG. 3. Quantitative computed tomography values for cancellous vertebral bone density in healthy Caucasian and African-American children in relation to Tanner stage of sexual development. Values represent the mean ± 1 SD, are expressed in milligrams per cubic centimeter, are valid for both boys and girls, and were, in part, obtained from Gilsanz *et al.* (46,47).

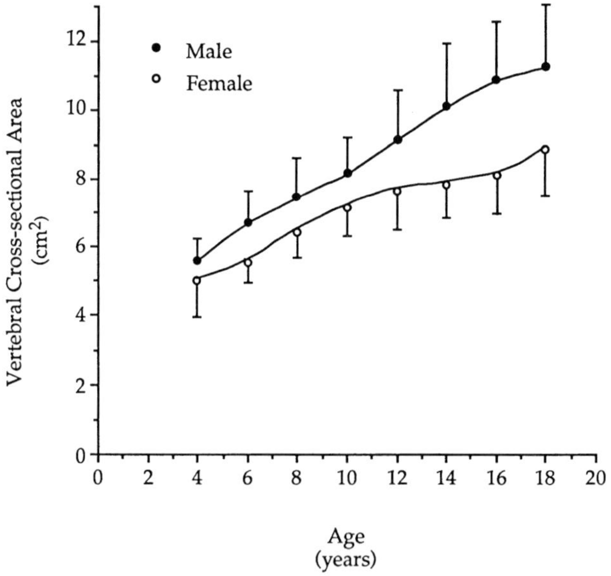

FIG. 4. Quantitative computed tomography values for cross-sectional area of the midportion of the vertebral body in healthy Caucasian boys and girls in relation to age. Values represent the mean ± 1 SD, are expressed in square centimeters, and were obtained from Gilsanz *et al.* (39,41).

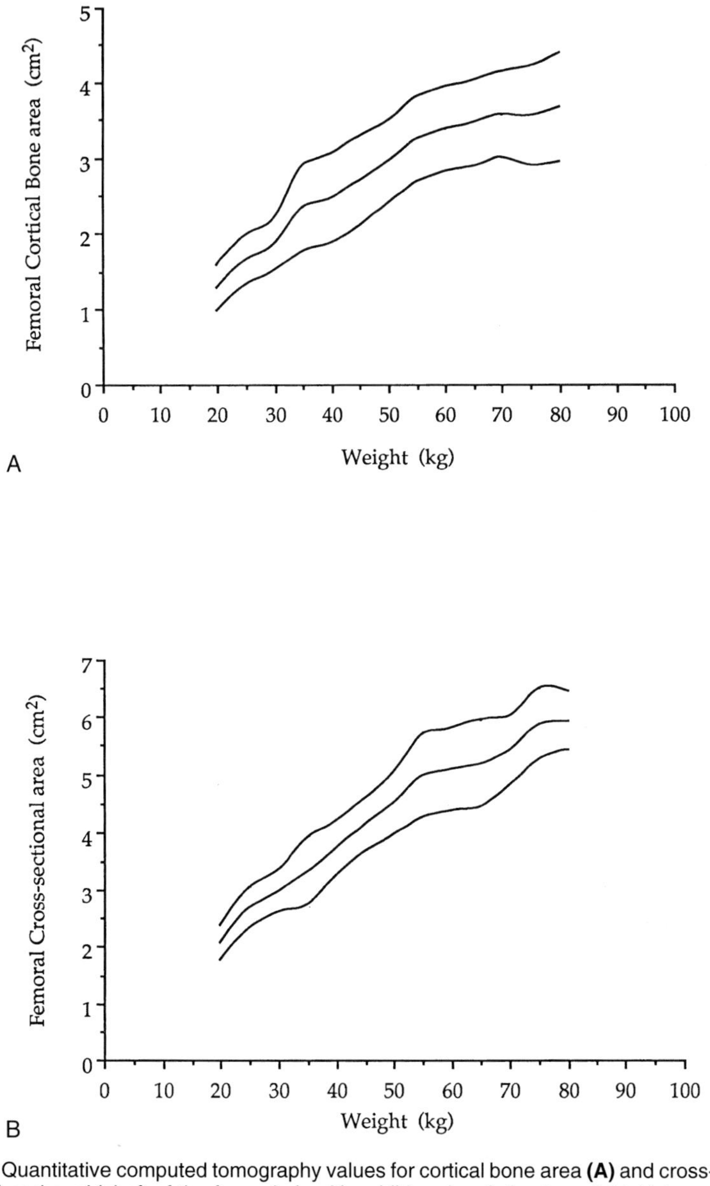

FIG. 5. Quantitative computed tomography values for cortical bone area **(A)** and cross-sectional area **(B)** at the midshaft of the femur in healthy children in relation to weight. Values represent the mean ± 1 SD, are expressed in square centimeters, are valid for both boys and girls, and were obtained, in part, from Gilsanz *et al.* (41).

In summary, the ability of QCT to assess both the volume and the density of bone in the axial and appendicular skeletons, without influence from body or skeletal size, is the major advantage of this method when used in children. Unfortunately, the cost and inaccessibility of CT scanners have markedly limited its use for bone measurements.

ULTRASOUND

Quantitative ultrasound (QUS) has recently been used to assess bone by measuring the changes that occur in the velocity and in the energy of ultrasound waves as they go through bone. Briefly, ultrasound equipment consists of two transducers, a transmitter and a receiver, that are placed on opposite sides of the bone of interest; most commonly the calcaneus, less frequently the patella, the tibia, or the phalanges. The ultrasound transmission velocity (also known as the speed of sound, SOS) is obtained by dividing the width of the region of interest by the transit time and is expressed in meters per second. The loss of acoustic energy that occurs when the ultrasound wave is absorbed or scattered by the medium through which it is being propagated results in a reduction in the amplitude of the wave and is referred to as broadband ultrasound attenuation (BUA). The ultrasound attenuation is a function of frequency, and for biological soft tissues this relationship is linear over the range of 200 to 600 kHz. The BUA is defined as the slope of attenuation versus the frequency in this range and is expressed in decibels per megahertz (dB/MHz).

It is generally believed that both BUA and SOS are determined not only by the number, the thickness, and the mineral content of the trabeculae but also by their three-dimensional arrangement. The BUA values are known to vary as much as 50% depending on the principal orientation of the trabeculae (37). It should be noted that ultrasound measurements are also influenced by the amount and composition of marrow in the bone and by other soft tissues in the path of the ultrasound waves (37). The generally poor precision of ultrasound has limited its usefulness for longitudinal monitoring of disease progression or response to treatment in adults (49). Numerous studies in adults have failed to find a strong correlation between ultrasound measurements of bone and values obtained using other bone measurement methods (37). Therefore, established relationships between techniques are not strong enough to allow ultrasound to be used as a surrogate for other methods.

Currently, all commercially available ultrasound equipment for bone measurements is designed for adults, and relatively large transducers are used. Smaller transducers are required for studying children to allow closer contact with the region of interest so that it can be scanned without interference from air. On average, the diameter of the specially designed transducers for pediatric studies has been 1 cm (50–53). As in adults, ultrasound studies in children require a coupling medium (a water bath or gel) between the transducers and the skin overlying the bone. The temperature of the coupling medium must be maintained constant to avoid inaccuracies in the velocity and attenuation of ultrasound measurements. Moreover, when

TABLE 3. *Ultrasound measurements of healthy Caucasian children*[a]

	Calcaneus		
Age (years)	BUA (dB/MHz)	SOS (m/sec)	Stiffness[b] (%)
6	83.1 ± 3.1	1,515 ± 13	59.5 ± 5.4
7	85.3 ± 3.7	1,527 ± 7	64.4 ± 4.0
8	87.8 ± 11.2	1,522 ± 22	64.7 ± 13.2
9	95.1 ± 5.6	1,526 ± 20	70.7 ± 8.2
10	98.9 ± 7.7	1,535 ± 21	75.7 ± 10.0
11	97.2 ± 6.9	1,531 ± 16	73.4 ± 6.4
12	100.3 ± 8.5	1,534 ± 23	76.2 ± 11.8
13	104.2 ± 5.7	1,554 ± 22	84.7 ± 8.7

[a] Data are expressed as mean ± SD and were obtained by Jaworski et al. (50) with an Achilles Ultrasound Densitometer (Lunar Corp., Madison, WI). Values at age 12 and 13 years are valid for girls only; all others are valid for both boys and girls.

[b] An index called "stiffness," derived from a combination of BUA and SOS, is also provided by this densitometer. Stiffness = (0.67 × BUA) + (0.28 × SOS) − 420.

examining children, specially developed foot pads or calipers for small feet are needed to maintain the correct position of the transducer near the bone to be scanned.

Ultrasound measurements of bone in children have been obtained at the calcaneus, the patella, and the phalanges of the thumb, although no device has been used to measure more than one skeletal site. The SOS is commonly measured in all sites, whereas BUA is mainly determined in the calcaneus. In children, SOS and BUA values increase with age, but they show considerable variability (Tables 3 and 4) (50,53). The influence of puberty on ultrasound indices has been investigated, and it has been shown that SOS values increase substantially between the second and third Tanner stages of sexual development in girls, whereas the increase is constant throughout all stages of puberty in boys (52). Reported intraobserver coefficients of variation in children range from 0.5% to 1.2% for SOS (50,51,53) and from 3% to 5% for BUA (50,52).

The attractiveness of QUS for bone measurements in children lies in its low cost,

TABLE 4. *Ultrasound measurements of healthy Caucasian children*[a]

Age (years)		Patella SOS (m/sec)	Thumb SOS (m/sec)
0–1	M	1,591–1,699	
	F	1,553–1,656	
1–6	M	1,696–1,794	1,594–1,770
	F	1,673–1,832	1,567–1,827
6–11	M	1,784–1,929	1,701–1,914
	F	1,781–2,014	1,762–1,980
11–17	M	1,805–1,993	1,748–2,029
	F	1,824–2,132	1,898–2,101
17–21	M	1,940–2,076	1,876–2,168
	F	1,954–2,063	2,002–2,197

[a] Data are expressed as a range of values and were obtained by Schönau et al. (53) with an Osteoson K4 (Minhorst, Wiesbaden, Germany).

portability, ease of use, and lack of ionizing radiation. Because in adults ultrasound can adequately predict fracture risk independently of bone mass determinations in patients with osteoporosis, QUS measurements must be related to some aspects of bone strength (54). Unfortunately, ultrasound values are dependent on so many structural variables, yet to be fully defined, that it is difficult to use this information in a meaningful way in children. Because these values seem to correlate more with bone size than with changes in the amount, density, or geometry of bone, increases seen during childhood may be related to changes in skeletal size (55).

REFERENCES

1. Weiner S, Traub W. Bone structure: from angstroms to microns. *FASEB J* 1992; 6: 879–885.
2. Lachman E. Osteoporosis: the potentialities and limitations of its radiologic diagnosis. *Am J Radiol* 1985; 4: 712–717.
3. Kovanlikaya A, Loro ML, Hangartner TN, Reynolds RA, Roe TF, Gilsanz V. Osteopenia in children: CT assessment. *Radiology* 1996; 198: 781–784.
4. Kreipe RE. Bones of today, bones of tomorrow. *Am J Dis Child* 1992; 146: 22–25.
5. Sartoris DJ, Resnick D. Dual-energy radiographic absorptiometry for bone densitometry: current status and perspective. *Am J Roentgenol* 1989; 152: 241–246.
6. del Rio L, Carrascosa A, Pons F, Gusinyé M, Yeste D, Domenech FM. Bone mineral density of the lumbar spine in white Mediterranean Spanish children and adolescents: changes related to age, sex, and puberty. *Pediatr Res* 1994; 35: 362–366.
7. Kröger H, Kotaniemi A, Kröger L, Alhava E. Development of bone mass and bone density of the spine and femoral neck—a prospective study of 65 children and adolescents. *Bone Miner* 1993; 23: 171–182.
8. Zanchetta JR, Plotkin H, Alvarez Filgueira ML. Bone mass in children: normative values for the 2–20-year-old population. *Bone* 1995; 14: 3S–399S.
9. Braillon PM, Salle BL, Brunet J, Glorieux FH, Delmas PD, Meunier PJ. Dual energy x-ray absorptiometry measurement of bone mineral content in newborns: validation of the technique. *Pediatr Res* 1992; 32: 77–80.
10. Koo WWK, Massom LR, Walters J. Validation of accuracy and precision of dual energy x-ray absorptiometry for infants. *J Bone Miner Res* 1995; 10: 1111–1115.
11. Venkataraman P, Ahluwalia BW. Total bone mineral content and body composition by x-ray densitometry in newborns. *Pediatrics* 1992; 90: 767–770.
12. Genant HK. Universal standardization for dual x-ray absorptiometry: patient and phantom cross-calibration results (letter). *J Bone Miner Res* 1995; 10: 997–998.
13. Kalender WA. Effective dose values in bone mineral measurements by photon absorptiometry and computed tomography. *Osteoporosis Int* 1992; 2: 82–87.
14. Lewis MK, Blake GM, Fogelman I. Patient dose in dual x-ray absorptiometry. *Osteoporosis Int* 1994; 4: 11–15.
15. Carter DR, Bouxsein ML, Marcus R, New approaches for interpreting projected bone densitometry data. *J Bone Miner Res* 1992; 7: 137–145.
16. Kröger H, Kotaniemi A, Vainio P, Alhava E. Bone densitometry of the spine and femur in children by dual-energy x-ray absorptiometry. *Bone Miner* 1992; 17: 75–85.
17. Katzman DK, Bachrach LK, Carter DR, Marcus R. Clinical and anthropometric correlates of bone mineral acquisition in healthy adolescent girls. *J Clin Endocrinol Metab* 1991; 73: 1332–1339.
18. Plotkin H, Núñez M, Alvarez-Filgueira ML, Zanchetta JR. Lumbar spine bone density in Argentine children. *Calcif Tissue Int* 1996; 58: 144–149.
19. Moro M, van der Meulen MCH, Kiratli BJ, Marcus R, Bachrach LK, Carter DR. Body mass is the primary determinant of midfemoral bone acquisition during adolescent growth. *Bone Miner* 1996; 19: 519–526.
20. Hangartner T. Influence of fat on bone measurements with dual-energy absorptiometry. *Bone Miner* 1990; 9: 71–78.
21. Koo WW, Walters J, Bush AJ. Technical considerations of dual-energy x-ray absorptiometry-based bone mineral measurements for pediatric subjects. *J Bone Miner Res* 1995; 10: 1998–2004.

22. Lapillonne AA, Glorieux FH, Salle BL, *et al.* Mineral balance and whole body bone mineral content in very low-birth-weight infants. *Acta Paediatr Suppl* 1994; 405: 117–122.
23. Chan GM. Performance of dual-energy x-ray absorptiometry in evaluating bone, lean body mass, and fat in pediatric subjects. *J Bone Miner Res* 1992; 7: 369–374.
24. Rupich RC, Specker BL, Lieuw-A-Fa M, Ho M. Gender and race differences in bone mass during infancy. *Calcif Tissue Int* 1996; 58: 395–397.
25. Bonjour J-P, Theintz G, Buchs B, Slosman D, Rizzoli R. Critical years and stages of puberty for spinal and femoral bone mass accumulation during adolescence. *J Clin Endocrinol Metab* 1991; 73: 555–563.
26. Faulkner RA, Bailey DA, Drinkwater DT, McKay HA, Arnold C, Wilkinson AA. Bone densitometry in Canadian children 8–17 years of age. *Calcif Tissue Int* 1996; 59: 344–351.
27. Faulkner RA, Bailey DA, Drinkwater DT, Wilkinson AA, Houston CS, McKay HA. Regional and total body bone mineral content, bone mineral density, and total body tissue composition in children 8–16 years of age. *Calcif Tissue Int* 1993; 53: 7–12.
28. Glastre C, Braillon P, David L, Cochat P, Meunier PJ, Delmas PD. Measurement of bone mineral content of the lumbar spine by dual energy x-ray absorptiometry in normal children: correlations with growth parameters. *J Clin Endocrinol Metab* 1990; 70: 1330–1333.
29. Lu PW, Briody JN, Ogle GD, *et al.* Bone mineral density of total body, spine, and femoral neck in children and young adults: a cross-sectional and longitudinal study. *J Bone Miner Res* 1994; 9: 1451–1458.
30. Moreira-Andrés MN, Cañizo FJ, Papapietro K, Rejas J, Hawkins FG. Comparison between spinal and radial bone mineral density in children measured by x-ray absorptiometry. *J Pediatr Endocrinol Metab* 1995; 8: 35–41.
31. Southard RN, Morris JD, Mahan JD, *et al.* Bone mass in healthy children: measurement with quantitative DXA. *Radiology* 1991; 179: 735–738.
32. Tsukahara H, Sudo M, Umezaki M, *et al.* Dual-energy x-ray absorptiometry in the lumbar spine, proximal femur and distal radius in children. *Pediatr Radiol* 1992; 22: 560–562.
33. Theintz G, Buchs B, Rizzoli R, *et al.* Longitudinal monitoring of bone mass accumulation in healthy adolescents: evidence for a marked reduction after 16 years of age at the levels of lumbar spine and femoral neck in female subjects. *J Clin Endocrinol Metab* 1992; 75: 1060–1065.
34. Bell NH, Shary J, Stevens J, Garza M, Gordon L, Edwards J. Demonstration that bone mass is greater in black than in white children. *J Bone Miner Res* 1991; 6: 719–723.
35. Bhudhikanok GS, Wang M-C, Eckert K, Matkin C, Marcus R, Bachrach L. Differences in bone mineral in young Asian and Caucasian Americans may reflect differences in bone size. *J Bone Miner Res* 1996; 11: 1545–1556.
36. Dyson ED, Jackson CK, Whitehouse WJ. Scanning electron microscope studies of human trabecular bone. *Nature* 1970; 225: 957–959.
37. Genant HK, Engelke K, Fuerst T. Noninvasive assessment of bone mineral and structure: state of the art. *J Bone Miner Res* 1996; 11: 707–730.
38. Gilsanz V. Quantitative computed tomography. In: Siegel M, ed. *Pediatric Body CT.* New York: Churchill Livingstone, 1988: 349–369.
39. Gilsanz V, Boechat MI, Roe TF, Loro ML, Sayre JW, Goodman WG. Gender differences in vertebral body sizes in children and adolescents. *Radiology* 1994; 190: 673–677.
40. Hangartner T, Gilsanz V. Evaluation of cortical bone by computed tomography. *J Bone Miner Res* 1996; 11: 1518–1525.
41. Gilsanz V, Kovanlikaya A, Costin G, Roe TF, Sayre J, Kaufman F. Differential effect of gender on the size of the bones in the axial and appendicular skeletons. *J Clin Endocrinol Metab* 1997; 82: 1603–1607.
42. Gong JK, Arnold JS, Cohn SH. Composition of trabecular and cortical bone. *Anat Rec* 1964; 149: 325–331.
43. Cann CE. Why, when and how to measure bone mass: a guide for the beginning user. In: Frey GD, Yester MV, eds. *Expanding the Role of Medical Physics in Nuclear Medicine.* Washington, DC: American Physics Institute, 1991: 250–279.
44. Mora S, Goodman WG, Loro ML, Roe TF, Sayre J, Gilsanz V. Age-related changes in cortical and cancellous vertebral bone density in girls: assessment with quantitative CT. *Am J Radiol* 1994; 162: 405–409.
45. Gilsanz V, Gibbens DT, Carlson M, Boechat MI, Cann CE, Schulz EE. Peak trabecular vertebral density: a comparison of adolescent and adult females. *Calcif Tissue Int* 1988; 43: 260–262.

46. Gilsanz V, Gibbens DT, Roe TF, *et al.* Vertebral bone density in children: effect of puberty. *Radiology* 1988; 166: 847–850.
47. Gilsanz V, Roe TF, Mora S, Costin G, Goodman WG. Changes in vertebral bone density in black girls and white girls during childhood and puberty. *N Engl J Med* 1991; 325: 1597–1600.
48. Gilsanz V, Boechat MI, Gilsanz R, Loro ML, Roe TF, Goodman WG. Gender differences in vertebral sizes in adults: biomechanical implications. *Radiology* 1994; 190: 678–682.
49. Genant HK, Faulkner KG, Fuerst T, Glüer CC. Controversies in the diagnosis of osteoporosis. *Radiology* 1996; 201: 28.
50. Jaworski M, Lebiedowski M, Lorenc RS, Trempe J. Ultrasound bone measurement in pediatric subjects. *Calcif Tissue Int* 1995; 56: 368–371.
51. Lappe JM, Recker RR, Malleck MK, Stegmane MR, Packard PP, Heaney RP. Patellar ultrasound transmission velocity in healthy children and adolescents. *Bone* 1995; 16: 251S–256S.
52. Mughal MZ, Langton CM, Utretch G, Morrison J, Specker BL. Comparison between broadband ultrasound attenuation of the calcaneum and total body bone mineral density in children. *Acta Paediatr* 1996; 85: 663–665.
53. Schönau E, Radermacher A, Wentzlik U, Klein K, Michalk D. The determination of ultrasound velocity in the os calcis, thumb and patella during childhood. *Eur J Pediatr* 1994; 153: 252–256.
54. Gluer CC, Cummings SR, Bauer DC, *et al.* Osteoporosis: association of recent fractures with quantitative US findings. *Radiology* 1996; 199: 725–732.
55. Serpe L, Rho J. Broadband ultrasound attenuation value dependence on bone width *in vitro*. *Phys Med Biol* 1996; 41: 197–202.

DISCUSSION

Dr. Specker: My question relates to the race differences that become apparent at puberty. Did you look at cross-sectional area of the whole bone, not just the cortical bone, and whether or not there were race differences before puberty in bone size?

Dr. Gilsanz: In the axial skeleton, racial differences in cancellous bone density are present only after puberty. In the appendicular skeleton, there are racial differences in the size of the bones before puberty.

Dr. Eisman: Do you think any of the change in QTC between 20 and 30 years is a shift between red marrow and fatty marrow rather than a change in the density of the actual bone within that area?

Dr. Gilsanz: Not all changes can be attributed to an increase in marrow. The approximate 10% decline in trabecular vertebral density among young women, relative to adolescent girls, is too large to be attributed to fat variation alone. The percentage of fat by weight in the vertebral body barely changes from 20 to 30 years of age and thereafter increases only at the rate of approximately 2% per decade (1).

Dr. Pettifor: Have you looked at longitudinal studies of calcium supplementation using QCT? What does it do to cortical area? What does it do to trabecular mass?

Dr. Gilsanz: We haven't done the calcium supplementation studies in humans. We did one study, however, which was published in the *American Journal of Physiology* many years ago with 24 rabbits (2). We did QCT and measured total bone density of the vertebrae. One-third of the animals were fed what was considered a normal-calcium diet for a rabbit, one-third were fed with three times that dose of calcium, and one-third with three times less, and we followed them from 8 weeks to the time when the rabbit reaches its peak bone density, which is at about 8 months. We pair-fed these animals, and after 6 months we saw no difference in the density of the vertebrae between the normal rabbits and the calcium-supplemented rabbits. At the end of the study we sacrificed the animals. The deprived group—the one that had one-third less calcium—had about a 4% decrease only. Vitamin D and PTH were lower in the calcium-supplemented animals.

Dr. Seeman: I know you are very tired, and that is probably why you can't remember your own data in the *American Journal of Physiology,* but let me refresh your memory! In fact, what you showed was that there was no benefit of calcium excess above the normal, but in those rabbits that had a deficiency there was a deficit in the trabeculae, but it was not in trabecular bone. I think it was a change in the cortical bone size or the density.

Dr. Gilsanz: The vertebra of a rabbit is a complex structure. It is very difficult to see a clear boundary between cortex and trabecula. So the QCT number was a representation of both cancellous and cortical bone. It was true that there was a difference in cortical thickness on histomorphometry, and it was somewhat decreased in the rabbits that were restricted.

Dr. Seeman: In a famous and often quoted 1979 paper in the *American Journal of Clinical Nutrition* (3), a group that lived in a high dietary calcium area had increased peak bone mass, and this was not a difference in the diameter of the metacarpal, which was the endpoint that was measured, but in the medullary area, so there were changes in the medullary surfaces of bone. There have been only two papers that have shown differences in bone size: one was by Philippe Bonjour *et al.* (4), and the other was a study in school children published in the 1920s in *Lancet* (5,6).

Dr. Seeman: You showed bone density increasing with weight, is that right?

Dr. Gilsanz: No. Cancellous bone density changes only with puberty. Cross-sectional area of the femur increases with weight, and the same is true for cortical bone area.

Dr. Seeman: What is the effect of height and age?

Dr. Gilsanz: They have no effect.

Dr. Seeman: How do you interpret that?

Dr. Gilsanz: It may be the stress of body mass.

Dr. Seeman: Do you believe that the correlation is causal?

Dr. Gilsanz: It is an association, and it is very strong!

Dr. Seeman: But is it causal? Everybody interprets it as being causal, but I think it is most unlikely to be. The association is genetically determined. Nature gives a monkey a bone and a muscle that are appropriate for the monkey's size; it doesn't give the bone of a monkey and the muscle of a elephant. We published a detailed explanation in the *American Journal of Physiology* some time ago (7) in which we looked at the association between muscle size and bone size in monozygotic and dizygotic twins. In identical twins, the correlation between muscle in twin A and bone in twin A is very similar to the correlation between muscle in twin A and bone in twin B, but with dizygotic twins the correlation is no different from that in any individual. After adjustment for differences in size, the correlation in monozygotic twins is lost; in other words, there are genes determining the size of these structures, and it is quite incorrect to infer that the correlation between muscle size and bone size means that if you exercise you will get more bone.

Dr. Specker: We have published in the last couple of months a study looking at prepubertal female athletes, both gymnasts and swimmers, and the gymnasts also had significantly higher bone mass but exactly same muscle mass as the swimmers (8). So even controlling for muscle mass, which in both cases was higher than in the control girls, you still had a significantly higher bone mass in the gymnasts. So I don't think we can say that physical activity doesn't have an effect once you control for muscle mass.

Dr. Seeman: I am not really saying that. You are talking about prepubertal children who are exercising vigorously. I don't believe that negates what I am saying at all.

Dr. Specker: But didn't you conclude that physical activity has no effect?

Dr. Seeman: No, I am saying that you cannot make the inference that the high correlation between muscle mass and bone mass implies a causal relationship. We know that in intervention trials there is very little effect of exercise in an adult. I think that in prepubertal children the strains imposed by the muscle are causing a larger bone mass. Muscle size in our gymnast children is normal; we don't see big muscles.

Dr. Gilsanz: You are talking about muscle; I was talking about weight. The correlation among weight and femoral size and cortical volume is very strong. The correlation among the femoral size, cortical bone volume, and the muscle we measured is not so strong, around 0.54.

Dr. Seeman: I am just suggesting to you that these associations are genetically determined. There are genes regulating size, and those genes to a large extent, though not totally perhaps, explain the high correlations you are getting.

REFERENCES

1. Cann CE, Ettinger B, Genant HK. Normal subjects versus osteoporotics: No evidence using dual energy computed tomography for disproportionate increase in vertebral marrow fat. *J Comput Assist Tomogr* 1985; 9: 617.
2. Gilsanz V, Roe TF, Antunes J, Carlson M, Duarte ML, Goodman WG. Effect of dietary calcium on bone density in growing rabbits. *Am J Physiol* 1991; 260: E471–E476.
3. Matkovic V, Kostial K, Simonovic I, Buzina R, Brodarec A, Nordin BEC. Bone status and fracture rates in two regions of Yugoslavia. *Am J Clin Nutr* 1979; 32: 540–549.
4. Bonjour JP, Carrie AL, Ferrari S, Clavien H, Slosman D, Theintz G, Rizzoli R. Calcium-enriched foods and bone mass growth in prepubertal girls: a randomized, double-blind, placebo-controlled trial. *J Clin Invest* 1997; 99: 1287–1294.
5. Orr JB. Milk consumption and the growth of school-children. *Lancet* 1928; 1: 202–203.
6. Leighton G, Clark ML. Milk consumption and the growth of school-children. *Lancet* 1929; 1: 40–43.
7. Seeman E, Hopper JL, Young NR, Formica C, Goss P, Tsalamandris C. Do genetic factors contribute to associations between muscle strength, fat-free mass and bone density? A twin study. *Am J Physiol* 1996; 270: E320–E327.
8. Cassell C, Benedict M, Specker B. Bone mineral density in elite 7–9 years old female gymnasts and swimmers. *Med Sci Sports Exerc* 1996:28(10); 1243–1246.

Nutrition and Bone Development, edited by
Jean-Philippe Bonjour and Reginald C. Tsang,
Nestlé Nutrition Workshop Series, Vol. 41, Nestec Ltd.,
Vevey/Lippincott–Raven Publishers,
Philadelphia © 1999.

Genetic Determinants of Peak Bone Mass

John A. Eisman

Garvan Institute of Medical Research, St. Vincent's Hospital, Sydney NSW 2010, Australia

Osteoporosis is a major and growing health care problem in all societies where the number and proportion of elderly people are steadily increasing as a result of better preventive health care and increasing life expectancy. This increasing impact may be greatest in those less developed societies where the projected increase in absolute numbers and proportion of elderly people is expected to be greatest (1). The increasing proportion of elderly people, combined with the exponential increase in the incidence of osteoporotic fractures with age, yields remarkable predictions for increasing numbers of all types of osteoporotic fractures. Some, particularly hip fractures, are projected to increase perhaps tenfold over the next few years worldwide (2–4).

Much epidemiologic research has concentrated on hip fractures and, to a lesser extent, vertebral fractures (1–4). This is largely because of the more straightforward recognition that these sorts of fractures are related to osteoporosis, at least in women. However, virtually any bone can fracture as a result of osteoporosis, though other types of fracture have not been so well documented. Furthermore, osteoporotic fractures in men have been relatively ignored. In more recent studies with more complete capture of all fractures and ascertainment of the forces involved in the fracture event, it is becoming clear that osteoporosis is more common in men than has been recognized in the past (5,6). Also, although hip fractures remain the most costly type of osteoporotic fracture, they are relatively uncommon in younger elderly people and only become the dominant fracture type from the ninth decade on. However, the numbers of individuals in any population declines fairly steeply from the ninth decade onward despite increasing life expectancies in both men and women. Thus, increasing emphasis is being applied to the wide range of other osteoporotic fractures. The remaining lifetime risk of a symptomatic osteoporotic fracture has been estimated to be 50% to 60% for a woman 60 years of age and to be 25% to 30% for a man at the same age (2). It is the scope of the problem that is leading to increasing concern about this condition internationally and to more intensive research on it. In view of the numbers potentially affected, population-based interventions are required rather than more narrow individual-based approaches. However, identifying what is most appropriate and what should be advised remains uncertain.

RISK OF FRACTURE

The risk of fracture relates to the strength of the bone, the forces applied to it, and the frequency and duration of such stresses on it. Recent research has examined falls (7–11) as a potentially major risk factor for fracture because falls can generate forces more than sufficient to fracture many bones, even in normal healthy young individuals. The avoidance reflexes, such as using the upper limbs to absorb some of the impact, and soft tissue "padding," which can dissipate much of the force of a fall and thus reduce the risk of fracture, become less effective in the elderly, particularly where muscle weakness and postural unsteadiness increase the likelihood and frequency of falls and slowed reflexes and muscle weakness limit protective actions. Despite the potential importance of these factors, they are not addressed further here. The focus is instead on factors that determine bone strength or its inverse, bone fragility.

Bone fragility has been difficult to assess until the availability of noninvasive techniques with low radiation dose, high precision, and high accuracy. These techniques, particularly dual-energy x-ray (DXA) or dual-photon bone (DPA) densitometry, measure the amount of bone within a given volume of bone tissue and relate the value obtained to the apparent area of bone scanned. Both DPA and DXA are particularly useful for examining the axial skeleton, such as the spine and hip, while comparable assessments of peripheral bones are possible using single-photon or single-energy x-ray absorptiometry (SPA or SXA). With all of these methods, the resultant values (g/cm^2) are compared to young normal reference ranges and to values for similarly aged individuals of the same sex. An adjustment is also often made for body weight but not for the third dimension of depth. Quantitative computerized tomographic (QCT) measurement of bone mineral density does take the third dimension into account, but the precision of this method is lower, offsetting the potential advantage. Recent work has used quantitative ultrasound (QUS) to probe bone mineral density and structure, with some studies suggesting that it provides information on fracture risk independent of bone mineral density. However, the majority of research in osteoporosis has used bone densitometry for assessment of bone strength. In fact, osteoporosis has recently been defined in bone mineral density terms as a value more than 2.5 standard deviations below young healthy normal values (12). This definition reflects the fact that the risk of fracture is determined to a large extent by bone strength or fragility. Moreover, most of the current data on the effects of either genetic or environmental factors on bone structure have been based on bone densitometry. The remainder of this review therefore deals with these studies.

BONE MINERAL DENSITY

Environmental and life-style factors, particularly skeletal loading and dietary calcium intake, have been extensively studied as potential determinants of bone mineral density. Dietary calcium intake has been shown in cross-sectional studies to predict bone mineral density in men (13), but perhaps not in women. Moreover, recent longitudinal studies show that calcium supplementation can induce increases in bone mineral density in adolescents and, combined with increased physical activity, can help maintain bone mineral density in postmenopausal women and elderly people (14–17). Although it has been suggested that high protein and salt intakes may affect bone adversely, these effects are weak. However, smoking and excessive alcohol intake are clearly harmful (18,19). Environmental factors appear to interact positively, such that increased physical activity and calcium supplementation may be more effective than either alone. However, other interactions, particularly with underlying genetic factors, have not been well studied.

Since low bone mineral density is necessary, if not sufficient on its own, for osteoporotic fracture, the critical question is what determines bone mineral density when fracture risk starts to increase. At each bone site, there is a wide normal range in peak bone mineral density, with similar values in men and women (4). In later life, bone mineral density at any site is the sum of the peak density achieved in young adulthood and the subsequent rate of bone loss. Although there may be some bone loss before the menopause, postmenopausal sex hormone deficiency occurs in all women and is probably the most important "environmental" factor in bone loss in women. Typically postmenopausal bone loss is about 2% per annum for 5 to 10 years after the menopause. Although this value decreases with advancing age, bone loss does continue at about 1% per annum for the remainder of life (11). It has been suggested that peak adult bone mineral density makes a greater contribution to bone mineral density than subsequent rates of bone loss until at least 15 years after the menopause. In men, without a menopausal acceleration of bone loss, the effect of peak bone mineral density is likely to extend even later into older age. Therefore, a "good" peak bone mineral density would appear to be the best prophylaxis against clinically relevant postmenopausal and even age-related osteoporosis. Based on these considerations, it seems clear that determinants of peak adult bone mineral density are of major significance in the prevention of osteoporosis.

GENETIC FACTORS

External factors that contribute to the development of peak bone mass have been extensively investigated, but genetic factors have been recognized to be of considerable if not greater importance. Almost 25 years ago, a key study reported greater similarity of bone mineral density in identical than in nonidentical male adult twins and in both male and female adolescent twins (20). This study of the radial midshaft was followed by similar studies using metacarpal morphometry in a smaller number of older twins (21). In these two studies the estimated heritability (h^2) ranged from 0.49 to 0.80. Interestingly, the lower of these estimates was obtained from the male twins (44 to 54 years) compared with the male and female sex twin pairs of adolescent (5 to 19 years) or older (64 to 75 years) age groups. About a decade ago this work on the peripheral skeleton was expanded with studies of the lumbar spine and femoral neck (22,23). In these studies of both genders and a wider age range of twins, similar heritability levels were calculated of 0.7 to 0.8. Of course, these heritability levels are estimated among twins selected to be similar for major factors known to affect bone, such as menopausal status. More recently, similar calculations have been made for heritability of total body bone mineral density (24).

These twin studies have been extensively supported by a wide range of family studies of both bone mineral density and osteoporosis. Asymptomatic relatives of patients with osteoporotic fractures were shown to have lower bone mineral density in the spine (by QCT) and, to a lesser extent, in the os calcis (25). Similarly, premenopausal daughters of women with osteoporotic vertebral fractures were found to have lower bone mineral density in their vertebrae and to a lesser extent in their femoral neck, and less so in the femoral shaft (26). Interestingly, premenopausal daughters of women with osteoporotic hip fractures had lower bone mineral density in the femoral neck or shaft and to a lesser extent in the spine (27). However, in another study, the daughters of women with various sorts of fractures had lower bone mineral density; the mother's bone mineral density explained about 16% of the daughter's bone mineral density at all sites, irrespective of the site of the mother's fracture (28). By contrast, in larger studies of family groups, including multigeneration groups, polygenic loci have been adduced to explain between 40% and 67% of bone mineral density components (29–33).

The reasons for these wide estimates are not clear, but in general, the higher estimates have come from the larger studies, perhaps because larger study numbers lessen the effect of unidentified external factors. Interestingly, in one of these studies of over 400 family members, low bone mineral density in the father increased the son's chance of low bone mineral density 3.8-fold, and low bone mineral density in the mother increased the daughter's risk 5.1-fold, with less predictive power for parents and children of opposite gender (32). Thus, as with the twin studies, it seems that somewhat different genetic factors may be operating in men and women. Similarly, in large epidemiologic studies, a family history of osteoporosis has been associated with low bone mineral density in both men and women (34,35). Again in one of these studies, there were gender differences in apparent heritability (34). In terms of fractures *per se,* army recruits were more likely to suffer stress fractures if they had a family history of osteoporosis (36).

Genetic factors may contribute to rates of bone loss, but results are conflicting. One study of radial bone mineral density in male twins over some 14 years showed no difference between the MZ and DZ twin pairs but rather similar rates of loss in both types of twins, consistent with shared environment rather than inherited factors (37). However, in another study of twins of both genders over a shorter time interval (3 years), there was evidence of heritability of lumbar spine bone loss (38). It is not clear whether these differences relate to the different sites measured (peripheral versus axial), the difference in gender of twins studied (male only versus both sexes), the difference in the time interval studied (mean of 14 versus 3 years), or as yet undefined variables.

The strength of the genetic effects on bone mineral density is considerably greater than the majority of environmental factors. However, the demonstration of the strength of such genetic factors in the determination of bone mineral density is only a first step in the identification of some of the involved genes by genome scanning or the candidate gene approach. In our group we took the candidate gene approach, examining the vitamin D receptor gene, which plays a role in virtually every step of bone and calcium homeostasis, from calcium absorption through parathyroid hormone regulation and regulation of its own renal activation pathway, to the function of osteoblasts and the recruitment of osteoclasts. The initial study of polymorphisms in the vitamin D receptor (VDR) gene showed an association between the genotypes at one locus and serum osteocalcin levels, which in other studies had been shown to be associated with bone mineral density (39–41). This led to a study of VDR alleles in twins and a population sample, both of which showed a strong relationship between VDR alleles and bone mineral density (42). One subsequent twin study in Indianapolis found no such relationship (43), and another study in United Kingdom twins found a similar if weaker effect (44). We have recently noted some errors in our twin genotyping in that original study. As a result of regenotyping and inclusion of further twins, the bone mineral density relationship with VDR alleles is weaker but still significant (45). Moreover, in the initial report (42) there were also differences of 1 SD between alternate homozygotes of the VDR alleles at the same polymorphic site in an independent population sample, not affected by genotyping errors.

Since the initial study, several studies across a wide range of ethnic and racial groups have examined this relationship. Similar VDR and bone mineral density relations have been found in several studies in Japan, Europe, and the United States (46–53). Overall, the significant gene effects have been of the order of 0.25 to 1.0 SD difference in bone mineral density at various skeletal sites between extreme homozygotes. The biological significance of such differences can be seen in the effect of a 1-SD decrease in bone mineral density, which effectively doubles fracture risk. However, various high quality studies have not found any relationship (43,54–59). Indeed, some have shown a significant but weak VDR bone mineral density relationship in the opposite sense to the earlier studies (47,49).

The reasons for these wide differences (60,61) are not yet clear, but several possibilities have been proposed. The suggestion of an ethnic limitation is not consistent with the reports of a relationship in Caucasian, black American, and Japanese sample populations. Variability in the association has been suggested to be related to variability in linkage disequilibrium between the VDR and a nearby causative gene. However, the wide range of racial/ethnic groups in which the association has been found, for example from Australia, Europe, Japan, and the United States, also makes this proposition rather unlikely. Thus, these possible explanations for spurious VDR allelic relations seem not to be valid. An alternate explanation may relate to gene–environment interactions. One possibility relates to effects of dietary calcium, as some studies show relations between VDR alleles and responses of bone mineral density over time to dietary calcium intake as well as to active vitamin D analogs (62–65). These showed differences in bone mineral density change over time, but only in some VDR alleles. The mechanism of these effects may be explained by other studies, which have shown relations between the VDR alleles and response of calcium absorption to change in dietary calcium intake. These results are particularly interesting, as they may suggest that gene–environment interactions could explain the lack of effect of VDR alleles in some studies in different environments, where there are differences in overall calcium intake and even in vitamin D levels. These are yet to be fully explored but do offer interesting possibilities. Interestingly, some studies in unrelated conditions have shown relationships between VDR alleles and clinical variables in primary hyperparathyroidism (66). A further study has shown a relationship between VDR alleles and the occurrence of prostatic malignancy (67).

There have now been other genes in which noncoding polymorphisms have been associated with differences in bone mineral density. These include the estrogen receptor gene, an intronic region of the collagen Ia1 gene, and the transforming growth factor (TGF) b1 gene (68–70). Each of these has been shown to have relations with bone mineral density, without any evidence of differences in the gene product *per se*. It remains to be shown if any of these polymorphic regions are in linkage with coding region differences or with regions that result in differences in the level of gene transcription or mRNA stability. Recently, polymorphisms in the apolipoprotein E gene have been associated with bone density, but again no mechanism has been defined (71). No clear mechanisms have been defined as yet for any of these genes. However, preliminary studies for the VDR suggest that different alleles may be associated with different steady-state levels of VDR mRNA (42,72), but another study did not find any relationship between VDR alleles and intestinal VDR protein levels in a small group of healthy individuals (73). Interestingly, the collagen Ia1 gene intronic polymorphism (68) appears to involve a binding site for the SpI transcription factor, which could theoretically be related to different rates of gene transcription.

Further work is continuing with both candidate gene approaches and with genome scanning in both human and primate models. These are likely to yield new polymorphic gene loci with associations with bone mineral density and sensitivity to bone loss in the early postmenopausal period as well as with aging. It is likely that similar allelic differences exist in other genes implicated in the determination of bone mass. Subtle functional differences in the gene product could be expected to contribute to each individual responding differently to different environmental "insults," depending on the underlying genetic makeup. The sum of these interactions throughout growth and early adulthood would eventually determine each individual's peak bone mass. Identification of each such gene offers important targets for both life-style and pharmacologic interventions. Understanding these gene–environment interactions may make it possible to provide individualized life-style and environmental factor prescriptions based on each individual's genetic predispositions.

SUMMARY

In summary, it is clear that genetic factors and environmental factors, such as dietary calcium and particularly physical activity, interact to contribute to the achievement and maintenance of adult bone mineral density. Strong genetic influences can be seen on peripheral and axial bone sites with respect to peak adult bone mineral density, bone turnover, and age-related changes in bone mass. Environmental and life-style factors, such as dietary calcium intake, weight-bearing physical activity, alcohol intake, and smoking, presumably interact to allow or inhibit expression of bone mineral density genotype. The operation of such factors throughout adolescence and adult life should influence achievement and maintenance of each individual's optimal genetic potential for bone mass. Optimization of bone mass should reduce an individual's risk of osteoporosis in later life. Although new treatments for osteoporosis have been and are being developed, preventive regimens still appear to be the most effective approach to minimize the overall community health impact of this growing public health problem.

REFERENCES

1. Cooper C, Campion G, Melton LJ. Hip fractures in the elderly: a world-wide projection. *Osteoporosis Int* 1992; 2: 285–289.
2. Jones G, Nguyen TV, Sambrook PN, Kelly PJ, Eisman JA. Symptomatic fracture incidence in elderly men and women: the Dubbo Osteoporosis Epidemiology Study. *Osteoporosis Int* 1994; 4: 277–282.
3. Kroger H, Tuppurainen M, Honkanen R, Alhava E, Saarikoski S. Bone mineral density and risk factors of osteoporosis a population based study of 1600 perimenopausal women. *Calif Tissue Int* 1994; 55: 1–7.
4. Cummings SR, Nevitt MC, Browner WS, *et al.* Risk factors for hip fracture in white women. *N Engl J Med* 1995; 332: 767–773.
5. Jones G, White C, Nguyen T, Sambrook P, Kelly P, Eisman J. Prevalent vertebral deformities: relationship to bone mineral density and spinal osteophytosis in elderly men and women. *Osteoporosis Int* 1996; 6: 233–239.
6. Nguyen TV, Eisman JA, Kelly PJ, Sambrook PN. Risk factors for osteoporotic fractures in men. *Am J Epidemiol* 1996; 144: 255–263.
7. Grisso JA, Kelsey JL, Strom BL, *et al.* Risk factors for falls as a cause of hip fracture in women. *N Engl J Med* 1991; 324: 1326–1331.
8. Nguyen TV, Sambrook PN, Kelly PJ, *et al.* Prediction of osteoporotic fractures by postural instability and bone density. *Br Med J* 1993; 307: 1111–1115.
9. Grisso JA, Kelsey JL, Strom BL, *et al.* and the Northeast Hip Fracture Study Group. Risk factors for hip fracture in black women. *N Engl J Med* 1994; 330: 1555–1559.
10. Hui SL, Slemenda CW, Johnston CC. The contribution of bone loss to postmenopausal osteoporosis. *Osteoporosis Int* 1990; 1: 30–34.
11. Jones G, Nguyen TV, Sambrook PN, Kelly PJ, Eisman JA. Progressive femoral neck bone loss: longitudinal findings from the Dubbo Osteoporosis Epidemiology Study. *Br Med J* 1994; 309: 691–695.
12. Kanis JA, and the WHO Study Group. Assessment of fracture risk and its application to screening for postmenopausal osteoporosis: synopsis of a WHO report. *Osteoporosis Int* 1994; 4: 368–381.
13. Kelly PJ, Pocock NA, Sambrook PN, Eisman JA. Dietary calcium, sex hormones, and bone mineral density in men. *Br Med J* 1990; 300: 1361–1364.
14. Prince RL, Smith M, Dick IM, *et al.* Prevention of postmenopausal osteoporosis. A comparative study of exercise, calcium supplementation, and hormone-replacement therapy. *N Engl J Med* 1991; 325: 1189–1195.
15. Johnston CC, Miller JZ, Slemenda CW, *et al.* Calcium supplementation and increases in bone mineral density in children. *N Engl J Med* 1992; 327: 119–120.
16. Chevalley T, Rizzoli R, Nydegger V, *et al.* Effects of calcium supplements on femoral bone mineral density and vertebral fracture rate in vitamin-D-replete elderly patients. *Osteoporosis Int* 1994; 4: 245–252.
17. Matkovic V, Heaney RP. Calcium balance during human growth: evidence for threshold behavior. *Am J Clin Nutr* 1992; 55: 992–996.

18. Pocock NA, Eisman JA, Kelly PJ, Sambrook PN, Yeates MG. Effects of tobacco use on axial and appendicular bone mineral density. *Bone* 1989; 10: 329–331.
19. Hopper JL, Seeman E. The bone density of female twins discordant for tobacco use. *N Engl J Med* 1994; 330: 387–392.
20. Smith DA, Nance WE, Won Kang K, Christian JC, Johnston CC. Genetic factors in determining bone mass. *J Clin Invest* 1973; 52: 2800–2808.
21. Moller M, Horman A, Harvarld B, Hauge M, Henningsen K, Nordin BEC. Metacarpal morphometry in monozygotic and dizygotic elderly twins. *Calcif Tissue Res* 1978; 25: 197–201
22. Pocock NA, Eisman JA, Hopper JL, Yeates MG, Sambrook PN, Eberl S. Genetic determinants of bone mass in adults: a twin study. *J Clin Invest* 1987; 80: 706–710.
23. Dequeker J, Nijs J, Verstaeten A, Geusens P, Gevers G. Genetic determinants of bone mineral content at the spine and the radius: a twin study. *Bone* 1987; 8: 207–209.
24. Young D, Hopper JL, Nowson CA, *et al.* Determinants of bone mass in 10- to 26-year old females: a twin study. *J Bone Min Res* 1995; 10: 558–567.
25. Evans RA, Marel GM, Lancaster EK, Kos S, Evans M, Wong SYP. Bone mass is low in relatives of osteoporotic patients. *Ann Intern Med* 1988; 109: 870–873.
26. Seeman E, Hopper JL, Bach LA, *et al.* Reduced bone mass in daughters of women with osteoporosis. *N Engl J Med* 1989; 320: 554–558.
27. Seeman E, Tsalamandris C, Formica C, Hopper JL, McKay J. Reduced femoral neck bone density in the daughters of women with hip fractures: the role of low bone density in the pathogenesis of osteoporosis. *J Bone Miner Res* 1994; 9: 739–743.
28. Hansen MA, Hassager C, Jensen SB, Christiansen C. Is heritability a risk factor for postmenopausal osteoporosis? *J Bone Miner Res* 1992; 7: 1037–1043.
29. Sowers MFR, Boehnke M, Jannausch ML, Crutchfield M, Corton G, Burns TL. Familiality and partitioning of the variability of femoral bone mineral density in women of child-bearing age. *Calcif Tissue Int* 1992; 50: 110–114.
30. McKay HA, Bailey DA, Wilkinson AA, Houston CS. Familial comparison of bone mineral density at the proximal femur and lumbar spine. *Bone Miner* 1994; 24: 95–110.
31. Krall EA, Dawson-Hughes B. Soft tissue body composition: familial resemblance and independent influences on bone mineral density. *J Bone Miner Res* 1995; 10: 1944–1950.
32. Jouanny P, Guillemin F, Kuntz C, Jeandel C, Pourel J. Environmental and genetic factors affecting bone mass: similarity of bone density among members of healthy families. *Arthritis Rheum* 1995; 38: 61–67.
33. Lonzer MD, Imrie R, Rogers D, Worley D, Licata A, Secic M. Effects of heredity, age, weight, puberty, activity and calcium intake on bone mineral density in children. *Clin Pediatr* 1996; 35: 185–189.
34. Soroko SB, Barrett-Connor E, Edelstein SL, Kritz-Siverstein D. Family history of osteoporosis and bone mineral density at the axial skeleton: the Rancho Bernardo study. *J Bone Miner Res* 1994; 9: 761–769.
35. Orwoll ES, Bauer DC, Vogt TM, Fox KM, and the Study of Osteoporotic Fractures Research Group. Axial bone mass in older women. *Ann Intern Med* 1996; 124: 187–196.
36. Friedl KE, Nuovo JA, Patience TH, Dettori JR. Factors associated with stress fracture in young Army women: indications for further research. *Military Med* 1992; 157: 334–338.
37. Slemenda CW, Christian JC, Reed T, Reister TK, Williams CJ, Johnston CC. Long-term bone loss in men: effects of genetic and environmental factors. *Ann Intern Med* 1992; 117: 286–291.
38. Kelly PJ, Nguyen T, Pocock N, Hopper J, Sambrook PN, Eisman JA. Genetic determination of changes in bone density with age: a twin study. *J Bone Miner Res* 1993; 8: 11–17.
39. Morrison NA, Yeoman R, Kelly PJ, Eisman JA. Contribution of *trans*-acting factor alleles to normal physiological variability: vitamin D receptor gene polymorphisms and circulating osteocalcin. *Proc Natl Acad Sci USA* 1992; 89: 6665–6669.
40. Kelly PJ, Hopper JL, Macaskill GT, Pocock NA, Sambrook PN, Eisman JA. Genetic factors in bone turnover. *J Clin Endocrinol Metab* 1991; 72: 808–813.
41. Tokita A, Kelly PJ, Nguyen TV, *et al.* Genetic determinants of type I collagen synthesis and degradation: further evidence for genetic regulation of bone turnover. *J Clin Endocrinol Metab* 1994; 78: 1461–1466.
42. Morrison NA, Qi JC, Tokita A, *et al.* Prediction of bone density by vitamin D receptor alleles. *Nature* 1994; 367: 284–287.

43. Hustmyer FG, Peacock M, Hui S, Johnston CC, Christian JC. Bone mineral density in relation to polymorphisms at the vitamin D receptor locus. *J Clin Invest* 1994; 94: 2130–2134.
44. Spector TD, Keen RW, Arden NK, *et al.* Vitamin D receptor gene (VDR) alleles and bone density in postmenopausal women; a UK twin study. *Br Med J* 1995; 310: 1357–1360.
45. Eisman JA. Genetics of osteoporosis. In: Papapoulos SE, Lips P, Pols HAP, Johnston CC, Delmas PD, eds: *Osteoporosis '96, International Congress Series 1118.* Amsterdam: Excerpta Medica, 1996: 131–135.
46. Riggs BL, Nguyen TV, Melton LJ, *et al.* Contribution of vitamin D receptor gene alleles to the determination of bone mineral density in normal and osteoporotic women. *J Bone Miner Res* 1995; 10: 991–996.
47. Salamone LM, Ferell R, Black DM, *et al.* The association between vitamin receptor gene polymorphisms and bone mineral density at the spine, hip and total body in premenopausal women. *Osteoporosis Int* 1996; 6: 63–68.
48. Tokita A, Matsumoto H, Morrison NA, *et al.* Vitamin D receptor alleles, bone mineral density and turnover in premenopausal Japanese women. *J Bone Miner Res* 1996; 11: 1003–1009.
49. Uitterlinden AG, Pols HAP, Burger H, *et al.* A large-scale population-based study of the association of vitamin D receptor gene polymorphisms with bone mineral density. *J Bone Miner Res* 1996; 11: 1241–1248.
50. Yamagata Z, Miyamura T, Iijima S, *et al.* Vitamin D receptor gene polymorphism and bone mineral density in healthy Japanese women. *Lancet* 1994; 344: 1027.
51. Fleet JC, Harris SS, Wood RJ, Dawson-Hughes B. The BsmI vitamin D receptor restriction length polymorphism (BB) predicts low bone density in premenopausal black and white women. *J Bone Miner Res* 1995; 10: 985–990.
52. Barger-Lux MJ, Heaney RP, Hayes J, DeLuca HF, Johnson ML, Gong G. Vitamin D receptor gene polymorphism, bone mass, body size, and vitamin D receptor density. *Calcif Tissue Int* 1995; 57: 161–162.
53. Houston LA, Grant SFA, Reid DM, Ralston SH. Vitamin D polymorphism, bone mineral density and osteoporotic vertebral fracture: studies in a UK population. *Bone* 1996; 18: 249–252.
54. Garnero P, Borel O, Sornay-Rendu E, Arlot MA, Delmas PD. Vitamin D receptor gene polymorphisms are not related to bone turnover, rate of bone loss and bone mass in postmenopausal women: the OFELY study. *J Bone Miner Res* 1996; 11: 827–834.
55. Garnero P, Borel O, Sornay-Rendu E, Delmas PD. Vitamin D receptor gene polymorphisms do not predict bone turnover and bone mass in healthy premenopausal women. *J Bone Miner Res* 1995; 10: 1283–1288.
56. Kroger H, Mahonen A, Ryhanen S, Turunen AM, Alhava E, Maenpaa P. Vitamin D receptor genotypes and bone mineral density. *Lancet* 1995; 345: 1239.
57. Looney JE, Yoon HK, Fischer M, *et al.* Lack of a high prevalence of the BB vitamin D receptor genotype in severely osteoporotic women. *J Clin Endocrinol Metab* 1995; 80: 2158–2162.
58. Melhus H, Kindmark A, Amer S, Wilen B, Lindh E, Ljunghall S. Vitamin D receptor genotypes in osteoporosis. *Lancet* 1994; 344: 949.
59. Scholler J, Jorgensen HL, Sand JC, Jensen M, Hassager C, Christiansen C. The impact of common allelic variation at the vitamin D receptor locus on bone mass is not clinically relevant. *J Bone Miner Res* 1995; 10 (Suppl).
60. Eisman JA. Vitamin D receptor gene alleles and osteoporosis: an affirmative view. *J Bone Miner Res* 1995; 10: 1289–1293.
61. Peacock M. Vitamin D receptor gene alleles and osteoporosis: contrasting view. *J Bone Miner Res* 1995; 10: 1294–1297.
62. Dawson-Hughes B, Harris SS, Finneran S. Calcium absorption on high and low calcium intakes in relation to vitamin D receptor genotype. *J Clin Endocrinol Metab* 1995; 80: 3657–3661.
63. Ferrari S, Rizzoli R, Chevalley T, Slosman D, Eisman JA, Bonjour J-P. Vitamin D receptor gene polymorphisms and the rate of change of lumbar spine bone mineral density in elderly men and women. *Lancet* 1995; 345: 423–424.
64. Krall EA, Parry P, Lichter JB, Dawson-Hughes B. Vitamin D receptor alleles and rates of bone loss: influence of years since menopause and calcium intake. *J Bone Miner Res* 1995; 10: 978–984.
65. Matsuyama T, Ishii S, Tokita A, *et al.* VDR gene polymorphisms and vitamin D analog treatment in Japanese. *Lancet* 1995; 345: 1238–1239.
66. Carling T, Kindmark A, Hellman P, *et al.* Vitamin D receptor genotypes in primary hyperparathyroidism. *Nature Med* 1995; 1: 1309–1311.

67. Taylor JA, Hirvonen A, Watson M, Pittman G, Mohler JL, Bell DA. Association of prostate cancer with vitamin D receptor gene polymorphism. *Cancer Res* 1996; 56: 4108–4110.
68. Sano M, Inoue S, Hosoi T, *et al.* Association of estrogen receptor dinucleotide repeat polymorphism with osteoporosis. *Biochem Biophys Res Commun* 1995; 217: 378–383.
69. Grant SFA, Reid DM, Blake G, Herd R, Fogelman I, Ralston SH. Reduced bone density and osteoporosis associated with a polymorphic Sp1 binding site in the collagen type Ia1 gene. *Nature Genet* 1996; 14: 203–205.
70. Langdahl BL, Loft AG, Moller N, Weeke J, Eriksen EF, Mosekilde L, Charles P. Skeletal responsiveness to thyroid hormone is not altered at menopause. *Bone* 1996; 19: 557–564.
71. Shiraki M, Shiraki Y, Aoki C, *et al.* Association of bone mineral density with apolipoprotein E phenotype (abstract). *J Bone Miner Res* 1996; 10: S436.
72. Ozono K, Yamagata M, Sakai N, Yabuta K, Tokita A, Nakajima S. Messenger RNA level of the allele with TaqI-digestive site is lower than that without the site in vitamin D receptor gene (abstract). *J Bone Miner Res* 1996; 10: S314.
73. Barger-Lux MJ, Heaney RP, Hayes J, DeLuca HF, Johnson ML, Gong G. Vitamin D receptor gene polymorphism, bone mass, body size, and vitamin D receptor density. *Calcif Tissue Int* 1995; 57: 161–162.

DISCUSSION

Dr. Tsang: Let me ask a statistical question. If the association of VDR allele is not particularly strong, and there is a bias toward publishing positive results, do you think there could be a whole lot of unpublished studies that are negative, and this is just a chance association? I am especially concerned because of the opposite conclusion from one of the studies you quoted. I never realized that there was an opposite finding. This makes the statistics even more contorted.

Dr. Eisman: There was a time when there would have been a bias against negative studies, but I am not sure that this is true in this area. It seems that the negative studies do get published, and rightly so. In particular, there is much less bias against negative results in abstracts of scientific meetings. At the ASBMR meeting last year there were perhaps 3,000 patient observations and 2,500 of those reported some association. There could be other small studies that aren't reported, and this can be examined as part of a meta-analysis. The finding of opposite results is telling us something about what these genes and their polymorphism mean in relation to the environment. A particular environment might mean that one allele gene is disadvantageous, and you have low bone density; in another environment the effects on calcium absorption could be such that the same allele is advantageous.

Dr. Guesry: For me the main interest of genetic studies would be to identify families at risk in order to institute prophylaxis. This would have a better chance of being followed for many years if a real risk were identified. From your talk I gather that you are still unable to identify at-risk families.

Dr. Eisman: Well, what sort of reliability would you have to have to identify an at-risk family? If you were right 50% of the time would you be satisfied?

Dr. Guesry: Yes. That is exactly what we do for allergy. If there is a 50% increased risk we suggest prophylaxis.

Dr. Eisman: Then you don't need to do any tests because half the people in this room are at risk of osteoporosis unless they are "fortunate enough" to die before it is a problem. Where I think it makes a greater difference to know the genotype is to enable you to say, if you are at risk or already have osteoporosis, you need to achieve a particular level of calcium intake, or if you are another, additional calcium won't make any difference.

Dr. Caverzasio: It is difficult to see a functional relationship between polymorphism and the reasons for these differences in bone mass. Is an animal model being developed to investigate that?

Dr. Eisman: We have been a bit simplistic about this. We are trapped to some extent by the mutational model, where you have a gene where the protein product suddenly doesn't work or is switched on all the time. That is very informative, but it is not a mechanism that we are likely to see in half the population. In fact, we see no coding differences in the actual gene. We have now sequenced a fairly large number of coding regions, about 90, and we have seen a few polymorphic changes, none of which changed the protein sequence. Thus, the likelihood is that any functional differences are going to be in relation to gene regulation. The argument that was made in relation to the collagen Iα1 is that the intronic polymorphism might interfere with an SP1 binding site. In other words, it could change the actual regulation of that gene. Now if you have something that changes the regulation of that gene, particularly if it is specific in one tissue or another, then you could get a subtle shift, say more receptor or less receptor in bone or in parathyroid, which could lead to an effect. You may be aware that there are now a couple of studies that have looked at the incidence of hyperparathyroidism, the size of the tumors, the PTH levels, and so forth, where there is a gene relationship with the VDR of the same polymorphism that we are talking about, so implying that there could be a functional change in the vitamin D endocrine system. It only needs to be a relatively small change biologically, and amplified over the 30-, 40-, 50-, or 80-year lifetime of an individual, to have the effect that we might be concerned about.

Dr. Potter: I am curious to know some more about the nature of this VDR polymorphism. You said it is not on a structural coding sequence, and you speculated that it's in the regulatory regions. Have you been able to identify whether it's in a promoter or an intron? You mentioned for collagen there was an SP1 binding site that was perturbed. Do you have any binding site for transcription factors that is perturbed in your VDR polymorphism?

Dr. Eisman: The polymorphisms arguably have to be in linkage disequilibrium with whatever might be causative, but there is nothing to suggest that they are.

Dr. Potter: So you are saying there could be some linked gene as well?

Dr. Eisman: There certainly could be something in that vicinity.

Dr. Potter: But you are arguing that it is that receptor, so if you could identify a functional cause, it would be helpful.

Dr. Eisman: I agree. What we have done is to look further at the 5′ and 3′ regions of those sites, and at this stage we haven't found anything more informative in the populations that we are looking at than the polymorphism we have already identified, though we certainly haven't identified every polymorphism that exists. Of course, the promoter of the vitamin D receptor is still unpublished. We have some evidence about where it is by direct sequencing, and it also seems that there are alternative promoters, but we have not yet determined whether there are any polymorphisms within those sites. We are setting up some transgenic models to look at subtle changes in receptor level, in this case, particularly in bone cells, to see whether that leads to any change in bone mass. We have some preliminary data to suggest that there are effects.

Dr. Seeman: I think all of these studies need to be redone. What is most seriously holding back progress in this field is the word "density," and we must not use this word, or if we are going to use it, we should use in with the greatest of care, at least use "apparent density" or "areal density" or "linear density" or volumetric density. If we use the term "apparent density," we might be lucky and find that our students might actually ask us what do you mean by "apparent density," and once they ask us a question we might be able to talk about it. Now I think the problem with these studies is that we have not taken size into account.

If the value of bone mass is, say, 1, 2, or 3 standard deviations away from the mean, and the amount of bone in that bone size is also 1, 2, or 3 standard deviations away from its mean, then the density will be the same. Low bone density results when there is disproportion, but disproportion relative to its own trait, so that if the bone size is of a given value but there is less bone present, we will end up with low volumetric density. Areal density measurements, which are the basis of all the VDR studies, do not take this into account. Bone size and bone mass are regulated differently, surely by different genes and different hormones. I believe this may contribute to some of the controversies that are seen.

Dr. Eisman: Your point may well be correct and I did allude to the fact that some studies suggested that there were differences in size that were related to the vitamin D receptor. And of course I am aware of this issue, and I think that there may well be size factors to be taken into account. However, I am not really convinced that correcting for area or for volume makes a lot of difference. I suspect that the only subset where you can reliably use bone mineral content, particularly on a comparative basis, is total body. When you start to divide up regions and then use bone mineral content, the values become very dubious. We went through this sort of analysis a long time ago, as I am sure you did too, to try to find the most reproducible values in an individual, and BMC is not as reproducible as any of these other measures.

Dr. Seeman: I think there is a great need for animal studies now, and for histomorphometric studies to look at what structural elements are associated with the different genotypes.

Dr. Gilsanz: In a small group of 100 prepubertal Mexican-American girls, we found that the VDR was not associated with size but seemed to be associated with apparent cancellous bone density and cortical bone density.

Dr. Eisman: I think there are two separate issues. One is, is there a vitamin D receptor genotype effect that has got anything to do with bone? I believe the answer is yes. The second question is, if there is such a difference, what exactly is it? There are a number of possible approaches. It could be a structural approach, where you say that it is actually this part of the bone or that part of the bone that is different. Our approach has been to see how people change in relation to their environment, because we consider it is a physiological difference, and that is where the interest lies. I think the future lies in being able to understand how people are likely to respond to, benefit or not benefit from, a particular intervention, particularly when you are talking about very long term interventions.

Nutrition and Bone Development, edited by
Jean-Philippe Bonjour and Reginald C. Tsang,
Nestlé Nutrition Workshop Series, Vol. 41, Nestec Ltd.,
Vevey/Lippincott–Raven Publishers,
Philadelphia © 1999.

Vitamin D and Bone Mass Development

Michèle Garabédian

CNRS URA 583, Université Paris V, Hôpital Saint Vincent de Paul, 75014 Paris, France

The spectacular deformations and major defects in the mineralization of the skeleton resulting from severe vitamin D deficiency are clear evidence that this vitamin plays a crucial role in cartilage and bone metabolism during postnatal growth. Numerous studies have unraveled most of the pathways whereby vitamin D promotes mineralization of the growing skeleton. However, few clinical investigations have so far focused on the possible long-term effects on bone mass of clinical or subclinical vitamin D deficiency during childhood.

VITAMIN D ACTIONS ON SKELETAL GROWTH AND MINERALIZATION

Clinical and experimental observations have taught us that vitamin D enhances the mineralization of the growing bone by direct and indirect routes (1,2). One of its major actions is to increase the efficiency of intestinal absorption of the calcium and phosphate present in the diet, thus increasing the availability of these ions in the vicinity of the newly formed bone and growth plate cartilage matrices (1–3). It also appears to increase the extracellular concentration of these ions by stimulation of the renal tubular reabsorption of phosphate and calcium (3,4), at least in situations of phosphate deficiency, vitamin D deficiency, or hyperparathyroidism. Finally, vitamin D stimulates the differentiation and fusion of osteoclast progenitors, indirectly activates mature osteoclasts, and mobilizes calcium and phosphate from the mineralized bone matrix (2,3,5,6). Although these latter effects enhance bone resorption and thus contribute to impaired bone mineralization, they may favor optimal mineralization of the newly formed bone matrix during growth by supplying some of the necessary calcium and phosphate locally.

Other actions of vitamin D indirectly enhance the mineralization of the skeleton. Thus, vitamin D inhibits the synthesis of parathyroid hormone (7), an effect that limits bone resorption, and it increases muscular strength by direct actions on the myocytes (8).

Vitamin D also directly modulates the differentiation and function of cells responsible for bone formation and mineralization. It stimulates the differentiation of growth plate chondrocytes and regulates their production of type II collagen and other cartilage matrix components (9–11). It influences the phenotypic maturation of osteoblasts and has complex effects on the bone-forming activity of these cells. Its local actions on bone cells are either direct or mediated through other actions because it modulates the production of local regulators of bone turnover as well as cell responses to these regulators (2,5). Finally, vitamin D may stimulate bone formation by controlling the deposition of bone morphogenic proteins on the matrix (12).

1,25-Dihydroxyvitamin D is responsible for most of the above effects. But other vitamin D metabolites, such as 24,25-dihydroxyvitamin D, may play a specific role in cartilage and bone cells (2,9,10,13). Their actions, in combination with those of 1,25-dihydroxyvitamin D, lead to increased volume and mineralizaton of bone.

SEVERE VITAMIN D DEFICIENCY AND SKELETAL MINERALIZATION IN CHILDREN AND ADOLESCENTS

Infants are particularly prone to develop severe vitamin D deficiency and to present with the typical skeletal signs of this deficiency—rickets, poor mineralization of the skeleton, bone deformities, and slow growth (14). Prophylactic measures, such as fortification of infant formulas with vitamin D and routine supplementation with daily or intermittent doses of vitamin D, have markedly decreased the incidence of this disease during the first 2 to 4 years of life. However, rickets can still be seen among unsupplemented breast-fed infants (15) or in infants fed macrobiotic (16) or strictly vegetarian diets (17).

Older children are classically less at risk of developing signs of vitamin D deficiency, but cases of rickets have been reported in school children, especially in adolescents during the growth spurt, in the tropics (14) as well as in Europe (18–26). Although the condition is rare in most temperate countries, investigations carried out in northern China showed an incidence of late-onset rickets as high as 5% to 15% among adolescents (27). Most of the cases are found in geographic areas with suboptimal solar irradiation or atmospheric pollution, particularly in communities with limited sunlight exposure for climatic, religious, or socioeconomic reasons and in subjects with heavy skin pigmentation.

Because of bone pain and bone deformities, vitamin D deficiency is usually diagnosed early and is not left untreated for long periods of time. Complete healing of the growth plate cartilage abnormalities that define rickets is usually obtained 3 to 6 months after the onset of vitamin D treatment. However, in the most severe cases, healing of rickets and correction of the bone deformities may take more than a year. Although severe osteopenia is associated with rickets, this sign is not commonly used as a marker of the efficacy of treatment, and measurement of bone mineral content is not the rule in the follow-up of children with rickets. Thus, no clear information is available on the time required to normalize bone mineralization under treatment. Information is also lacking on the long-term consequences on adult bone mass of the transient osteopenia induced by vitamin D deficiency, although sequelae such as permanent pelvic deformities have been related to vitamin D deficiency during puberty (25).

In addition, abnormalities of bone mass acquisition may be difficult to relate to vitamin D deficiency alone. Indeed, children with nutritional rickets often suffer from associated deficiencies of other nutrients, which increase the susceptibility to vitamin D deficiency or aggravate its effects on bone. For example, their diet may be deficient in calcium, protein, energy, magnesium, or vitamin A, or it may contain high concentrations of phytates, oxalates, or fiber, which impair the intestinal absorption of calcium (28).

SUBCLINICAL VITAMIN D DEFICIENCY AND SKELETAL MINERALIZATION IN CHILDREN AND ADOLESCENTS

If clinical vitamin D deficiency is seldom found in children and adolescents, low circulating levels of 25-hydroxyvitamin D suggestive of a low vitamin D status have been reported in at-risk populations of children living in northern European countries (20,21,23,29) and in a significant portion of unselected populations of European or South American children (30,31). In a recent investigation of 117 healthy children and adolescents aged 10 to 17 years living in northern France, we found that 14% of the children had circulating 25-hydroxyvitamin D concentrations below the reference range for healthy adult populations at the end of the winter (6 to 26 ng/ml) and that 6% of the children had very low levels, below 3 ng/ml (Table 1). The highest percentages of children with low or very low vitamin D status were found during winter and spring, particularly among adolescents at the end of pubertal maturation (32) (Table 1).

But the low levels of 25-hydroxyvitamin D found in adolescents does not necessarily imply true biological vitamin D deficiency. In elderly women (33) and neonates (34), 25-hydroxyvitamin D concentrations below 12 ng/ml (30 nmol/l) have been found to be associated with lower serum calcium and higher levels of parathyroid hormone. This value has therefore been proposed in these two extreme populations as a threshold for 25-hydroxyvitamin D concentrations below which vitamin D

TABLE 1. *Distribution of serum 25–(OH)D concentrations in 117 healthy children living in Paris*

	Percentage of children with 25–(OH)D concentrations			
	<3 ng/ml	3–5 ng/ml	6–10 ng/ml	>10 ng/ml
Total population (n = 117)	6	8	28	58
Population seen in winter/spring (n = 53)	9	13	45	33
Winter population at pubertal stages I to III (n = 24)	4	4	52	40
Winter population at pubertal stages IV and V (n = 29)	14	24	40	22

Some of these data have been published by Zeghoud et al. (32).

TABLE 2. *25-(OH)D threshold for vitamin D deficiency in 53 healthy adolescents*[a]

	Serum 25-(OH)D concentrations			
	<3 ng/ml	3–5 ng/ml	6–10 ng/ml	>10 ng/ml
Number of subjects	5	8	25	15 (28%)
Total calcium (mmol/liter)	2.28 ± 0.11	2.37 ± 0.15	2.36 ± 0.10	2.36 ± 0.12
Phosphate (mmol/liter)	1.42 ± 0.27	1.34 ± 0.19	1.72 ± 0.65	1.45 ± 0.10
PTH (pg/ml)	44 ± 28**	26 ± 12	21 ± 9	21 ± 10
1,25-$(OH)_2D$ (pg/ml)	44 ± 7	47 ± 9	48 ± 11	44 ± 12

[a] These data are mean ± 1 SD.
** Significantly different from PTH values in the three other groups of adolescents ($p < 0.001$).
Table adapted from Zeghoud et al. (32).

deficiency is defined. Results shown on Table 2 suggest that this threshold may be much lower in adolescent populations, 3 ng/ml (7.5 nmol/l). Above this level, no clear alterations in serum calcium, phosphate, or parathyroid hormone levels were found, and therefore no definite indication of vitamin D deficiency was obtained.

Low intakes of calcium or phosphate increase the production of 1,25-dihydroxyvitamin D and consequently activate the vitamin D metabolic clearance rate (1–3,35). Rapid skeletal growth may have similar effects, as it increases the demand of the organism for these ions (36). Thus, the pubertal growth spurt may result in a higher production rate of 1,25-dihydroxyvitamin D, although it is not consistently associated with high circulating levels of this metabolite (32,37). The resulting activation of vitamin D catabolism would explain the increased incidence of low serum 25-hydroxyvitamin D values in adolescents receiving no vitamin D supplements in late puberty, despite normal sunlight exposure. On the basis of the data presented in Table 2, 25-hydroxyvitamin D levels below the reference range for adults indicate low vitamin D status, but they may not necessarily have pathologic consequences in adolescents with adequate dietary intakes.

The situation may be different in children with poor calcium intakes. Dietary calcium restriction further increases the levels of circulating 1,25-dihydroxyvitamin D in children (38) and may thus aggravate hypovitaminosis D during rapid growth. Mild hypovitaminosis D may in turn impair the adaptation of 1,25-dihydroxyvitamin D production to low calcium intakes and therefore aggravate calcium deficiency.

Numerous studies have investigated the influence of spontaneous dietary calcium intakes on bone mass development and have evaluated the effects of calcium supplements on bone (39). However, more information is needed to determine the interactions between moderate hypovitaminosis D and calcium deficiency and the extent to which hypovitaminosis D could potentiate the effects of a low-calcium diet.

During a cross-sectional study of healthy chidren and adolescents living in northern France (40), we found that 67% of them had daily calcium intakes below 1,000 mg, the recommended dietary allowance in most European countries (41). Almost all (96%) of the children with calcium intakes above this level had a bone mineral density above -1 SD, when expressed as a z score, at the lumbar vertebral and upper femoral sites (40). In contrast, up to 26% of the children with calcium intakes below 1,000 mg/day had low bone mineral density, between −1 SD and −2 SD. It is possible that some of these children with low bone mineral density had been unable to adapt to the low-calcium diet because of associated subclinical vitamin D deficiency.

If the consequences of moderately low levels of 25-hydroxyvitamin D are not clear, very low levels during puberty below 3 ng/ml (7.5 nmol/l) may alter bone metabolism, as they are associated with some degree of secondary hyperparathyroidism. Moreover, this subclinical vitamin D deficiency may remain unrecognized for long periods of time. As an example, it was found in a significant proportion (6%) of apparently healthy adolescents living in the Paris area (Table 1). However, as with severe vitamin D deficiency, there has been no systematic investigation of the effects of transient or chronic subclinical deficiency on bone mass development during puberty nor of its long-term effects on adult bone mass. The few reports published at present have not shown a clear relationship between bone mineral content and vitamin D metabolites during puberty, at least in boys with 25-hydroxyvitamin D values above deficiency levels (37), nor have they found a significant association between metacarpal mass and a high incidence of low 25-hydroxyvitamin D levels in prepubertal and pubertal children (31).

GENETIC VARIATIONS IN THE GENE ENCODING THE VITAMIN D RECEPTOR AND BONE MASS DEVELOPMENT

Common allelic variations in the gene encoding the 1,25-dihydroxyvitamin D receptor (VDR) represent one of the genetic determinants of bone mass or bone mass variance with age, although the contribution of VDR polymorphism is not as important as proposed originally. Of interest, a recent meta-analysis of the published studies suggests a stronger association of the VDR polymorphism with bone mineral density in young adult women than during postmenopausal life (42). Three recent reports suggest that the VDR genotype may influence bone mass in girls (43–45) and their response to calcium supplements (45) from prepubertal life.

CONCLUSION

Vitamin D is one of the main regulators of bone mineralization, and the consequences of severe vitamin D deficiency on the skeleton are well recognized. But the long-term effects of severe vitamin D deficiency on adult bone mass, as well as the short- and long-term effects of more subtle depletion, have not been fully investigated. Further investigation should take into account other related environmental or genetic determinants of bone mass, such as dietary calcium and the VDR genotype.

REFERENCES

1. Fraser DR. Regulation of the metabolism of vitamin D. *Physiol Rev* 1980; 60: 551–613.
2. Bouillon R, Okamura WH, Norman AW. Structure–function relationships in the vitamin D endocrine system. *Endocr Rev* 1995; 16: 200–257.

3. Kumar R. The metabolism and mechanism of action of 1,25-dihydroxyvitamin D_3. *Kidney Int* 1986; 30: 793–803.
4. Kawashima H, Kurokawa K. Metabolism and sites of action of vitamin D in the kidney. *Kidney Int* 1986; 29: 98–107.
5. Lowe KE, Maiyar AC, Norman AW. Vitamin D-mediated gene expression. *Crit Rev Eukaryot Gene Expr* 1992; 2: 65–109.
6. Suda T, Takahashi N, Martin TJ. Modulation of osteoclast differentiation. *Endocr Rev* 1992; 13: 66–80.
7. Silver J, Naveh-Many T, Mayer H, Schmelzer HJ, Popovtzer MM. Regulation by vitamin D metabolites of parathyroid hormone gene transcription in the rat. *J Clin Invest* 1986; 78: 1296–1301.
8. Boland R. Role of vitamin D in skeletal muscle function. *Endocr Rev* 1986; 7: 434–448.
9. Corvol MT, Dumontier MF, Garabédian M, Rappaport R. Vitamin D and cartilage. II. Biological activity of 25-hydroxycholecalciferol, and 24,25- and 1,25-dihydroxycholecalciferols on cultured growth plate chondrocytes. *Endocrinology* 1978; 102: 1269–1274.
10. Schwartz Z, Brooks B, Swain L, Del Toro F, Norman A, Boyan B. Production of 1,25-dihydroxyvitamin D_3 and 24,25-dihydroxyvitamin D_3 by growth zone and resting zone chondrocytes is dependent on cell maturation and is regulated by hormones and growth factors. *Endocrinology* 1992; 130: 2495–2504.
11. Walters MR. Newly identified actions of the vitamin D endocrine system. *Endocr Rev* 1992; 13: 719–764.
12. Finkelman RD, Linkhart TA, Mohan S, Lau KHW, Baylink DJ, Bell NH. Vitamin D deficiency causes a selective reduction in deposition of transforming growth factor β in rat bone: possible mechanism for impaired osteoinduction. *Proc Natl Acad Sci USA* 1991; 88: 3657–3660.
13. Nakamura T, Suzuki K, Hirai T, Kurokawa T, Orimo H. Increased bone volume and reduced bone turnover in vitamin D-replete rabbits by the administration of 24*R*,25-dihydroxyvitamin D_3. *Bone* 1992; 13: 229–236.
14. Bhattacharrya AK. Nutritional rickets in the tropics. *World Rev Nutr Diet* 1992; 62: 140–197.
15. Edidin D, Levitsky L, Schey W, Dumbovic N, Campos A. Resurgences of nutritional rickets associated with breast-feeding and special dietary practices. *Pediatrics* 1980; 65: 232–235.
16. Dagnelie PC, Vergote F, Van Staveren WA, van den Berg H, Dingjan PG, Hautvast JGAJ. High prevalence of rickets in infants on macrobiotic diets. *Am J Clin Nutr* 1990; 51: 202–208.
17. Key LL. Nutritional rickets. *Trends Endocrinol Metab* 1991; 2: 81–85.
18. Ford JA, Colhoun EM, McIntosh WB, Dunnigan MG. Rickets and osteomalacia in the Glasgow Pakistani community 1961–1971. *Br Med J* 1972; ii: 677–680.
19. Dayras JC, Gold F, Hartmann O, See G. Rachitisme carentiel familial tardif: quatre observations dans une même fratrie. *Ann Pediatr* 1972; 19: 765–773.
20. Moncrieff MW, Lunt HRW, Arthur LJH. Nutritional rickets at puberty. *Arch Dis Child* 1973; 48: 221–224.
21. Cooke WT, Asquith P, Ruck N, Melikian V, Swan CHJ. Rickets, growth, and alkaline phosphatase in urban adolescents. *Br Med J* 1974; ii: 293–297.
22. Corbeel L, Bouillon R, Deschamps L, Geussens H. Vitamin D sensitive rickets in puberty. *Acta Paediatr Belg* 1976; 29: 103–108.
23. Ford JA, McIntosh WB, Butterfield R, *et al.* Clinical and subclinical vitamin D deficiency in Bradford children. *Arch Dis Child* 1976; 51: 939–943.
24. Freycon MT, Pouyau G, Abeille A, *et al.* Rachitisme carentiel chez le grand enfant. A propos de deux observations. *Pediatrie* 1983; 38: 485–490.
25. O'Hare AE, Uttley WS, Belton NR, *et al.* Persisting vitamin D deficiency in the Asian adolescent. *Arch Dis Child* 1984; 59: 766–770.
26. Bénichou JJ, Sallière D, Labrune B. Rachitisme carentiel chez une adolescente. *Arch Fr Pediatr* 1985; 42: 443–445.
27. Zhou H. Rickets in China. In: Glorieux FH, ed. *Rickets. Nestlé Nutrition Workshop Series, vol 21.* New York: Raven Press, 1991: 253–261.
28. Allen LH. Calcium bioavailability and absorption, a review. *Am J Clin Nutr* 1982; 35: 783–808.
29. Colmant A, Freycon MT, Serio AM, *et al.* Déficit plasmatique en 25-(OH)D chez les enfants maghrébins de plus de 10 ans immigrés en France. *Pediatrie* 1985; 40: 17–25.
30. Vainsel M. Facteurs influençant le capital osseux de la vie foetale à l'adolescence. *Tempo Med* 1994; 147: 9–16.
31. Oliveri B, Ladizesky M, Sotelo A, Griffo S, Ballesteros G, Mautalen C. Nutritional rickets in Argen-

tina. In: Glorieux FH, ed. *Rickets. Nestlé Nutrition Workshop Series, vol 21.* New York: Raven Press, 1991: 233–245.
32. Zeghoud F, Delaveyne R, Rehel P, Chalas J, Garabédian M, Odièvre M. Vitamine D et maturation pubertaire. Intérêt et tolérance d'une supplémentation vitaminique D en période hivernale. *Arch Pediatr* 1995; 2: 221–226.
33. Ooms ME, Roos JC, Bezemer PD, Van der Vijgh WJF, Bouter LM, Lips P. Prevention of bone loss by vitamin D supplementation in elderly women: a randomized double-blind trial. *J Clin Endocrinol Metab* 1995; 80: 1052–1058.
34. Zeghoud F, Vervel C, Guillozo H, Walrant-Debray O, Boutignon H, Garabédian M. Subclinical vitamin D deficiency in neonates: definition and response to vitamin D supplements. *Am J Clin Nutr* 1997; 65: 771–778.
35. Halloran BP, Bikle DD, Levens MJ, Castro ME, Globus RK, Holton E. Chronic 1,25-dihydroxyvitamin D_3 administration in the rat reduces the serum concentration of 25-hydroxyvitamin D by increasing metabolic clearance rate. *J Clin Invest* 1986; 78: 622–628.
36. Lund BJ, Clausen N, Lund B, Andersen E, Sorensen OH. Age-dependent variations in serum 1,25-dihydroxyvitamin D in childhood. *Acta Endocrinol* 1980; 94: 426–429.
37. Krabbe S, Christiansen C, Hummer L. Serum vitamin D metabolites are not related to growth rate, bone mineral content, or serum alkaline phosphatase in male puberty. *Calcif Tissue Int* 1986; 38: 127–129.
38. Belon C, Dumas R, Tau C, Sabatier R, Bourdeau A, Garabédian M. Dysrégulation du 1,25(OH)2D plasmatique au cours d'une restriction calcique chez des enfants hypercalciuriques. *Arch Fr Pediatr* 1992; 49: 519–524.
39. Bonjour JP, Rizzoli R. Bone acquisition in adolescence. In: Marcus R, Feldman D, Kelsey J, eds. *Osteoporosis.* New York: Academic Press, 1996: 465–476.
40. Ruiz JC, Mandel C, Garabédian M. Influence of spontaneous calcium intake and physical exercise on the vertebral and femoral bone mineral density of children and adolescents. *J Bone Miner Res* 1995; 10: 675–682.
41. Trichopoulou A, Vassilakou T. Recommended dietary intakes in the European community member states: an overview. *Eur J Clin Nutr* 1990; 44 (Suppl 2): 51–125.
42. Cooper GS, Umbach DM. Are vitamin D receptor polymorphisms associated with bone mineral density? A meta-analysis. *J Bone Miner Res* 1996; 11: 1841–1849.
43. Klisovic D, Young AP, Ilich JZ, Skugor M, Badentrop N, Matkovic V. Vitamin D receptor gene polymorphism (VDR) and bone mineral density (BMD) in prepubertal females (P 243) (abstract). *J Bone Miner Res* 1995; 10 (Suppl 1): S189.
44. Kovanlikaya A, Sainz J, Loro ML, Savre J, Roe T, Gilsanz V. Relationship between vitamin D receptor alleles and the volume and density of cortical bone in children (S 475) (abstract). *J Bone Miner Res* 1996; 11 (Suppl 1): S208.
45. Ferrari SL, Rizzoli R, Theintz G, Siosman DO, Bonjour JP. Vitamin D receptor (VDR) gene polymorphism and the effects of calcium supplementation on bone mass accumulation in prepubertal girls (P235) (abstract). J Bone Miner Res 1995; 10 (suppl 1): S187.

DISCUSSION

Dr. Mughal: You cited 12 publications on adolescent rickets, and four of those were from English workers. The first was by Ford, who was the first person to describe adolescent rickets among Asian immigrants in the United Kingdom. I see quite a few of these problems in adolescent Asian girls, though not in the black Afro-Caribbean population. I think it is a problem of vitamin D deficiency resulting from little sunlight exposure and a culture of not going out very much. You said that you didn't see biological signs of vitamin D deficiency in your 53 adolescents who had very low 25-hydroxyvitamin D levels?

Dr. Garabédian: The Asian girls with clinical signs of rickets and vitamin D deficiency that have been reported by the English authors belong to a specific at-risk population. I agree with you that this deficiency likely resulted from lack of sun exposure, linked to sociocultural habits, in addition to the low intensity of the UV irradiation present in the solar light at the end of winter in northern Europe. The results that I presented concern an unselected population of healthy schoolchildren living in France, in the same geographic area, but with habitual outdoors activities. As you noted, 25-hydroxyvitamin D levels were low, below 10 ng/ml, in the majority of the 53 children seen during the winter (72%). But biological signs of vitamin D deficiency were found only in those with very low 25-hydroxyvitamin D levels, below 3 ng/ml, that is, in 9% of the total population.

Dr. Mughal: The point I was going to make is that the adolescents who have subclinical vitamin D deficiency don't often come in with genu valgum or genu varum. The key sign is bone pain, and they are often labeled as malingerers. They also often have proximal myopathy, and that improves when you treat their vitamin D deficiency.

Dr. Garabédian: That is not what I call subclinical vitamin D deficiency. Subclinical deficiency is when there are no patent manifestations of muscle weakness or bone pain or anything else.

Dr. Mughal: What you didn't tell us was whether you specifically looked for the signs of proximal myopathy in these children. Unless you do tests for evidence of myopathy, you will miss it.

Dr. Specker: A recent paper in the *American Journal of Clinical Nutrition* (1) showed that in the adults a PTH response occurred at 25-hydroxyvitamin D values of 30 to 35 ng/ml. Why do you think the level of PTH response was so much higher than you see in France?

Dr. Garabédian: This may be related to differences in the age of the subjects, to the nature of the PTH response (above or within normal range), or to assay methods. When comparing results of studies dealing with 25-hydroxyvitamin D levels, you first have to verify that the different assay methods used give comparable data. Unless they belong to a multicenter quality control system, such a comparison between results from different groups may be difficult.

Dr. Specker: But don't you think this is important when you are setting normative ranges or, in your case, threshold levels? If you start reporting threshold levels of 3 ng/ml, you are, as you just said, talking about a very specific assay, which might not be relevant to an assay run in Boston.

Dr. Garabédian: The assay that we use is a classical in-house chromatographic protein-binding assay and not a "very specific assay," and results obtained with this method are comparable to those obtained in the several other laboratories throughout the world belonging to the same quality control system (the 25-hydroxyvitamin D EQAS in London). As for the value of 25-hydroxyvitamin D levels as markers of vitamin D deficiency, you cannot base the diagnosis of vitamin D deficiency only on these levels. In my view, in order to say that there is vitamin D deficiency, you need a low 25-OHD, a high PTH, and, if possible, a low serum calcium. The point I wanted to make is that there seem to be many adolescents with low 25-OHD levels. Yet, they may have only low vitamin D status but not real deficiency; that is, there are no detectable pathologic consequences, long-term or short-term, of the low level of vitamin D. Below 3 ng/ml I assume there may be deficiency because in the short term I can already see biological signs of secondary hyperparathyroidism. But above 3 ng/ml I am not able to assure you that vitamin D deficiency is present.

Dr. Oliveri: We have recently studied a group from the southernmost part of Argentina, and a high percentage of healthy children and adolescents had very low levels of 25-hydroxyvitamin D in winter and increased PTH levels. We did bone mineral density measurements at the distal radius and found no difference between that group and a control group of similar age and sex from Buenos Aires, who had adequate levels of 25-hydroxyvitamin D in winter.

Dr. Garabédian: Unless it is very severe, vitamin D deficiency may well not affect bone unless there is coexisting calcium deficiency, protein deficiency, or whatever. In order to find a difference in bone mass, you may need to separate the children according to their 25-OHD levels within the same population. It is not sufficient to compare one group with a mean level of 10 ng/ml with another group with a mean level of 5 ng/ml in a different population. It would be better to select the children with 25-OHD levels below 3 ng/ml in your southern population and compare those with the remainder, for example.

Dr. Pettifor: Your data can be interpreted in two ways: one is to say that we needn't worry about low levels of vitamin D in Europe at all; the other is to say that we should worry if there is a 25-OHD of less than 3 ng/ml because this represents possible vitamin D deficiency. My concern is from a public health point of view. If one says that the vast majority of the population have a 25-OHD level greater than 3 ng/ml, and therefore you needn't worry about vitamin D fortification or supplementation, you may well run into problems. I think it would be better to use the figure of 10 or 12 ng/ml that you used for neonates and old people as being an indicator of marginal vitamin D status. If your calcium intake falls or is relatively low in these circumstances, you may well run into clinical vitamin D deficiency.

Dr. Garabédian: I think that what we have to do now is to take the population of children with 25-OHD between 3 and 10 ng/ml and put them on a no-milk and no-milk-products diet for 5 days to see if they are able to increase their 1,25-$(OH)_2D$ to adapt to their low-calcium diet. That is the only way to tell whether there is a potential problem.

Dr. Pettifor: I think 5 days may be too short because, if you put them on a low-calcium diet, you are going to increase 1,25-$(OH)_2D$ and reduce the 25-OHD levels. So you are increasing the rapidity of development of vitamin D deficiency, but you may not see that within the 5 days of your calcium deprivation.

Dr. Garabédian: A preliminary prospective study of eight children suggests that a 5-day dietary calcium restriction is sufficient to detect a marked increase in the serum 1,25-$(OH)_2D$ levels of children with no vitamin D deficiency (mean values: 45 pg/ml on day 0 and 74 pg/ml on day 5) (2). Moreover, if the calcium deprivation lasts longer, it may completely deplete the vitamin D pool.

Dr. Pettifor: There is a risk of depleting your vitamin D pool if you reduce your calcium intake.

Dr. Garabédian: That is why I would confine the low calcium intake to 5 days, so as not to deplete the pool.

Dr. Haschke: My concern is with your interpretation of the RDA. You measured calcium intake and compared it with the RDA value, and you found that 66% of French adolescent girls had intakes below the RDA. Do you interpret this as meaning that these intakes are inadequate?

Dr. Garabédian: No, I just said it was below the recommended reference.

Dr. Haschke: This is a misinterpretation of the RDA values. The RDA value is the 95th centile of the calcium intake of a healthy reference population, and 95% of the population therefore have values below that figure and are healthy. The European Union has now focused on this because it is very often interpreted in the way you have done. When an intake is below the RDA, there could be a problem. The RDAs are not produced for this kind of comparison. We now have a new value, first proposed by the United Kingdom and now taken up by the European Union: the lower population threshold level. This could be used for your comparison instead of the RDA.

Dr. Garabédian: I was not speaking about RDAs. I just wanted to show you that there may be some difference in the children taking more than 1 g of calcium per day and those taking less than 1 g of calcium per day. Not all the children taking less than 1 g have altered bone mineralization: only about 20% in our population. What I am saying is that the risk of having an alteration in apparent bone mineral density is less evident in children who consume more than 1 g of calcium per day, and I pointed out that 1 g of calcium per day is the recommended dietary allowance.

Dr. Prentice: Are we now setting vitamin D requirements in terms of PTH levels? If that is the case, how do we then interpret data like ours in The Gambia, where the women, both postmenopausally and premenopausally, have raised parathyroid hormone levels but their 25-OHD status would not traditionally give rise to concern. Do you think that we should be looking at PTH levels on a population basis rather than 25-OHD to set vitamin D requirements?

Dr. Garabédian: I think you have to look at both. If PTH levels are increased but the 25-OHD levels are apparently in the sufficient range, then it may have nothing to do with vitamin D; but if it is associated with very low levels of the 25-OHD, then it is likely that the two things are linked.

Dr. Tsang: With regard to the issue of PTH, I should hope that we would not be using PTH as an indicator of vitamin D deficiency. I have always found PTH concentrations to be the most variable of all the things that we do measure, and I would be hesitant to rely on a fairly variable response to define a condition. I would be more in favor of Dr. Pettifor s view that from a public health viewpoint a 25-OHD values of 10 or 12 ng/ml is more useful. This value has been a remarkably constant lower limit across many studies. We don't need to use the term vitamin D deficiency but simply say that they are borderline.

Dr. Garabédian: What I was saying is that the adolescent population is very different from the adult population or the younger child population, in the sense that there is a greater incidence of low levels in the adolescent population. The distribution I showed is very specific to adolescents. Work published in Belgium shows the same thing: there are large numbers of adolescents with low levels of 25-OHD (3). So this is not a difference between countries; it is a difference specifically related to adolescents. Now the question is, do these adolescents with low levels of 25-OHD have vitamin D deficiency? If we say they should have 25-OHD values of 10 or 12 ng/ml, that means that 40% of French adolescents are vitamin D deficient. However, on the basis of PTH values, only about 6% of the population appear to have a degree of vitamin D deficiency.

Dr. Tsang: I have trouble using a response marker as a definition of disease.

Dr. Schofer: I am interested in your group of adolescents with very low 25-OHD levels and raised PTH. Do you have any follow-up data on these? If you again found very low vitamin D levels and increased PTH on follow-up 3 or 4 months later, would you recommend treatment, even in the absence of clinical signs.

Dr. Garabédian: We do not have sufficient follow up data yet, but you are right, our findings ask the question of the prevention of vitamin D deficiency during winter–spring, at least in adolescents who appear to be the more at risk, that is, those at pubertal stages IV and V. We performed a very preliminary double-blind interventional study in nine adolescents to analyze the biological effects of one oral dose of 2.5 mg of vitamin D_3 and obtained data that suggest that this supplementation does not induce significant vitamin D overload (4). We are right now doing a double-blind prospective follow-up of adolescents from October to May, receiving or not receiving intermittent oral doses of 2.5 mg of vitamin D_3 every 3 months, in order to analyze the biological effects of this supplementation on a larger scale.

Dr. Schofer: Did you look at alkaline phosphatase levels in those children?

Dr. Garabédian: Although an elevation of the serum alkaline phosphatase activity is the rule in children with overt vitamin D deficiency, we have been unable so far to find a relationship between alkaline phosphatase activities and 25-hydroxyvitamin D levels in healthy children, whether or not presenting with biological signs of subclinical vitamin D deficiency. But there is a problem with alkaline phosphatase during adolescence because of its wide variations at that time.

REFERENCES

1. Dawson-Hughes B, Harris SS, Dallal GE. Plasma calcidiol, season, and serum parathyroid hormone concentrations in healthy elderly men and women. *Am J Clin Nutr* 1993; 65: 67–71.
2. Belon C, Dumas R, Tau C, Sabatier R, Bourdeau A, Garabédian M. Dysrégulation du 1,25-(OH)2D plasmatique au cours d'une restriction calcique chez des enfants hypercalciuriques. *Arch Fr Pediatr* 1992; 49: 519–524.
3. Vainsel M. Facteurs influençant le capital osseux de la vie foetale à l'adolescence. *Tempo Méd.* 1994; 147: 9–16.
4. Zeghoud F, Delaveyne R, Rehel P, Chalas J, Garabédian M, Odièvre M. Vitamin D and pubertal maturation. Interest and tolerance of vitamin D supplementation during the winter (in French). *Arch Pediatr* 1995; 2: 221–226.

Nutrition and Bone Development, edited by
Jean-Philippe Bonjour and Reginald C. Tsang,
Nestlé Nutrition Workshop Series, Vol. 41, Nestec Ltd.,
Vevey/Lippincott–Raven Publishers,
Philadelphia © 1999.

Calcium and Bone Growth

Jean-Philippe Bonjour, Serge Ferrari, Daniel Slosman,
and René Rizzoli

Division of Bone Diseases (formerly Division of Clinical Pathophysiology), WHO Collaborating Center for Osteoporosis and Bone Diseases, Department of Internal Medicine, University Hospital, 1211 Geneva 14, Switzerland

Over the last 10 years much has been published on the relationship between calcium intake and bone mass acquisition during childhood and adolescence. Among observational—that is, noninterventional—studies, some but not all suggest that increasing the calcium intake promotes greater bone mass gain and thereby a higher peak bone mass [reviewed by Bonjour and Rizzoli (1)]. Obviously, only prospective interventional studies can determine to what extent calcium supplementation can influence bone mass growth and, in the case of a positive response, investigate how such an intervention may interfere with the processes of bone formation and resorption. Only a few prospective randomized, double-blind, placebo-controlled intervention trials have examined the effects of calcium supplements in children and adolescents (2–5). Overall they indicate that calcium supplementation can increase bone mass gain, although the magnitude of the effect appears to be highly variable, being affected by the skeletal sites examined and the stage of pubertal maturation at the time of the intervention (2–5). Other factors may influence the response to calcium supplementation. It is possible that the type of response observed at various skeletal sites may also depend on the chemical composition of the calcium salt. As described below, our own recent prospective randomized, double-blind, placebo-controlled study in prepubertal girls (6) indicates that spontaneous calcium intake is important in determining the magnitude of the response. It also suggests that the calcium effect could be modulated by an interaction with the vitamin D receptor genotype (7).

The positive effects of calcium supplementation have so far been ascribed to a reduction in bone remodeling. In two of the studies cited above, the positive effect of calcium given as either citrate malate or carbonate salts on bone mass was not associated with a significant change in either the scanned bone area (a reliable estimate of bone size) or standing height (3,5). Furthermore, in one study the plasma concentration of osteocalcin, a biochemical marker of bone remodeling in adults, was significantly reduced in calcium-supplemented subjects, suggesting an inhibition of bone remodeling (3). This interpretation is in keeping with the currently favored mechanism for the inhibitory effect of calcium on age-related bone loss. In elderly people, the calcium effect on bone remodeling is usually ascribed to inhibition of secretion of parathyroid hormone (PTH), plasma concentrations of which tend to increase with aging. Whether in healthy children lowering the plasma level of PTH from normal to low values is central to the calcium-induced inhibition of bone remodeling remains to be determined.

In addition to this inhibitory effect on bone remodeling, the possibility that milk calcium salt may positively influence bone modeling and longitudinal growth has been suspected for several decades (8–10). In those earlier studies it was not possible to discriminate between the effects of calcium and those of milk proteins or of energy. The effects of socioeconomic factors, which markedly influence nutrient intakes, on the physical growth of children in developing countries have been and continue to be well documented (11,12). However, observations made in both the United Kingdom and Japan indicated that under these circumstances the increase in calcium intake is much greater than that of protein or energy. Thus, it has been suggested that calcium *per se* may play a role in the well-known growth-promoting effect of milk by positively affecting skeletal modeling as well as by its inhibitory effect on remodeling.

The relationship between calcium intake and bone growth remains a fundamental issue because the reason cross-cultural variation in the prevalence of osteoporotic fracture is poorly related to calcium consumption is still not understood (13). It is well known that environmental factors strongly influence body size. Adjustment of the bone size growth in relation to the availability of dietary calcium may represent a key adaptive process in human evolution.

Anthropologic observations suggested that changes in nutritional status could explain the change in body size estimated from skeletal remains (14–16). A decrease in physical size during the early stages of animal domestication has been attributed to a necessary adaptation to an insufficient diet. Nickens (14) considered that there was a geographic and temporal differentiation in stature and, based on the examination of skeletal data available in Mexico, proposed the following hypothesis:

> . . . man's body size is reduced as a result of a shift from a hunting and gathering to an intensive agricultural way of life. It can be further posited that as man learns to cope with a diet lacking the necessary nutritive requirements—carbohydrates, lipids, amino acids (ingested as protein), vitamins and minerals—his body size will again increase. A similar occurrence is seen in the physical size of domesticated animals. Finally, a relationship between the average size of a population in Mesoamerica and the carrying capacity of its environment (expressed as mode of subsistence) is seen as being biologically adaptive.

In a more recent review, Eaton and Nelson (16) developed a provocative hypothesis on the secular trend in height in relation to calcium intake. Part of their argument is as follows:

> The earliest human species, *Homo habilis,* appears to have been appreciably shorter than we are at present, but by 1.5 million years their successors, *Homo erectus,* had become as tall as contemporary humans. Thereafter, as far as is now known, height remained relatively constant, and in the late Paleolithic era (30,000–20,000 years ago)

> Eurasian Cro-Magnon men averaged 177.2 cm, and women 165.7 cm. Shortly thereafter, in the Mesolithic period (20,000–10,000 years ago), average height began to decline, reaching a nadir 5.0–15.2 cm below prior values in the Bronze age (about 2,000 BC). In the Americas there was an analogous but later decline as well. In Eurasia height reduction began as big-game hunting shifted to what has been called broad-spectrum hunting and gathering (probably because large game animals became scarce while human population density was increasing). This phase of human evolutionary experience immediately preceded and was probably causally related to the Neolithic Revolution during which agriculture became established in the Old World beginning about 10,000 years ago. Thereafter, several factors operated jointly to accelerate the diminution in human-stature. These included a general decrease in dietary protein, increased frequency of nutritional stress (i.e., periodic food shortages up to and including famine), more exposure to epidemic infectious diseases, and the emergence of cereal grains as dietary staples. Before about 20,000 years ago cereal grains were infrequently used by humans, but for most people living after the adoption of agriculture they provided a major proportion of the diet. Grains, however, are a poor source of calcium for several reasons: they contain much less calcium than do uncultivated vegetable foods; some (especially wheat) contain phytate, which avidly binds calcium *in vitro* and which may reduce its absorption from the human intestinal tract; and their proportions of calcium and phosphorus are highly disadvantageous. Uncultivated plant foods generally provide more calcium than phosphorus, but grains have 10 times more phosphorus than calcium. The relative importance of these factors—less protein, more infection, more nutritional stress, and less calcium—in reducing human height after the beginning of agriculture is currently unclear, but availability of dietary calcium was almost certainly a contributory influence.

Thus, these considerations, based on anthropological investigations (14–16), suggest that fluctuations in the availability of dietary calcium may have played a role in the secular variations in height, which obviously is directly dependent on the longitudinal growth of the bones.

Animal experiments also suggest that calcium may be a limiting nutrient in growth. Rat experiments indicated that calcium could affect not only bone resorption through its impact on PTH secretion but also bone formation by a PTH-independent mechanism. Earlier histomorphometric studies in thyroparathyroidectomized (TPTX) rats showed that the decrease in bone formation, as assessed by measuring a reduction in both matrix and mineral deposition rates, can be corrected by increasing the intake of calcium and thereby its extracellular concentration (17). Calcium balance and kinetics studies in TPTX rats receiving a constant infusion of PTH also indicated that bone formation was dependent on calcium intake and on the resulting intestinal absorption and extracellular concentration of calcium (18). More recently we also observed that calcium and calciotropic hormones such as PTH and 1,25-dihydroxyvitamin D could affect, at least in some well-defined experimental conditions, the hepatic production of insulin-like growth factor 1 (IGF-1) (19), a factor that exerts positive effects on phosphate economy and bone mass growth (20–22).

Calcium has been shown to control the proliferation of various nontumorigenic cells *in vitro* and *in vivo* (23,24). In osteoblastic MC3T3E1 cells, more recent *in vitro* experiments showed that an increase in extracellular calcium caused a stimulation of DNA synthesis and cell proliferation (25). Calcium could react with a G-protein-coupled cation-sensing mechanism (26), which may be related to the recently cloned parathyroid calcium receptor (27). Evidence has been obtained indicating that the stimulatory effect of calcium observed *in vitro* on osteoblastic cells may be mediated by an increase in the production and secretion of IGF-1 (28). *In vivo,* it is possible that calcium may either directly or indirectly—through a cascade of events involving calciotropic hormones and growth factors—stimulate longitudinal growth by favoring the proliferation rather than the differentiation of epiphyseal chondrocytes. This calcium effect could be mediated by an interaction with PTH-related protein (PTHrP), which plays an important role in the rate of cartilage differentiation at the level of the epiphyseal plate (29).

STUDIES IN CHILDREN AND ADOLESCENTS

Observational Studies

Our first noninterventional studies in children and adolescents (30,31) allowed us to examine cross-sectionally and then longitudinally the relationships between skeletal growth and some putative determinants of peak bone mass, such as pubertal maturation, nutrition, physical exercise, and genetics [reviewed by Bonjour and Rizzoli (1)]. The nutrient intake was assessed by two 5-day diaries in about 200 female and male subjects aged 9 to 19 years (32). The tight relationship found between the energy intake and the number of weekly hours spent in physical activity provides an estimate of the good reliability of the diary method used in this study. As expected, the calcium intake was significantly greater in boys than in girls, at any pubertal stage. In the whole cohort, which included subjects of both sexes from Tanner stage P1 to P5, the gain in bone mass as assessed by dual-energy x-ray absorptiometry (DXA) in determining the areal bone mineral density or content at spinal and femoral levels was not statistically significant after adjustment for sex, age, or pubertal stage. The same negative results were obtained with the P2-to-P4 subgroup. However, a positive relationship between calcium intake and bone mass accrual was obtained in the prepubertal (P1) boys and girls. At the lumbar spine (L2 to L4) level of P1 subjects, the association was significant not only for the gain in bone mineral content and bone mineral density but also for the gain in bone area, suggesting a positive effect on bone size. Interestingly, the pattern of the relationship between calcium and the gain in standing height was similar to that of the L2 to L4 bone mineral content, bone mineral density, and area—that is, it was significant in P1 but not in the whole cohort or in the P2 to P4 subjects.

Thus, these observational studies suggested that calcium supplementation could be particularly effective before puberty for stimulating bone mass gain. Furthermore, in prepubertal children, the calcium effect on bone mass could be mediated, at least in part, by an increase in bone size and longitudinal growth.

Interventional Studies

Very recently we examined the effects of calcium supplements on bone mass accrual at various sites of the skeleton in prepubertal girls. With the objective of increasing calcium intake at population level, we used a set of calcium-enriched foods rather than a single pharmaceutical calcium supplement (6).

In a double-blind, placebo-controlled study, 149 healthy prepubertal girls aged 7.9 $\pm$ 0.1 years (mean $\pm$ SEM, range 7 to 9 years) were randomly allocated to receive on a daily basis one set of two food products containing or not containing (placebo) 850 mg of milk-extracted calcium for 1 year. The food products contained the same amount of energy and protein; bone mineral content, bone mineral density, and bone size were determined by dual-energy x-ray absorptiometry after 1 and 2 years.

The two groups were similar at baseline in terms of age, statural height, body weight, bone mineral density and content at all sites, and spontaneous calcium intake. Among the girls who completed the 12-month intervention study (active treatment cohort, $n = 108$), bone mineral density gains at radial (metaphysis and diaphysis) and femoral sites (neck, trochanter, and diaphysis) but not at the lumbar spine level were 7 to 12 mg/cm^2 per year greater in the calcium-supplemented group ($n = 55$) than in the placebo group ($n = 53$). This difference was significant. The difference in bone mineral density gains between the calcium-supplemented and placebo groups was greater in girls with a spontaneous calcium intake below the median of 880 mg/day (mean bone mineral density gain of the six sites: 30 $\pm$ 3 versus 19 $\pm$ 3 mg/cm^2 per year, $p = 0.01$, and 28 $\pm$ 2 versus 23 $\pm$ 2, $p < 0.1$, in spontaneously low and high calcium consumers, respectively). The increase in mean bone mineral density at the six sites in the low calcium consumers was accompanied by significantly greater gains in both mean bone mineral content and bone area ($p < 0.05$). Examination of the changes in scanned bone area and in standing height suggests that calcium supplementation, as provided in our study, could affect bone modeling. Indeed, in the group of spontaneously low calcium consumers, calcium-enriched foods enhanced the gain of both mean scanned bone area and stature to the level achieved by the spontaneously high calcium consumers. Morphometric analysis of the changes observed in lumbar spine and femoral diaphysis suggests that calcium could enhance both the longitudinal and cross-sectional growth of the bones. Part of the difference in bone mass and bone size was still present 1 year after the end of the intervention study. Thus, this study (6) suggests that milk calcium supplementation may affect not only the remodeling but also the modeling of the skeleton.

The tested foods were enriched with calcium from milk extract and thus contained phosphate. The mean increase in phosphorus intake on the active supplement was 386 mg/day as compared to 870 mg/day for calcium. On the basis of previous dietary diary records in prepubertal girls of that age (32), we estimate that the enriched foods increased the intake of phosphorus by 30% to 35%, as compared to a 100% increase for calcium. To what extent this increase in the phosphorus intake played a contributing role in the stimulation of bone mass accrual reported in this study remains to be determined. It is also possible that the ratio of calcium to phosphate present in the milk extract could be particularly effective at enhancing the growth factors involved in bone modeling.

In these prepubertal girls, we also observed a statistically significant association between polymorphisms of the vitamin D receptor (VDR) gene and the baseline values of both spinal and femoral bone mineral density (7). Note that we did not find this association in a cohort of premenopausal women, the large majority of whom were the mothers of these prepubertal girls. Interestingly, in the girls who had the VDR genotype "BB," calcium supplementation appeared to increase the bone mass gain up to the level of those having the "bb" VDR genotype (7). Such a differential response suggests an interaction among the VDR genotype, calcium metabolism, and bone mass accrual. These results could explain discrepancies relating to the association between VDR genotype and bone mass in adult subjects because environmental factors such as dietary calcium could abolish genetic differences in peak bone mass potential. Whether, in response to calcium supplementation, the VDR genotype influences bone mass accrual by a greater effect on the modeling process than on the remodeling process remains to be determined.

CONCLUSIONS

The possibility that calcium might be a limiting factor in growth has been suspected for many years, but to our knowledge this has never been adequately tested. The relationship between calcium intake and bone growth remains a fundamental issue because we still do not understand the reasons why cross-cultural variations in the prevalence of osteoporotic fracture are poorly related to calcium consumption. Environmental factors strongly influence body size, explaining the secular trend in height observed in several ethnic groups. Both *in vitro* and *in vivo* experiments have clearly identified calcium as a stimulator of bone formation. It is conceivable that survival of mammalian species in a low-calcium environment requires the operation of several adaptive mechanisms that would not only increase intestinal absorptive and renal reabsorptive capacity to transport calcium toward the extracellular compartment but also curb the demand for calcium by reducing bone growth. This latter adaptive mechanism would contribute to the avoidance of osteopenia and osteoporosis in the presence of a low-calcium environment. The study on bone mass gain we have just completed in prepubertal girls (6) suggests that milk-extracted calcium salt may not only increase bone mass by reducing bone resorption but also enhance the longitudinal growth of the lumbar spine and increase the external cross-sectional diameter of the long bones. So far, there has been no randomized, placebo-controlled trial with the primary objective of testing the effect of calcium on bone growth at several levels of the skeleton and on stature. Further studies should therefore be aimed at testing the hypothesis that calcium affects the longitudinal and transverse sizes of bones and thereby influences not only bone mass accrual but also linear growth of children.

REFERENCES

1. Bonjour JP, Rizzoli R. Bone acquisition in adolescence. In: Marcus R, Feldman D, Kelsey J, eds. *Osteoporosis.* San Diego: Academic Press, 1996: 465–476.

2. Matkovic V, Fontana D, Tominac C, Goel P, Chesnut CH. Factors that influence peak bone mass formation: a study of calcium balance and the inheritance of bone mass in adolescent females. *Am J Clin Nutr* 1990; 52: 878–888.
3. Johnston CC, Miller JZ, Slemenda CW, *et al.* Calcium supplementation and increases in bone mineral density in children. *N Engl J Med* 1992; 327: 82–87.
4. Lloyd T, Andon MB, Rollings N, *et al.* Calcium supplementation and bone mineral density in adolescent girls. *JAMA* 1993; 270: 841–844.
5. Lee WTK, Leung SSF, Wang SH, *et al.* Double-blind, controlled calcium supplementation and bone mineral accretion in children accustomed to a low-calcium diet. *Am J Clin Nutr* 1994; 60: 744–750.
6. Bonjour JP, Carrié AL, Ferrari S, *et al.* Calcium-enriched foods and bone mass growth in prepubertal girls: a randomized, double-blind, placebo-controlled trial. *J Clin Invest* 1997; 99: 1287–1294.
7. Ferrari SL, Rizzoli R, Slosman DO, Bonjour J-Ph. Do dietary calcium and age explain the controversy surrounding the relationship between bone mineral density and vitamin D receptor gene polymorphisms? *J Bone Miner Res* 1998; 13: 358–561.
8. Corry-Mann HC. *Diets for Boys During the School Age. Medical Research Council Special Report Series No 105.* London: HMSO, 1926.
9. Orr JB. Milk consumption and the growth of school children. *Lancet* 1928; i: 202–203.
10. Leighton G, Clark ML. Milk consumption and growth of school children: second preliminary report on test to Scottish Board of Health. *Lancet* 1929; i: 40–43.
11. Martorell R, Habicht JP. Growth in early childhood in developing countries. In: Falkner F, Tanner JM, eds. *Human Growth. A Comprehensive Treatise, 2nd ed.* New York: Plenum Press, 1987: 241–262.
12. Shen T, Habicht JP, Chang Y. Effect of economic reforms on child growth in urban and rural areas of China. *N Engl J Med* 1996; 335: 400–406.
13. Abelow BJ, Holford TR, Insogna KL. Cross-cultural association between dietary animal protein and hip fracture-a hypothesis. *Calcif Tissue Int* 1992; 50: 14–18.
14. Nickens PR. Stature reduction as an adaptive response to food production in Mesoamerica. *J Archaeol Sci* 1976; 3: 31–41.
15. Frayer D. Body size, weapon use, and natural selection in the European Upper Paleolithic and Mesolithic. *Am Anthropologist* 1981; 83: 57–73.
16. Eaton SB, Nelson DA. Calcium in evolutionary perspective. *Am J Clin Nutr* 1991; 54: 281S–287S.
17. Wergedal J, Stauffer M, Baylink D, Rich C. Inhibition of bone matrix formation, mineralization, and resorption in thyroparathyroidectomized rats. *J Clin Invest* 1973; 32: 1052–1058.
18. Haldimann B, Bonjour JP, Fleisch H. Role of parathyroid hormone in the regulation of main calcium fluxes in rats. *Am J Physiol* 1977; 232: E535–E541.
19. Caverzasio J, Shigematsu T, Rizzoli R, Bonjour JP. Potential role of IGF-1 in parathyroid hormone-related renal growth induced by high protein diet in uninephrectomized rats. *Kidney Int* 1995; 48: 33–38.
20. Froesch ER, Schmid C, Schwander J, Zapf J. Actions of insulin-like growth factors. *Annu Rev Physiol* 1985; 47: 443–467.
21. Caverzasio J, Bonjour JP. IGF-I, a key regulator of renal phosphate transport and 1,25-dihydroxyvitamin D_3 production during growth. *News Physiol Sci* 1991; 6: 206–210.
22. Ammann P, Rizzoli R, Meyer JM, Slosman D, Bonjour JP. Bone density and shape as determinants of bone strength in IGF-1 and/or pamidronate-treated ovariectomized rats. *Osteoporosis Int* 1996; 6: 219–227.
23. Whitfield JF, Boynton JP, MacManus JP, Sikorsma M, Tsang BK. The regulation of cell proliferation by calcium and cyclic AMP. *Mol Cell Biochem* 1979; 27: 155–179.
24. Jobin JR, Bonjour JP. Compensatory renal growth: modulation by calcium, PTH and 1,25-$(OH)_2D_3$. *Kidney Int* 1986; 29: 1124–1130.
25. Kanatani M, Sugimoto T, Fukase M, Fujita T. Effect of elevated extracellular calcium on the proliferation of osteoblastic MC3T3-E1 cells: its direct and indirect effects via monocytes. *Biochem Biophys Res Commun* 1991; 181: 1425–1430.
26. Quarles LD, Hartle JE II, Middleton JP, Zhang J, Athur JM, Raymond JR. Aluminum-induced DNA synthesis in osteoblasts: mediation by a G-protein coupled cation sensing mechanism. *J Cell Biochem* 1994; 56: 106–117.
27. Brown EM, Gamba G, Ricardi D, *et al.* Cloning, expression, and characterization of a G-protein-coupled bovine parathyroid Ca^{2+} receptor. *Nature* 1993; 366: 575–580.
28. Sugimoto T, Kanatani M, Kano J, *et al.* IGF-I mediates the stimulatory effect of high calcium concentration on osteoblastic cell proliferation. *Am J Physiol* 1994; 266: E709–E716.

29. Vortkamp A, Lee K, Lanske B, Segre GV, Kronenberg HM, Tabin CJ. Regulation of rate of cartilage differentiation by Indian Hedgehog and PTH-related protein. *Science* 1996; 273: 613–622.
30. Bonjour JP, Theintz G, Buchs B, Slosman D, Rizzoli R. Critical years and stages of puberty for spinal and femoral bone mass accumulation during adolescence. *J Clin Endocrinol Metab* 1991; 73: 555–563.
31. Theintz G, Buchs B, Rizzoli R, *et al.* Longitudinal monitoring of bone mass accumulation in healthy adolescents: evidence for a marked reduction after 16 years of age at the levels of lumbar spine and femoral neck in female subjects. *J Clin Endocrinol Metab* 1992; 75: 1060–1065.
32. Clavien H, Theintz G, Rizzoli R, Bonjour JP. Does puberty alter dietary habit in adolescents living in a western society? *J Adolesc Health* 1996; 19: 68–75.

DISCUSSION

Dr. Specker: Because these girls were enrolled around age 9, could they have gone into puberty through the follow-up period? That could lead to increased variability 3 years on and may be why you don't see an effect. Did you control for pubertal status at 3 years?

Dr. Bonjour: All the girls remained prepubertal during the intervention period, so for the second measurement they were definitely prepubertal. In the follow-up a few girls were at stage P2, so this increased the variability. If I were to do the study again, I would choose girls who would definitely still be prepubertal after 3 years. This is what we would like to do now in boys, starting at the age of 7 so that we are sure that we will have at least 3 or 4 years before a certain percentage enter puberty.

Dr. Prentice: I wonder to what extent you really feel convinced that what you are seeing is a calcium effect. The other calcium supplementation studies that have been reported with calcium carbonate and calcium citrate malate do not show the same anabolic effects on bone as you have seen, and in the old literature it was milk supplementation that seemed to have effects on stature and so forth in developing countries. I wonder whether there is something else in your supplement, the phosphate or some other component of milk, that may be having these effects, and not calcium itself.

Dr. Bonjour: The calcium supplementation was a milk extract, so the salt was calcium phosphate mainly. We doubled the mean calcium of these girls. For phosphate we increased the basal intake by 30%, so it is less remarkable, but it could be that calcium phosphate is particularly active in bone modeling as compared to other calcium salts.

Dr. Bachrach: I wonder how you explain the differences between your results and those of Lee in Hong Kong (1), where the girls were of similar age and where, because of the background low dietary calcium intake in that Hong Kong population, the supplement really did produce a dramatic increase in calcium intake. Even so the effects in that study were short-lived.

Dr. Bonjour: Perhaps it is calcium phosphate that really influences the modeling; or maybe the effect of calcium is modulated by other factors in the diet such as the protein intake.

Dr. Seeman: In the children with a spontaneously high calcium intake, was the height different at the onset of the study?

Dr. Bonjour: Yes, but don't try to make me say that this was caused by calcium alone! It is clear that they also had an increase in protein and energy intakes. Whether that was because they were growing faster than the others we don't know. You cannot draw conclusions from this kind of observational study that could enable you to relate one nutrient causally to anthropometric or bone differences.

Dr. Seeman: The other question I have is that you have looked at the data dichotomously, control versus case. But what if you looked across the whole sample, do you see a dose response? Have you looked at the changes in the bone density in the whole sample versus some index of total calcium intake during the study, for example?

Dr. Bonjour: When we analyzed the intention to treat a cohort, we had a certain number of girls who dropped out of the study. We assessed the cumulative amount of calcium taken by these girls and obtained a dose response. This dose response is also reflected by the fact that the calcium-supplemented girls of the intention-to-treat group gained less than the active cohort.

Dr. Tsang: Could you clarify the placebo group? What really were they taking?

Dr. Bonjour: The placebo was a piece of chocolate looking exactly like the active supplement and tasting like it, but with no calcium added. The lipids and proteins were the same, but of course you cannot give calcium unless as a salt, so it was given calcium phosphate.

Dr. Pettifor: What happened to the basal calcium intake in the group that were not getting the calcium supplement? Did their calcium intakes drop because they were no longer taking dairy products and were eating the relatively calcium-free chocolate and the relatively calcium-free whatever else was in the supplement that you were giving?

Dr. Bonjour: The baseline spontaneous calcium intake at the beginning, at 6 months, at 12 months, and at 24 months remained pretty constant. There was no evidence for a reduction in the spontaneous calcium intake up to the end of the intervention study and after that.

Dr. Haschke: The results that were obtained 1 year after discontinuation of the supplement showed that there were still small differences in height velocity and bone mineral content, but neither difference was significant. Is that right?

Dr. Bonjour: Yes.

Dr. Haschke: Have you done analyses in the subgroups as well?

Dr. Bonjour: The study was not designed to have an analysis of this follow-up period, so it is not a perfect study in that respect. It is clear we should have started with younger girls or younger boys, where we could be sure that none of them would enter puberty before the end of the study because the variability increases so much under those circumstances. Also, by the end of the study we had only 24 or 25 subjects in each group, and we needed about 50 in each group to see a 5% difference. So the statistical power was much reduced. However, at some sites such as the lumbar spine, the change in the height was maintained and remained statistically significant in spite of the small numbers, so I believe this was not just a kind of statistical artifact.

Dr. Eisman: I was interested in your change in cortical area. Was this because the bones were wider in diameter or because the cortex itself was thicker?

Dr. Bonjour: We still have some difficulty with detecting the inner cortical edge on the DXA measurement, so I can't say for sure.

Dr. Seeman: I think metacarpal morphometry is a very simple and precise way of looking at cortical thickness.

Dr. Bonjour: But we have no x-rays of these girls. The ethics committee in Geneva is very strict, and if x-rays or blood samples are proposed there is a real risk that the study will never be accepted. That is why we were totally noninvasive.

REFERENCE

1. Lee WTK, Leung SSF, Leung DMY, Cheng JCY. A follow-up study on the effects of calcium-supplement withdrawal and puberty on bone acquisition of children. *Am J Clin Nutr* 1996; 64: 71–77.

Nutrition and Bone Development, edited by
Jean-Philippe Bonjour and Reginald C. Tsang,
Nestlé Nutrition Workshop Series, Vol. 41, Nestec Ltd.,
Vevey/Lippincott–Raven Publishers,
Philadelphia © 1999.

Calcium Deficiency and Impaired Bone Mass Acquisition

John M. Pettifor

MRC Mineral Metabolism Research Unit, Department of Paediatrics, University of the Witwatersrand and Baragwanath Hospital, Johannesburg 2013, South Africa

Over the past several decades, considerable attention has been paid to the role of habitual dietary calcium intakes in determining bone mass, not only in the adult but also during the period of rapid bone growth that occurs during adolescence (1,2). The impetus for this interest has been prompted by the growing concern over the high prevalence of fractures associated with postmenopausal and senile osteoporosis, which has reached epidemic proportions in many developed countries (3) and is consuming an increasing proportion of the national health expenditure in these countries.

There is general agreement that the dietary calcium intake together with a number of other environmental factors plays a permissive role in determining peak bone mass and the rate of bone loss during the perimenopausal and postmenopausal years (1). In another chapter in this volume, Bonjour discusses the effect of dietary calcium on bone mass during childhood and adolescence at levels generally found in countries in the developed world. In this chapter, I discuss the effect of pathologically low dietary calcium intakes on appendicular bone mass.

DIETARY CALCIUM DEFICIENCY

Since our group's description of rickets and bone deformities caused by dietary calcium deficiency in rural black children in South Africa some 15 years ago (4–6), a number of other researchers have reported their findings on similar children from other parts of Africa (7–9). The clinical and biochemical presentations of the disease in the different reports are very similar: typically, the children are older than those suspected of having vitamin D deficiency, lower limb deformities predominate, and dietary calcium intakes are estimated to be approximately 150 to 200 mg/day. Biochemically, serum calcium values are low or low normal; serum phosphorus concentrations are very variable, with both low and high values being reported; serum alkaline phosphatase values are raised; and serum 25-hydroxyvitamin D concentrations are within the normal range, although they may be lower than those of control children living in the same area. As would be expected in a situation of calcium deprivation, serum parathyroid hormone values are increased, and 1,25-dihydroxyvitamin D concentrations are either normal or high. The characteristic features of the diet are a lack of dairy products and a consumption of high-fiber, high-phytate staples such as maize and cassava.

Isolated cases of rickets caused by or aggravated by low dietary calcium intakes have been reported from industrialized countries (10–14). In the majority of reports, the diets had been manipulated because of gastrointestinal problems. However, the studies by Dagnelie *et al.* (13) and Rudolf *et al.* (10) highlight the risks of macrobiotic or vegetarian diets in infants. It is also believed that the high-phytate, low-calcium diet, which is common in the Asian community in the United Kingdom, plays a role in predisposing both children and adults to rickets and osteomalacia in a situation of marginal vitamin D status (15,16).

In the symptomatic child with rickets caused by dietary calcium deficiency, radiographic and histomorphometric evidence of osteopenia is a universal finding (4,17). Radiographically and on histomorphometric analysis of bone biopsies, there is an improvement in the osteomalacia and bone volume during recovery. However, as far as I am aware, there are no long-term studies of the quantitative changes in bone mass following treatment and during recovery. Thus, it is unclear whether or not the acquisition of bone during childhood or the achievement of peak bone mass is influenced by an episode of clinical rickets in a young child.

Of more relevance from a public health point of view is an evaluation of the effect of asymptomatic habitual low dietary calcium intakes during childhood on bone acquisition and peak bone mass, as a failure to achieve optimal peak bone mass during the third decade of life might lead to a greater prevalence of symptomatic osteoporosis in later life with the resultant increase in morbidity and mortality.

In a study of rural black children living in a community in which biochemical evidence of low dietary calcium intakes had been found to be common (18), we were able to show that children selected on the basis of the presence of biochemical abnormalities suggestive of altered mineral homeostasis linked to dietary calcium deficiency (low serum calcium and raised alkaline phosphatase concentrations) had significantly lower bone mineral density at the distal third of the radius than age-matched controls living in the same area (Table 1) (19). The difference in bone mineral density between the study and control groups varied between 17% and 22%. Mean calcium intakes in the study groups ranged between 199 and 229 mg/day compared with 338 and 378 mg/day in the control groups. It should be stressed that the children participating in the study were clinically well, with no stigmata of rickets or bone deformities.

Following on these initial studies, we have now measured appendicular bone mass by single-photon absorptiometry (Norland 278, Norland Corporation, Fort Atkinson, Wisconsin, USA) in a large random sample of black children between the ages of 6 and 20 years living in the same rural community and have compared the results with those obtained from a sample of school children living in a rural area in which dietary calcium deficiency rickets has not been observed. As is typical of children

TABLE 1. *Bone mineral density and calcium intakes in study and control children living in a community with a high prevalence of low dietary calcium intakes*[a]

	Age group 8–10 years		Age group 13–16 years	
	Study	Control	Study	Control
Number of subjects	15	15	13	13
Age (years)	9.3 ± 1.6	9.2 ± 1.3	14.7 ± 1.1	15.0 ± 1.2
Serum calcium (mmol/liter)	2.11 ± 0.19*	2.42 ± 0.12	2.08 ± 0.21*	2.31 ± 0.11
Alkaline phosphatase (IU/liter)	364 ± 50*	186 ± 51	500 ± 181*	214 ± 84
Bone mineral density (g/cm^2)	0.34 ± 0.10*	0.41 ± 0.06	0.42 ± 0.08*	0.54 ± 0.06
Dietary calcium intake (mg/kg body weight)	7.1 ± 3.2*	14.9 ± 8.0	5.5 ± 4.2*	8.6 ± 5.6

[a] The children were grouped into study or control groups depending on the presence or absence of low serum calcium and raised alkaline phosphatase values.
* Values significantly different from age-matched controls ($p < 0.05$).
Table modified from Eyberg et al. (19).

in developing countries, the children in both communities tended to be both underweight for age and stunted when compared to the NCHS reference ranges, but there were no consistent significant differences in the weight or height z scores between children of the same ages in the two communities (Table 2). Between 4% and 5% of the boys and girls were hypoalbuminemic (serum albumin <35 g/l).

After correction for differences in age, height, and weight by covariant analysis, both boys and girls in the study community had similar mean bone mineral content but significantly greater bone width and hence significantly lower bone mineral density than the children in the control community (Table 3). In an attempt to correct for the influence of body size on bone mass, a volumetric measure of bone density—bone mineral apparent density (BMAD)—was calculated according to the method of Katzman and co-workers (20). Unlike bone mineral content, bone width, and bone mineral density, BMAD did not correlate with age, weight, or height and remained fairly constant across the age range of the children studied. The BMAD was significantly lower in both boys and girls in the study area than in the control area (Table 3). The difference between the two areas was approximately 20% in both sexes.

Stepwise regression analysis was used to determine the interrelated effects of

TABLE 2. *Weight and height* z *scores of boys and girls in the study and control communities*

	Mean weight z score		Mean height z score	
	Control	Study	Control	Study
Males	−1.28 ± 0.63	−1.40 ± 0.55	−1.59 ± 1.11	−1.75 ± 0.99
Females	−0.79 ± 0.70	−1.09 ± 0.60	−1.04 ± 0.93	−1.50 ± 1.24

TABLE 3. *Least squares means of appendicular bone mass variables in children between the ages of 6 and 20 years in the study and control communities*

	Male		Female	
	Control	Study	Control	Study
Bone mineral content (g/cm)	0.554	0.567	0.540	0.570*
Bone width (cm)	1.074	1.221*	1.019	1.169*
Bone mineral density (g/cm^2)	0.504	0.454*	0.518	0.479*
Bone mineral apparent density (g/cm^3)	0.608	0.478*	0.656	0.523*

* Statistically significant differences between study and control children of the same sex ($p < 0.0001$).

anthropometric and biochemical variables on appendicular bone mass. As expected, weight and height were the variables accounting for the majority of the explained variance in bone mineral content, bone width, and bone mineral density in both boys and girls. Nevertheless, in children of both sexes, serum calcium contributed positively and alkaline phosphatase negatively to the explained variance in bone mineral content and bone mineral density, and serum calcium had a significant but small negative effect on bone width in boys. The BMAD in both boys and girls was directly correlated with serum calcium values ($r = 0.309$, $p < 0.0001$; and $r = 0.218$, $p < 0.001$, respectively) and inversely related to alkaline phosphatase values ($r = -0.266$, $p = 0.0002$; and $r = -0.273$, $p < 0.0001$, respectively).

Thus, these studies have documented that children living in a community in which low dietary calcium intakes are prevalent have nearly similar appendicular bone mineral content, greater bone width, lower bone mineral density, and lower BMAD than similarly nourished children in a rural community in which biochemical features of pathologically low dietary calcium intakes were not found. That the pathogenesis of the altered appendicular bone mass measurements is related to low dietary calcium intakes is supported by the finding of positive correlations of bone mineral content, bone mineral density, and BMAD with serum calcium concentrations and an inverse relationship between the same bone mass variables and serum alkaline phosphatase values.

It might be argued that the alterations in bone mass measurements are a consequence of generalized undernutrition, which was prevalent in both the study and control populations, rather than dietary calcium deficiency. Against this hypothesis are, first, the lack of a consistent difference in mean weight or height z scores between children from the two communities, and second, the finding of a greater bone width in the study children than in the control children. If generalized malnutrition were responsible for the differences in bone mass measurements, bone width would be expected to be reduced and not increased, as found in the study population (21). Further, protein-energy malnutrition is associated with a fall in both serum total calcium and alkaline phosphatase values. Thus, if malnutrition were responsible for the lower bone density measurements, bone mineral content, bone mineral density, and BMAD should have been positively related to both serum calcium and alkaline phosphatase and not positively related to serum calcium but inversely related to alkaline phosphatase, as was found in the study. The combination of these latter relationships points strongly to the pathogenesis being related to altered bone and mineral homeostasis, possibly as a consequence of an inadequate calcium supply to meet the needs of the growing skeleton.

The mechanisms by which asymptomatic dietary calcium deficiency causes a decrease in bone mass are unclear. Symptomatic children have increased serum parathyroid hormone and 1,25-dihydroxyvitamin D concentrations (5), which would increase bone turnover and thus the remodeling space. Further, symptomatic children have radiologic rickets and a marked increase in the extent and volume of osteoid at the trabecular bone surfaces (17). Thus, osteopenia and a reduction in bone mineral content and bone density would be expected. In asymptomatic children, the finding of a high prevalence of hypocalcemia and raised alkaline phosphatase concentrations suggests that similar mechanisms may be operating but at a reduced level. Support for this hypothesis is provided by a study conducted on a heterogeneous group of black teenagers being investigated for genu valgum or genu varum (22). Although the children had no radiologic features of rickets, bone histology revealed osteomalacia in 20% and features of increased bone turnover or hyperparathyroidism in another 34%. The remaining patients had osteopenia with normal or decreased bone turnover. Serum calcium values were inversely related to features of osteomalacia, and 1,25-dihydroxyvitamin D levels were positively correlated to the degree of eroded surfaces and osteoid thickness and volume.

Studies of children in other communities of the world where low dietary calcium intakes are common have also documented low appendicular bone mass. In a study of 5-year-old Chinese children (23), those living in Jiangmen, China (mean calcium intake 244 mg/day) had a 14% lower appendicular bone mineral content and lower bone mineral density than similar-aged children living in Hong Kong (mean calcium intake 542 mg/day). In Africa, a study of young Gambian children aged less than 36 months found reduced bone mineral content at the radius compared to British children of the same age even after adjustment for differences in body size and weight (24). The authors postulate that differences in calcium intake might explain the residual differences found.

In these and other studies of the influence of dietary calcium intakes on bone mass in children, it is difficult to separate the role of dietary calcium content from other environmental factors such a differences in growth rates, other nutrient intakes, physical activity, infection rates, and vitamin D status. Nevertheless, it would be surprising if calcium intakes did not influence bone mass at the lower extreme of intake, as adaptation to a low intake by improving intestinal calcium absorption and reducing urinary calcium loss is finite and limited and may not be adequate to ensure the necessary positive balance to maintain mineralization of the growing skeleton.

Whether these reported effects of low dietary calcium intakes in children are of any clinical consequence in the long term is unclear. Although data on fracture rates in the adult population living in the community in which the studies on children were performed are not available, fracture rates in black adults in South Africa are among the lowest in the world (25,26). Calcium intakes in South African black adults have been estimated to range between 175 and 475 mg/day (27), which are similar to those reported in the children living in the community in which biochemical evidence of dietary calcium deficiency was found. Despite low calcium intakes in the adult black population, Walker and co-workers, in a number of studies conducted over 25 years ago (27–29), were unable to show major differences in metacarpal indices of bone mass between black and white South African adults. They concluded that there was little or no evidence to show that the habitually low calcium intakes of black South Africans were detrimental to bone health.

In a more recent study of both appendicular and axial bone mass in premenopausal and perimenopausal black and white women (30), we found no statistical differences between the two racial groups in bone mineral density at the radial or lumbar sites (Table 4). Femoral neck bone mineral density was significantly greater in the black than in white women. From this study it was concluded that the increased femoral bone mass in black women probably reflects the effect of physical activity and possibly increased adiposity.

Irrespective of the conclusions drawn about the relationship between dietary calcium intake and bone mass, it is clear that bone mineral content is not the only determinant of fracture risk in the elderly. Aspray and co-workers (31) have found a 42% reduction in lumbar bone mineral content and a 31% reduction in bone mineral density in Gambian women over 64 years of age when compared to similarly aged British white women, yet minimal trauma fractures are almost unknown in Gambian women.

At the present time, our data on dietary calcium deficiency in black children suggest that at very low levels of intake rickets and bone deformities might result. However, the vast majority of children on low intakes are asymptomatic, even though

TABLE 4. *Bone mineral density in black and white women in South Africa*

	Premenopausal			Perimenopausal		
	Blacks	Whites	p^a	Blacks	Whites	p
Spinal bone mineral density (g/cm^2)	1.016 ± 0.118	1.042 ± 0.096	0.16	1.097 ± 0.142	1.053 ± 0.133	0.05
Femoral neck bone mineral density (g/cm^2)	1.031 ± 0.109	0.959 ± 0.107	0.0001	1.089 ± 0.108	0.963 ± 0.118	0.0001
Radial bone mineral density (g/cm^2)	0.637 ± 0.074	0.651 ± 0.068	0.24	0.663 ± 0.071	0.669 ± 0.080	0.74

[a] Significance of difference between black and white women of the same menopausal status.
Adapted from Daniels et al. (30).

they might have biochemical evidence of altered calcium and bone homeostasis and lower appendicular bone mass. It appears that there are few long-term consequences of low dietary calcium intakes during childhood, as fracture rates in the black population of South Africa are low and bone mass measurements of adult black women are similar or better than those of their white peers. However, further studies are required to assess the effect of changes in lifestyle and dietary patterns on bone mass in the urbanizing black community before conclusions can be drawn about the lack of sequelae related to low dietary intakes, as changes in protein, fiber, and other nutrient intakes might alter the adaptive response.

DIETARY CALCIUM INTAKE AND ENDEMIC FLUOROSIS IN CHILDREN

Endemic fluorosis in children has been described from several countries, in particular from India (32,33), Tanzania (34,35), China (36), and South Africa (37,38). At a previous Nestlé Nutrition Workshop (4), I presented our studies and those of others, which suggest that low dietary calcium intakes might hasten the onset and aggravate the severity of symptoms and clinical signs of endemic fluorosis in children because of the increased demands for calcium placed on the children by the increased osteoid formation.

More recently we have measured appendicular bone mass and serum calcium, phosphorus, and alkaline phosphatase concentrations in school children (between 6 and 22 years of age) living in an area with high water fluoride levels (8.8 to 9.4 ppm) and compared them to age-matched controls living in a similar environment, but with normal water fluoride concentrations (1.6 to 2.0 ppm) (R. Greeff and J.M. Pettifor, *unpublished data*). Approximately 600 children spread evenly between the sexes and over the age range were studied in each of the areas.

Clinically none of the children suffered from crippling fluorosis. However, 25% of the study group had genu valgum deformities compared to 14% in the control area. In both areas the deformities were more common in girls. Mean serum calcium values were very similar between the two groups and fell within the normal reference range, but 10% of the study group were hypocalcemic (<2.25 mmol/liter) compared to only 3% in the control group. Mean serum phosphorus and alkaline phosphatase concentrations were significantly higher in the study children than in the control children. Thirteen percent of children in the study group had alkaline phosphatase values above the upper limit of normal (400 IU/l) compared to 0.8% in the control group.

Appendicular bone mass measurements in the two groups are summarized in Table 5. Male and female subjects in the high-fluoride area had similar bone mineral content but greater bone width and thus lower bone mineral density and BMAD than children living in the control area. The finding of osteopenia of the appendicular skeleton is supported by a study from China, in which osteoporosis of the long bones was considered to be the earliest radiographic sign of skeletal fluorosis (36). The pattern of appendicular bone mass changes is very similar to that found in the

TABLE 5. *Mean values for appendicular bone mass measurements in children living in an area with high water fluoride concentrations compared to those of control children*

	Male			Female		
	Study	Control	p	Study	Control	p
Bone width (cm)	1.23 ± 0.25	1.13 ± 0.23	0.0001	1.18 ± 0.24	1.05 ± 0.21	0.0001
Bone mineral content (g/cm)	0.61 ± 0.25	0.60 ± 0.22	0.88	0.58 ± 0.21	0.58 ± 0.20	0.59
Bone mineral density (g/cm^2)	0.48 ± 0.12	0.52 ± 0.10	0.0001	0.48 ± 0.12	0.53 ± 0.11	0.001
Bone mineral apparent density (g/cm^3)	0.50 ± 0.11	0.60 ± 0.12	0.0001	0.54 ± 0.14	0.65 ± 0.13	0.0001

asymptomatic children on low dietary calcium intakes. However, unlike the findings in the dietary calcium-deficient children reported earlier in this chapter, there were no correlations between the bone mass and biochemical variables in the children living in the study area. Nevertheless, the finding of a higher prevalence of hypocalcemia and elevated alkaline phosphatase concentrations in children living in the endemic fluorosis area suggests an alteration in bone and mineral homeostasis similar to that postulated to be occurring in the children on low dietary calcium intakes. The biochemical changes are also similar but of a less severe degree to those described in children suffering from clinical symptoms related to high fluoride intakes (38). As in dietary calcium deficiency, the increased radial bone width in endemic fluorosis is thought to be a manifestation of chronic secondary hyperparathyroidism stimulating endosteal bone resorption. Raised levels of immunoreactive parathyroid hormone have been found in individuals suffering from skeletal fluorosis (39).

Dietary calcium intakes were measured in a small sample of children included in the study. Their mean intakes were similar to those of other estimates for children living in rural areas of South Africa and ranged between 190 and 319 mg/day.

Thus, it is postulated that the biochemical abnormalities and lower appendicular bone mineral density in the children living in the high-fluoride area are caused by low dietary calcium intakes that do not meet the extra demands for calcium placed on the body by the altered bone metabolism as a result of increased fluoride ingestion. This hypothesis will be confirmed only when calcium supplementation studies are conducted in children living in areas of high water fluoride concentrations.

CONCLUSIONS

We have presented data that suggest that extremely low dietary calcium intakes in black children in a number of situations result in alterations of bone and mineral homeostasis with consequent osteopenia in the appendicular skeleton. However, it is unclear whether these changes have long-term detrimental effects on bone health in the adult. Further studies are required to clarify a number of questions before recommendations can be made concerning the need for interventions to increase calcium intakes in at-risk populations.

REFERENCES

1. Heaney RP. Calcium, bone health, and osteoporosis. In: Peck WA, ed. *Bone and Mineral, vol 4.* Amsterdam: Elsevier Science Publishers, 1986: 255–301.
2. Marcus R. The relationship of dietary calcium to the maintenance of skeletal integrity in man an interface of endocrinology and nutrition. *Metabolism* 1982; 31: 93–102.
3. Melton LJ, Chrischilles EA, Cooper C, Lane AW, Riggs BL. How many women have osteoporosis? *J Bone Miner Res* 1992; 7: 1005–1010.
4. Pettifor JM. Dietary calcium deficiency. In: Glorieux FH, ed. *Rickets. Nestlé Nutrition Workshop No 21.* New York: Raven Press, 1991: 123–143.
5. Pettifor JM, Ross FP, Travers R, Glorieux FH, DeLuca HF. Dietary calcium deficiency: a syndrome associated with bone deformities and elevated serum 1,25-dihydroxyvitamin D concentrations. *Metab Bone Rel Res* 1981; 2: 301–305.
6. Pettifor JM, Ross P, Wang J, Moodley G, Couper-Smith J. Rickets in children of rural origin in South Africa: is low dietary calcium a factor? *J Pediatr* 1978; 92: 320–324.
7. Bhimma R, Pettifor JM, Coovadia HM, Moodley M, Adhikari M. Rickets in black children beyond infancy in Natal. *S Afr Med J* 1995; 85: 668–672.
8. Okonofua F, Gill DS, Alabi ZO, Thomas M, Bell JL, Dandona P. Rickets in Nigerian children: a consequence of calcium malnutrition. *Metabolism* 1991; 40: 209–213.
9. Oginni LM, Worsfold M, Oyelami OA, Sharp CA, Powell DE, Davie MWJ. Etiology of rickets in Nigerian children. *J Pediatr* 1996; 128: 692–694.
10. Rudolf M, Arulanantham K, Greenstein RM. Unsuspected nutritional rickets. *Pediatrics* 1980; 66: 72–76.
11. Davidovits M, Levy Y, Avramovitz T, Eisenstein B. Calcium-deficiency rickets in a four-year-old boy with milk allergy. *J Pediatr* 1993; 122: 249–251.
12. Kooh SW, Fraser D, Reilly BJ, Hamilton JR, Gall D, Bell L. Rickets due to calcium deficiency. *N Engl J Med* 1977; 297: 1264–1266.
13. Dagnelie PC, Vergote FJVRA, van Staveren WA, van den Berg H, Dingjan PG, Hautvast JGAJ. High prevalence of rickets in infants on macrobiotic diets. *Am J Clin Nutr* 1990; 51: 202–208.
14. Proesman W, Legius E, Eggermont E. Rickets due to calcium deficiency. In: *Proceedings of the Symposium on Clinical Disorders of Bone and Mineral Metabolism.* New York: Mary Ann Liebert, 1988: 15.
15. Clements MR, Johnson L, Fraser DR. A new mechanism for induced vitamin D deficiency in calcium deprivation. *Nature* 1987; 325: 62–65.
16. Pettifor JM. Privational rickets: a modern perspective. *J R Soc Med* 1994; 87: 723–725.
17. Marie PJ, Pettifor JM, Ross FP, Glorieux FH. Histological osteomalacia due to dietary calcium deficiency in children. *N Engl J Med* 1982; 307: 584–588.
18. Pettifor JM, Ross FP, Moodley GP, Shuenyane E. Calcium deficiency in rural black children in South Africa a comparison between rural and urban communities. *Am J Clin Nutr* 1979; 32: 2477–2483.
19. Eyberg C, Pettifor JM, Moodley G. Dietary calcium intake in rural black South African children. The relationship between calcium intake and calcium nutritional status. *Hum Nutr Clin Nutr* 1986; 40C: 69–74.
20. Katzman DK, Bachrach LK, Carter DR, Marcus R. Clinical and anthropometric correlates of bone mineral acquisition in healthy adolescent girls. *J Clin Endocrinol Metab* 1991; 73: 1332–1339.
21. Pettifor JM, Roussouw JE. Protein energy malnutrition. In: Cohen RD, Lewis B, Alberti KGMM, Denman AM, eds. *The Metabolic and Molecular Basis of Acquired Disease.* London: Baillière Tindall, 1990: 514–530.
22. Schnitzler CM, Pettifor JM, Patel D, Mesquita JM, Moodley GP, Zachen D. Metabolic bone disease in black teenagers with genu valgum or varum without radiologic rickets: a bone histomorphometric study. *J Bone Miner Res* 1994; 9: 479–486.

23. Lee WT, Leung SS, Ng MY, *et al.* Bone mineral content of two populations of Chinese children with different calcium intakes. *Bone Miner* 1993; 23: 195–206.
24. Prentice A, Laskey MA, Shaw J, Cole TJ, Fraser DR. Bone mineral content of Gambian and British children aged 0–36 months. *Bone Miner* 1990; 10: 211–224.
25. Pollitzer WS, Anderson JJB. Ethnic and genetic differences in bone mass: a review with a hereditary vs environmental perspective. *Am J Clin Nutr* 1989; 50: 1244–1259.
26. Solomon L. Osteoporosis and fracture of the femoral neck in South African blacks. *J Bone Joint Surg [Br]* 1968; 50B: 2–13.
27. Walker ARP. The human requirement of calcium: should low intakes be supplemented? *Am J Clin Nutr* 1972; 25: 518–530.
28. Walker ARP, Richardson B, Walker F. The influence of numerous pregnancies and lactations on bone dimensions in South African Bantu and Caucasian mothers. *Clin Sci* 1972; 42: 189–196.
29. Walker ARP. Osteoporosis and calcium deficiency. *Am J Clin Nutr* 1965; 16: 327–336.
30. Daniels ED, Pettifor JM, Schnitzler CM, Russell SW, Patel DN. Ethnic differences in bone density in female South African nurses. *J Bone Miner Res* 1995; 10: 359–367.
31. Aspray TJ, Prentice A, Cole TJ, Sawo Y, Reeve J, Francis RM. Low bone mineral content is common but osteoporotic fractures are rare in elderly rural Gambian women. *J Bone Miner Res* 1996; 11: 1019–1025.
32. Teotia M, Teotia SPS, Kunwar KB. Endemic skeletal fluorosis. *Arch Dis Child* 1971; 46: 686–691.
33. Teotia M, Teotia SPS, Singh RK. Skeletal fluoride toxicity in children. *Ind J Pediatr* 1979; 46: 389–396.
34. Wenzel A, Thylstrup A, Melsen B, Fejerskov O. The relationship between water-borne fluoride, dental fluorosis and skeletal development in 11–15 year old Tanzanian girls. *Arch Oral Biol* 1982; 27: 1007–1011.
35. Christie DP. The spectrum of radiographic bone changes in children with fluorosis. *Pediatr Radiol* 1980; 136: 85–90.
36. Zong-Cheng L, En-Huei W. Osteoporosis an early radiographic sign of endemic fluorosis. *Skel Radiol* 1986; 15: 350–353.
37. Jackson WPU. Further observations on the Kenhardt bone disease and its relation to fluorosis. *S Afr Med J* 1962; 36: 932–936.
38. Pettifor JM, Schnitzler CM, Ross FP, Moodley GP. Endemic skeletal fluorosis in children: hypocalcemia and the presence of renal resistance to parathyroid hormone. *Bone Miner* 1989; 7: 275–288.
39. Sivakumar B, Krishnamachari KAVR. Circulating levels of immunoreactive parathyroid hormone in endemic genu valgum. *Horm Metab Res* 1976; 8: 317–319.

DISCUSSION

Dr. Seeman: You have a total of about 50 cases. Do you really believe that dietary calcium deficiency is producing 50 cases among presumably thousands of children?

Dr. Pettifor: I believe that the children who present with bone deformities are the tip of the iceberg. The vast majority of children with low calcium intakes are asymptomatic. They are running around at school with no clinical features at all of calcium deficiency. If you measure them biochemically they tend to have elevated alkaline phosphatase values and lower serum calcium values than the control group.

Dr. Seeman: I want to make another comment. Blacks have got longer legs than whites; therefore, if you only adjust for height and fail to adjust for the length of the region you are measuring, you will make an error.

Dr. Pettifor: We actually measured the femoral neck axis length in black and white adults, and they tend to be shorter in blacks than in whites.

Dr. Seeman: You make the inference, I think, that dietary calcium deficiency is present at an intake of 200 mg or less?

Dr. Pettifor: No, I don't have those data. All I am saying is that the children who present clinically with rickets have an intake between 125 and 250 mg/day, as compared with a control group with normal biochemistry, where the intake was between 300 and 400 mg/day. I am not saying that there is a cutoff point.

Dr. Seeman: Do you believe that we know what dietary calcium deficiency is? It has never been studied to my knowledge.

Dr. Pettifor: No. The whole problem is that we don't know what is an adequate calcium intake, particularly when there is a chronic low intake with adaptation. These children have habitually elevated $1{,}25(OH)_2D$ levels, and although we haven't measured PTH on large numbers, we presume that their PTH is elevated as well.

Dr. Seeman: Do you think the bigger bones are caused by delayed skeletal maturation with open epiphyses and continuing growth?

Dr. Pettifor: We do have bone age data, but they are not yet analyzed. Preliminary analysis shows that compared with whites there is about a year to a year and a half delay in bone age. When we compare the dietary deficient group with the rural control group, nutritional status is similar, and delay in puberty is similar. So I don't believe the increase in bone width is related to a difference in puberty but rather to an effect of chronic hyperparathyroidism.

Dr. Gilsanz: Correct me if I am wrong. I thought that increase of radial width was a hallmark of rickets. Is not the widening you showed just a further indication that maybe the children have rickets? And is it not probably independent of the level of parathyroid hormone, as we know that older cases of rickets don't have elevated PTH?

Dr. Pettifor: I am not sure that that is actually true because if one looks at the metacarpals, one sees widening of the midshaft of the metacarpals as well, and that is not a feature that one sees in rickets. We were measuring the diaphysis, not the epiphysis.

Dr. Frenk: Regarding rickets in a zone of endemic fluorosis, you may remember an epidemic of knock knees in such a zone that occurred in the central part of India as a consequence of building a huge dam. This was not caused by fluoride itself but by a sudden increase in the concentration of molybdenum in the water. This competed with copper and in some way influenced collagen formation. The disorder was not really rickets because it occurred in young adults, and the epidemic was very well studied by the Indian Nutrition Institute. The "epidemic" resolved when sufficient copper was supplied in the diet. What, then, really is the significance of raised activity of alkaline phosphatase? In a study we did to try to find out whether air contamination could cause rickets, 12% of the infants had a high alkaline phosphatase but a normal concentration of 25-hydroxyvitamin D. What exactly is the meaning of this high alkaline phosphatase in the presence of apparently normal vitamin D? These were not children or school-age children, as you showed, but infants.

Dr. Pettifor: I am not sure that anybody knows. I think alkaline phosphatase is a reasonable marker for bone activity, but what it is measuring I am not sure. We have a similar problem with osteocalcin. In children with all forms of rickets, whether hypophosphatemic or vitamin D deficient, we have been unable to show an elevation of osteocalcin despite an elevation of alkaline phosphatase. So I must admit, I don't know what we are measuring.

Dr. Mithal: About the molybdenum hypothesis: the NIN group from Hyderabad subsequently reviewed the data, and they could not substantiate this hypothesis that molybdenum was the cause of the problem. The only consistent factor they could come up with was poor calcium intakes, which seemed to be determining the prevalence of endemic genu valgum in areas of fluorosis.

Dr. Eisman: The sort of differences that you are picking up in bone width are probably well below the level that would trigger radiologists to say, this is a widened epiphysis or metaphysis; this indicates rickets. It doesn't have to be that gross. As you said yourself, you are looking at a continuum of effect. The implication for me is that the wider radius found in these children now was once the widened epiphysis of rickets.

Dr. Pettifor: I accept that there is abnormal modeling. However, the issue is that if you have hyperparathyroidism, you get increased endosteal bone resorption, and you also get an increase in periosteal new bone formation, so the bone actually widens.

Dr. Eisman: I think what you have to explain is that these children don't have less bone. They have the same amount of bone, but it is differently distributed. For some reason they have as much bone but spread out over a larger area.

Dr. Pettifor: The way I would interpret it is that one has a wider bone but a thinner cortex.

Dr. Eisman: But why would the bone remodel like that? If there was enough calcium to do the smaller version, why do the bigger version? It doesn't make sense when there is actually the same amount of bone there.

Dr. Pettifor: The bone mineral content is the same, but the bones tend to be wider, and therefore, if you measure volumetric bone density, the bone density is lower. If you took a bit of bone out of the cortex, I believe that the density of that bone would be the same as in a normal individual, and I believe this is due to hyperparathyroidism.

Dr. Jüppner: There are probably two different disorders going on at the same time. One is a remodeling problem, and the other is a bone-forming problem taking place at the metaphysis, where, presumably because of the secondary hyperparathyroidism, you have inhibition of chondrocyte maturation and therefore get the widened metaphysis. So it would perhaps be helpful to measure type 2 collagen degradation products to differentiate between bone remodeling and abnormalities in the growth plate.

Dr. Pettifor: If one looks at bone histology in children who present with radiologic abnormalities or with genu valgum or varum, with or without radiologic evidence of rickets, there is a spectrum of abnormality from hyperparathyroidism right through to frank osteomalacia. Children who have radiologic evidence of rickets have frank osteomalacia on bone histology, so this is not the type of bone disease that one sees with renal osteodystrophy, for instance; it is not pure hyperparathyroidic bone disease that one sees at the metaphysis.

Dr. Jüppner: All I am saying is that there are probably two distinct areas where elevated PTH levels have different consequences.

Dr. Mithal: Do you think that the group with fluorosis requires a less severe degree of calcium deficiency to develop the same picture as the severely calcium deficient group without fluorosis?

Dr. Pettifor: That would be my hypothesis, but we don't have good data to support it. We have calcium intake data, which are as reliable as we can get, showing that calcium intake in the children in the endemic fluorosis area was about 350 to 450 mg/day, very similar to the control group, and this is slightly higher than the calcium intakes of the children with dietary calcium deficiency.

Dr Tsang: Did you give calcium supplements?

Dr. Pettifor: No, we didn't treat anybody with calcium. We treated children with calcium in a separate study, which we presented some time ago (1). We gave a group of children 500 mg of calcium per day, but we could continue this for only 3 months because of unrest in the area that disrupted the study. But in that 3-month period, we were able to show a significant fall in alkaline phosphatase values and rise in serum calcium.

Dr. Pohlandt: In your case presentation of one child with calcium deficiency, you showed that after starting calcium supplementation the phosphorus increased. How could you explain that? The opposite would be expected.

Dr. Pettifor: No, I think this is because there was also a concomitant fall in parathyroid hormone and fall in urinary cyclic AMP, so what we had was decreased urinary excretion of phosphate and an increase in serum phosphorus.

Dr. Pohlandt: But you would need more phosphate to form apatite if you supplement with calcium. That is what we see in preterm infants fed on preterm formula. If you supplement them with calcium, the plasma phosphorus falls.

Dr. Pettifor: I think that depends on the amount of available phosphate present in the diet. These children have very adequate phosphate intakes of about 900 to 1,000 mg/day, and in fact some of the children are hyperphosphatemic on presentation and have evidence of renal resistance to parathyroid hormone.

REFERENCE

1. Pettifor JM, Ross FP, Moodley GP, Shuenyane E. The effect of dietary calcium supplementation on serum calcium, phosphorus and alkaline phosphatase concentrations in a rural black population. *Am J Clin Nutr* 1981; 34: 2187–2191.

Nutrition and Bone Development, edited by
Jean-Philippe Bonjour and Reginald C. Tsang,
Nestlé Nutrition Workshop Series, Vol. 41, Nestec Ltd.,
Vevey/Lippincott–Raven Publishers,
Philadelphia © 1999.

Endemic Fluorosis and Calcium Intake

Ambrish Mithal and Anil K. Singh

Department of Medical Endocrinology, Sanjay Gandhi Postgraduate Institute of Medical Sciences, Lucknow 226014, India

Fluorine is a trace element that is essential for many enzymatic actions in the human body. Although widely distributed in nature, it is rarely found in its free form, as it is highly reactive. In low doses, fluoride is known to help prevent dental caries. Recently, low doses and slow-release preparations of fluoride have been shown to be beneficial in the treatment of spinal osteoporosis (1). Prolonged exposure to excess fluoride can, however, lead to adverse effects on several body tissues, especially the dental and skeletal systems, leading to a condition known as fluorosis. The most widespread form of fluorosis is hydric fluorosis, which occurs with chronic consumption of large amounts of fluoride in drinking water. The first reports of skeletal fluorosis appeared more than half a century ago from India (2). This condition, which leads to considerable morbidity and loss of human resources, continues to be endemic in many parts of the world, particularly in Asia and Africa.

Because of the vital role of calcium in building and maintaining the skeletal framework, it is not surprising that the calcium status of an individual modifies and modulates skeletal fluoride toxicity. In this chapter we attempt to provide a brief overview of endemic skeletal fluorosis and the importance of calcium intake in the expression of skeletal manifestations of this disorder.

FLUORIDE KINETICS

Fluoride is absorbed in the stomach (a pH-dependent process) and intestine. There is almost complete absorption under fasting conditions. Urinary and fecal excretion and deposition in bones are the most important elements in the physiological handling of fluoride. Fluoride excretion in the urine is the primary route of elimination. Fluoride is filtered freely through the kidneys, and renal fluoride clearance is dependent on glomerular filtration rate (GFR) and urine flow. Renal clearance is also positively correlated with urinary pH (3). Patients with reduced GFR have higher plasma fluoride concentrations. In areas of fluorosis, even mild decreases in renal function lead to a marked increase in skeletal fluoride toxicity. Although plasma fluoride reflects ongoing levels of fluoride exposure, urinary fluoride excretion reflects present as well as past fluoride exposure because fluoride released during bone remodeling continues to be eliminated by the renal route long after fluoride exposure has ceased (4).

Fecal fluoride, which forms 10% to 30% of the amount ingested, has traditionally been believed to be unabsorbed fluoride. However, in an elegant study on rats, Whitford (5) showed that raised plasma fluoride concentrations increased fecal fluoride excretion and thereby reduced the net absorption balance of ingested fluoride. Most importantly, he showed for the first time that fluoride does not move passively and unidirectionally from the gastrointestinal tract but could actually be secreted into the gut when plasma fluoride concentrations are increased. According to the model proposed, almost 100% of the dietary fluoride is absorbed in the proximal gastrointestinal tract. Most of the fluoride in feces is that which reenters the distal gastrointestinal tract along the diffusion gradient between the interstitial and luminal fluid and subsequently becomes associated with unabsorbed cations such as calcium and magnesium (5). In another study, Whitford and his colleagues showed that short-term fluoride kinetics differ in various species and that young adult dogs resemble young adult humans most closely in this respect (6).

Deposition of fluoride in the skeleton is a major factor in the metabolism of absorbed fluoride. Experimental studies using radiofluorine showed that the skeletal distribution pattern of fluoride was the same as for calcium: in long bones there is a preferential deposition in the primary spongiosa beneath the cartilage, a generalized patchy distribution in trabeculae, and a linear distribution on endosteal and periosteal surfaces (7). Fluoride binds to bone in a nonlinear fashion, and a lesser percentage of fluoride is bound as the intake increases (8).

Using this and other existing evidence, Turner *et al.* developed a mathematical model for fluoride uptake by the skeleton and showed that it was positively associated with the bone-remodeling rate and also that fluoride clearance from the skeleton takes over four times longer than uptake (9). Boivin *et al.* measured bone fluoride content in iliac bone biopsies from normal controls, untreated osteoporosis subjects, osteoporosis subjects treated with fluoride, and patients with skeletal fluorosis. They showed that during prolonged exposure of adult bone tissue to fluoride, the early bone fluoride uptake is variable and depends on the remodeling activity; it subsequently increases rapidly before becoming more or less stable at a maximum level (10).

There is a progressive increase in bone fluoride with age, but this does not merely reflect cumulative passive sequestration of fluoride in bone. Guo *et al.* studied skeletal fluoride kinetics in growing rats (11). They found that 60% of fluoride mobilized during bone resorption was redeposited in the skeleton and that this redeposition showed a positive correlation with mineral deposition. This led to their conclusion that retention of fluoride in the growing skeleton of rats results mainly from redeposition of resorbed fluoride.

MODE OF ACTION OF FLUORIDE ON BONE CELLS

Effect on Osteoblasts

Fluoride enhances osteoblast proliferation. However, the molecular mechanisms of action of fluoride on osteoblast proliferation and activity are still incompletely understood. The interaction of fluoride with various growth factors involved in bone formation is thought to be important in mediating its effects on bone-forming cells. Fluoride potentiates the mitogenic actions of growth factors with tyrosyl kinase receptors. This is probably mediated by inhibition of phosphotyrosyl phosphatase and enhancement of tyrosyl phosphorylation of cellular proteins (12,13). It has been suggested that a fluoride-induced increase in intracellular calcium via activation of the phosphatidylinositol pathway, increase in sensitivity to TGF-α, and enhancement of the *ras* signal transduction pathway are possible mechanisms of fluoride action on osteoblasts (14–17).

Depending on its concentration, fluoride has a biphasic action on bone-forming cells. Though it stimulates osteoblasts at low concentrations, at high concentrations it can cause their suppression. Moreover, high doses of fluoride may lead to formation of cross-link-deficient collagen and impairment of mineralization (18).

Effect on Osteoclasts

Very little is understood about the effect of fluoride on osteoclastic activity. There is a dichotomy between *in vivo* bone resorptive indices and *in vitro* experimental and biophysical data. Though histomorphometric and biochemical evidence indicates increased bone resorption in subjects with fluorosis, *in vitro* studies on osteoclasts have paradoxically shown a fluoride-induced decrease in resorptive activity (19). Moreover, in the presence of fluoride, there is a preferential formation of fluoroapatite over hydroxyapatite. Fluoroapatite has a large crystal size and is less soluble (20). Fluoride also inhibits dissolution of preformed hydroxyapatite (21). The functional quality of bone is affected by fluoride in a biphasic manner, with improvement at low doses but deleterious effects at high doses.

FLUOROSIS

The term ‘‘fluorosis’’ describes the syndrome that results from chronic exposure to excess fluoride. The predominant effects are on the skeleton and teeth. Recent reports have highlighted metabolic and soft tissue manifestations such as glucose intolerance (22). Traditional descriptions of fluorosis have emphasized the presence of osteosclerosis, particularly of the axial skeleton (23). However, it is now recognized that osteosclerosis is not necessarily the predominant feature in skeletal fluorosis.

Causes

Hydric Fluorosis

Hydric fluorosis results from consumption of drinking water containing toxic amounts of fluoride. Excessive amounts of fluoride present in the soil leach into well water, which is subsequently consumed. Hydric fluorosis unfortunately continues to be endemic in vast areas of the developing world, particularly in Asia and Africa. In India alone, 25 million people are though to be at risk for development of fluoride toxicity.

Inhalational Fluorosis

Inhalational (airborne) fluorosis could be telluric fluorosis caused by inhalation of fluoride-rich dusts or industrial fluorosis caused by inhalation of fluorinated gases, first described in cryolite workers. Recent studies have shown that fluorosis occurs with coal burning in China (24).

Iatrogenic Fluorosis

Iatrogenic fluorosis may occur with the prolonged consumption of fluoride-containing drugs, for example, niflumic acid, or sodium fluoride for the treatment of osteoporosis.

Other Causes

Other causes described include wine fluorosis (described from Spain, where fluoride was added to stop the fermentation process in certain local wines) and dentifrice-induced fluorosis.

Clinical Features

Often only mild or nonspecific musculoskeletal symptoms are present in the initial stages of skeletal fluorosis despite definite radiologic changes in the skeleton. Clinically, overt skeletal fluorosis manifests with generalized bone and joint pains and with stiffness and restriction of movement of large joints and the spine. Moreover, fixed deformities, especially of the spine, hips, and knees, may appear in the late stages and can ultimately lead to incapacitation, either from the deformities themselves or because of complicating compressive myeloradiculopathy. Some of these patients may present with bowing of the femur, tibia, radius, or ulna, and others present with genu valgum or varum deformities (25,26). Traditionally, skeletal fluorosis was known to cause deformities of the spine in adults. However, it has now been shown that very young children can also suffer from severe skeletal fluorosis. The toxic effects of fluoride may in fact be more deleterious on the growing skeleton because of the rapid turnover of bone. Long bone involvement may lead to crippling deformities in children and adolescents (4,26). Most patients with fluorosis, especially of the endemic hydric variety, also show evidence of dental involvement, which is characterized (in increasing severity) by chalky white opaque areas over the enamel surface, marked attrition of surfaces subjected to wear, brown staining, and discrete or confluent pitting and hypoplasia of enamel.

Relationship to Calcium Intake

Modeling defects resulting in genu varum and valgum deformities typically occur in fluorotic children with poor calcium intake and have been described primarily from regions and populations where calcium undernutrition is common, such as parts of India, Tanzania, China, and South Africa (4,26). Krishnamachari (4) showed that 2% to 4% of the susceptible population develop genu valgum in some villages known for severe endemic fluorosis. The age at manifestation varies from 6 to 15 years. In a given village, nutritionally deprived individuals develop genu valgum. He analyzed the diets of patients suffering from the genu valgum type of endemic fluorosis and reported very low calcium intakes, less than 300 mg/day. In addition he found high phosphate contents in the diet. He also found that genu valgum did not occur in nonfluorotic populations with similar dietary calcium intakes, confirming the importance of fluoride calcium interactions in producing adverse skeletal effects. He concluded that low calcium intake predisposes to genu valgum in a fluorosis area. One study actually suggested that a calcium-depleted diet could improve the crippling clinical deformities associated with fluorosis and showed clinical evidence to this effect (27)! However, the same authors later made a case for high calcium intakes being protective against the adverse effects of skeletal fluorosis (28).

The combination of chronic fluoride excess in the drinking water and a nutritionally poor diet containing very little calcium may be responsible for the earlier onset and greater severity of skeletal fluorosis, along with frequent long bone deformities, seen in many parts of the world.

Radiologic Findings

Traditionally, osteosclerosis (especially spinal) and calcification of the interosseous membrane of the forearm have been described as the hallmarks of skeletal fluorosis (Fig. 1). A marked tendency for calcification of ligaments and muscular attachments, irregular osteophytoses, and exostoses is also characteristic (23). Later descriptions have, however, highlighted the wide spectrum of radiologic findings, including bowing of long bones and simultaneous presence of osteosclerosis, osteoporosis, and osteomalacia (29–31) (Fig. 2). A report from India showed that in addition to osteosclerosis there may be evidence of a coarse trabecular pattern, axial osteosclerosis with distal osteopenia, and diffuse osteopenia. Occasional patients show changes of hyperparathyroidism and rickets or osteomalacia (30). Despite clinical abnormalities of the long bones suggesting rachitic deformities, radiology does not commonly reveal typical features of rickets.

Calcium Intake and Radiologic Changes in Fluorosis

An important finding in the report mentioned above was that subjects with osteopenic changes had a significantly lower dietary calcium and protein intake than those with typical osteosclerosis (30). None of the patients with adequate calcium intakes showed an osteopenic picture. Therefore, it seems that osteosclerosis is the predominant lesion in fluorosis patients with adequate dietary calcium intake, whereas the osteopenic/osteomalacic picture predominates in people with suboptimal or poor calcium intake. The absence of osteopenic varieties of fluorosis in earlier reports from India can be attributed to the fact that these were mainly from the nutritionally rich regions of India, that is, the Punjab, which is known for its abundance of dairy products and high calcium intakes. However, apart from dietary calcium intake,

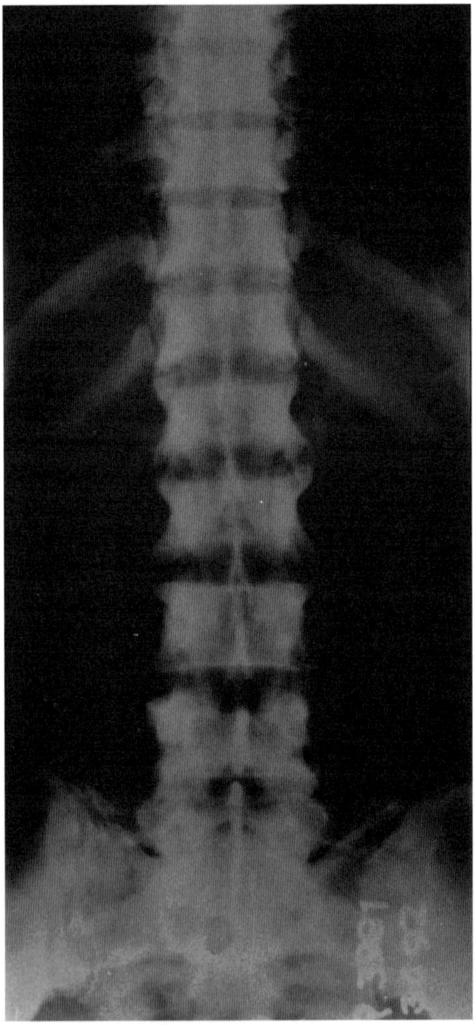

FIG. 1. Spinal osteosclerosis and ligamentous calcification in a 35-year-old woman with skeletal fluorosis.

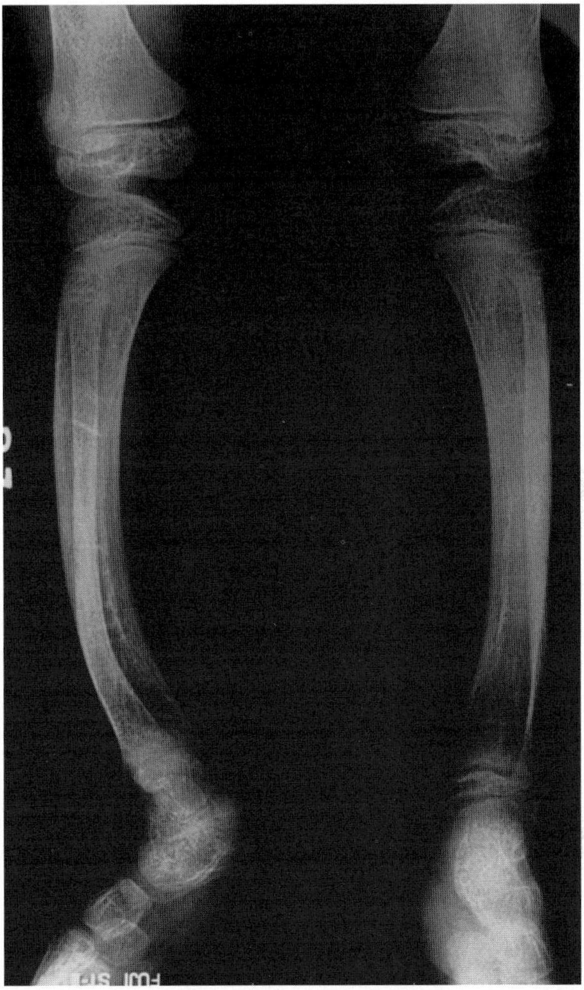

FIG. 2. Osteopenia and bowing of tibia and fibula in a 9-year-old boy with skeletal fluorosis.

there may be yet other undefined factors, including toxins or nutrients, that could also be modifying the skeletal changes in fluorosis.

Bone Metabolism Indices

Apart from a study from South Africa in which hypocalcemia was reported in school children, most studies have found essentially normal levels of calcium (total and ionized) and phosphate in fluorosis (32). There is no agreement among various studies on the state of parathyroid function in fluorosis. Some workers have reported cases of hyperparathyrodism, but others have found normal parathyroid function in most patients (33–35). Recent data, using the intact PTH assay, suggest that hyperparathyroidism may be less common than previously thought (36). When given to osteoporosis patients for 1 year, fluoride did not induce any changes in circulating PTH level (37). In thyroparathyroidectomized as well as sham-operated rats, fluoride increased periosteal new bone formation and increased endosteal resorption without any effect on PTH levels, suggesting that effects of fluoride on bone are not mediated by PTH (38).

There is consensus on the existence of increased bone turnover in fluorosis, regardless of the state of parathyroid function. Bone scans show evidence of increased tracer uptake and turnover in virtually all patients with overt skeletal fluorosis (39). Bone formation markers such as serum alkaline phosphatase and osteocalcin are increased, as are markers of resorption such as urinary hydroxyproline and tartarate-resistant acid phosphatase (4,34,36).

Serum 25-hydroxyvitamin D concentrations have generally been found to be normal in fluorosis (4,34,36). There are reports of radiologic osteomalacia in patients with fluorosis, but in these patients the 25-hydroxyvitamin D level was not estimated (29). Interestingly, a patient with osteoporosis treated with fluoride, vitamin D, and calcium developed osteomalacia despite high circulating levels of 25-hydroxyvitamin D (40). There is also a report of elevated serum 1,25-dihydroxycholecalciferol concentrations in children with endemic fluorosis (32). Thus, contrary to speculations by some workers, vitamin D deficiency is not the major determining factor in skeletal changes of fluorosis (41).

There does not seem to be a major alteration in serum calcitonin levels in skeletal fluorosis, although reports of both high and low values are available (4,36).

Calcium Intake and Bone Metabolism Indices

It has been shown that low calcium intakes further enhance the increased bone turnover in fluorosis. It has also been suggested that patients with calcium-deficient genu valgum may show a greater degree of secondary hyperparathyroidism (4). A study of nine children with skeletal fluorosis, six of whom had hypocalcemia, showed that renal responsiveness to exogenously administered PTH was impaired and that there was a direct correlation between serum calcium values and the degree of the phosphaturic response (32). Dietary correction of hypocalcemia resulted in a restoration of renal responsiveness to PTH. The authors suggested that hypocalcemia may directly modify the renal responsiveness to PTH, especially with regard to phosphate, which resulted in hyperphosphatemia rather than hypophosphatemia in four children.

Histology/Histomorphometry

Histomorphometric analysis of bone from patients with skeletal fluorosis has shown that in the typical osteosclerotic pattern of involvement there is a significant increase in cortical thickness and porosity but no reduction in compact bone mass. Trabecular bone volume is significantly increased. Parameters reflecting bone formation (trabecular osteoid volume, trabecular osteoid surfaces, and thickness of osteoid seams) are markedly increased. Compared to the effect on increase in osteoid surfaces, the effect on resorption is much less. The number of osteoblasts increases, although there is a greater proportion of flat osteoblasts. Thus, there is evidence of an unbalanced coupling in favor of bone formation (18). One study, however, has shown enhanced bone resorptive activity in severe skeletal fluorosis. Evidence of mineralization defects in the form of mottled periosteocytic lacunae has also been shown (42).

Calcium Intake and Bone Histology in Fluorosis

In a study on school children with skeletal fluorosis, histomorphometry revealed an inverse relationship between serum calcium values and osteoid volume, surface and seam thickness, and mineralization lag time, suggesting that serum and dietary calcium may be important in the development of osteomalacia in these patients. This study provided further evidence that the mineralization defects seen in patients with skeletal fluorosis are related to fluoride *per se,* combined with the effects of a low calcium intake (32). In fluoride-treated osteoporotics, an inverse relationship has been found between the amount of calcium and the extent of resorption surface in iliac bone samples (43).

CALCIUM–FLUORIDE INTERACTIONS

Metabolic Studies in Humans

Calcium balance studies in humans with endemic fluorosis have found low urinary and fecal calcium excretion and showed that fluorosis patients retain significantly higher amounts of calcium. In one study, when placed on a dietary calcium intake of 800 mg daily, six patients with fluorosis retained a mean of 405 mg calcium/day, whereas the controls retained only 139 mg (44). In another study, 53% retention of calcium was found in fluorosis patients given 800 mg calcium daily (45). Using calcium infusion studies, Rao *et al.* (46) studied calcium retention in fluorosis patients who were maintained on a metabolic diet supplying 800 mg of calcium, 40 mg of phosphorus, and 150 mg of magnesium per day; 15 mg/kg of calcium gluconate was infused over a 4-hour period, and the total output of calcium during the following 12 hours was measured. A remarkably low output was found (mean value 5.49% of administered dose) (46). These studies confirmed that patients with the classic osteosclerotic form of fluorosis show a high avidity for calcium.

The administration of fluoride to osteoporotic patients also results in a low urinary calcium excretion as well as enhanced calcium absorption from the gut. The average plasma fluoride concentration of osteoporotic patients in one study increased by 54% when their supplemental calcium and vitamin D were discontinued (47).

Narasingarao *et al.* (48) determined ^{47}Ca turnover in patients with endemic fluorosis and age-matched controls. They found that total calcium turnover was significantly greater in younger subjects and subjects with fluorosis. Bone mineralization rates were also significantly higher in patients with fluorosis than in age-matched controls. Interestingly, total body calcium turnover and bone mineralization rates were significantly higher in fluorosis patients with genu valgum (who are known to have poorer calcium intakes) than in classical forms of fluorosis. It was surprising that in genu valgum where osteopenia was the dominant lesion, the bone mineralization rate was higher than in classical fluorosis. It is likely that this just reflects the markedly enhanced bone turnover in these patients, and the increase in resorption rate may actually be much greater than the increase in formation rate.

Not only can dietary calcium adequacy alter the skeletal response to fluoride, but a recent study by Dure-Smith *et al.* showed that the skeletal response to fluoride can itself alter the state of adequacy of body calcium (49). They studied calcium retention, serum PTH, and spinal bone density in three groups of osteoporotic subjects, two of which had been treated with calcium and fluoride for 32 ± 19 months while the third group served as a control. Of the two groups treated with calcium and fluoride, one showed rapid increases in spinal bone density, but the other showed decreases or only slow increases in spinal bone density. They found a positive correlation among the increase in spinal density, serum intact PTH, and calcium retention, indicating that fluoride administration can induce a state of calcium deficiency and secondary hyperparathyroidism in proportion to the increase in bone formation. Administration of calcitriol in seven of their subjects resulted in a significant amelioration of calcium deficiency caused by fluoride.

Metabolic Studies in Animals

One of the earliest studies on fluorosis suggested that supplements of dietary calcium prolonged the survival period of rats exposed to toxic levels of fluoride (50). Whitford's study on rats (5) showed that increased calcium intake reduced the urinary fluoride excretion but increased the fecal and total excretion of fluoride. This resulted in lower, or even negative, balances of ingested fluoride, thus highlighting the influence of dietary calcium intake on fluoride kinetics. This could have important implications in determining skeletal responses to fluoride.

Reddy and Srikantia induced experimental fluorosis in growing monkeys and found that adequate dietary calcium mitigated the toxic effects of fluoride and that higher amounts of fluoride were retained in the bones of animals on low-calcium diets (51). In another study in which experimental fluorosis was produced in monkeys by intragastric feeding of sodium fluoride, it was observed that calcium-deficient animals had increased retention of ^{45}Ca. High fluoride, when fed to monkeys on a low-calcium diet, resulted in highest retention of ^{45}Ca ($>90\%$ on the tenth day) (52). The role of calcium deficiency in modifying the skeletal manifestations of fluorosis is supported by another study on Rhesus monkeys. When they were given fluoride alone, there was an increase in bone formation and density, which the authors labeled as mild fluorosis. Administration of a low-calcium diet resulted in osteoporosis with increased resorption evident on histology. When a high-fluoride intake was combined with a calcium-deficient diet, osteoporosis could be prevented, but there was evidence of defective mineralization leading to osteomalacia (53).

Mechanism of Calcium–Fluoride Interaction

Clinical and experimental data (some of which have been discussed above) provide ample evidence that there is a close interaction between calcium and fluoride kinetics and their effects on the skeleton. This interaction is of crucial importance in determining the severity and nature of the skeletal response to toxic and therapeutic levels of fluoride. However, the exact mechanism of such an interaction is not definitively known. The interaction is probably at multiple levels such as gastrointestinal absorption and skeletal uptake of fluoride as well as modulation of bone turnover and mineralization. Higher dietary calcium intake reduces net fluoride absorption from the gastrointestinal tract. This was traditionally believed to reflect nonabsorption of a proportion of the ingested fluoride because of formation of insoluble calcium fluoride. However, it could also be caused by an increase in fluoride secretion in the distal gastrointestinal tract along the interstitial fluid–intestinal luminal gradient, caused by a lowering of luminal fluoride ion concentration because of formation of insoluble complexes with cations such as calcium and magnesium. Thus, higher dietary calcium decreases the bioavailability of fluoride.

Exposure to fluoride increases the rate of bone turnover, with unbalanced coupling in favor of bone formation, through its action on the bone-forming cells. High bone turnover induced by calcium deficiency, on the other hand, has a resorptive bias. Hence, when fluoride exposure is combined with calcium deficiency, osteopenia accompanies or replaces osteosclerosis. The high-turnover state induced by calcium deficiency also increases the skeletal uptake of fluoride. Fluoride exposure can by itself induce a state of relative calcium deficiency by increasing the calcium demand resulting from fluoride-stimulated bone turnover and formation.

In addition to the above, calcium deficiency aggravates fluoride-induced mineralization defects. Undermineralized soft bones may be responsible for the greater incidence of long bone deformities seen in calcium-deficient fluorotic children.

CONCLUSIONS

In conclusion, low dietary intake of calcium in subjects with endemic fluorosis causes not only an earlier onset but a greater severity of the disease. Long bone involvement and deformities are seen more frequently. Osteopenia, especially of the long bones, is often seen. There is a greater enhancement of bone turnover with more avid calcium retention and possibly greater frequency of secondary hyperparathyroidism. The effects of low calcium intake on endemic fluorosis are as follows:

1. Increased severity and earlier (childhood) onset of disease manifestations
2. Higher prevalence of long bone involvement and deformity
3. Increased likelihood of osteopenia, especially of long bones
4. Further enhancement of bone turnover; more avid calcium retention
5. Higher prevalence of secondary hyperparathyroidism

However, much still remains to be understood about the intricacies of calcium-fluoride interaction. Delineation of the exact mechanism of their interaction at the cellular and molecular level will not only help greatly in understanding the skeletal effects of fluoride but will also provide insights into the processes of normal bone formation and remodeling.

ACKNOWLEDGMENTS

We gratefully acknowledge the contributions of Sushil K. Gupta, M.D., D.M. and Nitin Trivedi, M.D., D.M., as well as all other members of the Fluoride Collaborative Study Group. Grant support received from Japan International Cooperation Agency (India) and from Sanjay Gandhi Postgraduate Institute of Medical Sciences is also gratefully acknowledged. Most of all, however, thanks are due to residents of endemic villages from Unnao District, Uttar Pradesh, who willingly allow themselves to be subjected to tedious investigations for the sake of science.

REFERENCES

1. Pak CYC, Sakhaee K, Adams-Huet B, Piziak V, Peterson RB, Poindexter JR. Treatment of post menopausal osteoporosis with slow-release sodium fluoride. Final update of a randomized controlled trial. *Ann Intern Med* 1995; 123: 401–408.
2. Shortt HE, Pandit CC, Raghavachari TNS. Endemic fluorosis in the Nellore district of South India. *Ind Med Gaz* 1937; 72: 396–403.
3. Whitford GM. The metabolism and toxicity of fluoride. In: Myers HM, ed. *Monographs in Oral Science 13.* Basel: S Karger, 1989.
4. Krishnamachari KAVR. Skeletal fluorosis in humans: a review of the recent progress in the understanding of the disease. *Prog Food Nutr Sci* 1986; 10: 279–314.
5. Whitford GM. Effect of plasma fluoride and dietary calcium concentrations on GI absorption and secretion of fluoride in the rat. *Calcif Tissue Int* 1994; 54: 421–425.
6. Whitford GM, Biles ED, Birdsong-Whitford NL. A comparative study of fluoride pharmacokinetics in five species. *J Dent Res* 1991; 70: 948–951.
7. Faccini JM. Fluoride and bone. *Calcif Tissue Res* 1969; 3: 1–16.
8. Kekki M, Lampainen E, Kauranen P, Hoikka V, Alhava EM, Pasternack A. The non linear tissue binding character of fluoride kinetics in normal and anephric subjects. *Nephron* 1982; 31: 129–134.
9. Turner CH, Boivin G, Meunier PJ. A mathematical model for fluoride uptake by the skeleton. *Calcif Tissue Int* 1993; 52: 130–138.
10. Boivin G, Chapuy M-L, Baud CA, Meunier PJ. Fluoride content in human iliac bone: results in controls, patients with fluorosis, and osteoporotic patients treated with fluoride. *J Bone Miner Res* 1988; 3: 497–502.
11. Guo MK, Nopakun J, Messer HH, Ophaug R, Singer L. Retention of skeletal fluoride during bone turnover in rats. *J Nutr* 1988; 118: 362–366.
12. Lau WKH, Farley JR, Freeman TK, Baylink DJ. A proposed mechanism of the mitogenic action of fluoride on bone cells: Inhibition of the activity of osteoblastic acid phosphatase. *Metabolism* 1989; 38: 858–863.
13. Thomas AB, Hashimoto H, Baylink DJ, Lau WKH. Fluoride at mitogenic concentrations increases

the steady state phosphotyrosyl phosphorylation level of cellular proteins in human bone cells. *J Clin Endocrinol Metab* 1996; 81: 2570–2578.

14. Zerwekh JE, Morris AC, Padalino PK, Gottschalk F, Pak CYC. Fluoride rapidly and transiently increases intracellular calcium in human osteoblasts. *J Bone Miner Res* 1990; 5 (Suppl 1): 131–136.
15. Reed BY, Zerwekh JE, Antich PP, Pak CYC. Fluoride stimulated ^{3}H thymidine uptake in a human osteoblastic osteosarcoma cell line is dependent on transforming growth factor beta. *J Bone Miner Res* 1993; 8: 19–25.
16. Caverzasio J, Imai T, Ammann P, Burgener D, Bonjour J-P. Mitogenic signaling process induced by fluoride in osteoblast-like cells involves focal adhesion kinase, GRB2, and mitogen activated protein kinase (abstract). *J Bone Miner Res* 1995; 10 (Suppl 1): S143.
17. Caverzasio J, Imai T, Ammann P, Burgener D, Bonjour J-P. Aluminum potentiates the effects of fluoride on tyrosine phosphorylation and osteoblast replication *in vitro* and bone mass *in vivo*. *J Bone Miner Res* 1996; 11: 46–55.
18. Boivin G, Chavassieux P, Chapuy MC, Baud CA, Meunier PJ. Skeletal fluorosis: histomorphometric analysis of bone changes and bone fluoride content in 29 patients. *Bone* 1989; 10: 89–99.
19. Okuda A, Kanehisa J, Heersche JNM. The effects of sodium fluoride on resorptive activity of isolated osteoclasts. *J Bone Miner Res* 1990; 5 (Suppl 1): 115–118.
20. Eanes ED, Reddi AH. The effect of fluoride on bone mineral apatite. *Metab Bone Dis Rel Res* 1979; 2: 3–10.
21. Christofferson J, Christofferson MR. The effect of bendroflumethazide and hydrochlorothiazide on the rate of dissolution of calcium hydroxyapatite. *Calcif Tiss Int* 1984; 36: 431–434.
22. Trivedi N, Mithal A, Gupta SK, Godbole MM. Reversible impairment of glucose intolerance in endemic fluorosis. *Diabetologia* 1993; 36: 826–830.
23. Singh A, Jolly SS, Bansal BC, Mathur CC. Endemic fluorosis. Epidemiological, clinical and biochemical study of chronic fluorine intoxication in Punjab (India). *Medicine* 1963; 42: 229–249.
24. Jianxue L, Cao S. Recent studies on endemic fluorosis in China. *Fluoride* 1994; 27: 125–128.
25. Krishnamachari KAVR, Krishnaswamy K. Genu valgum and osteoporosis in an area of endemic fluorosis. *Lancet* 1973; ii: 877–879.
26. Mithal A, Trivedi N, Gupta SK, for the Fluoride Collaborative Study Group. Endocrinology of fluorosis: an overview and a preliminary study of one hundred patients. In: Kochupillai N, ed. *Endocrinology, Metabolism and Diabetes, vol I.* Delhi: Macmillan India, 1992: 308–316.
27. Teotia SPS, Kunwar KB, Teotia M. Metabolic studies on skeletal fluorosis with a new approach to its treatment. *Fluoride* 1969; 2: 142–152.
28. Teotia SPS, Teotia M. Endemic fluorosis in India: a challenging national health problem. *J Assoc Physicians India* 1984; 32: 347–352.
29. Christie DP. The spectrum of radiographic bone changes in children with fluorosis. *Radiology* 1980; 136: 85–90.
30. Mithal A, Trivedi N, Gupta SK, Kumar S, Gupta RK. Radiological spectrum of endemic fluorosis: relationship with calcium intake. *Skel Radiol* 1993; 22: 257–261.
31. Wang Y, Yuming Y, Gilula LA, Wilson AJ. Endemic fluorosis of the skeleton: radiographic features in 127 patients. *Am J Radiol* 1994; 162: 93–98.
32. Pettifor JM, Schnitzler CM, Ross FP, Moodley GP. Endemic skeletal fluorosis in children: hypocalcemia and the presence of renal resistance to parathyroid hormone. *Bone Miner* 1989; 7: 275–288.
33. Teotia SPS, Teotia M. Secondary hyperparathyroidism in patients with endemic skeletal fluorosis. *Br Med J* 1973; i: 637–640.
34. Srivastava RN, Gill DS, Moudgil A, Menon RK, Thomas M, Dandona P. Normal ionized calcium, parathyroid hypersecretion, and elevated osteocalcin in a family with fluorosis. *Metabolism* 1989; 38: 120–124.
35. Boillat MA, Garcia J, Dettweiler W, Burckhardt P, Courvoisier B. Clinical aspects of industrial fluorosis. In: Courvoisier B, Donath A, Baud CA, eds. *Fluoride and Bone.* Bern: Huber, 1978: 155–162.
36. Mithal A, Trivedi N, Gupta SK, Dabadghao P, Godbole MM, Zaidi M. Skeletal fluoride toxicity in children: clinical, radiologic and metabolic profile (abstract). *J Bone Miner Res* 1995; 10 (Suppl): 246.
37. Manzke E, Rawley R, Vose G, Roginsky M, Rader JI, Baylink DJ. Effect of fluoride therapy on nondialyzable urinary hydroxyproline, serum alkaline phosphatase, parathyroid hormone and 25-hydroxyvitamin D. *Metabolism* 1977; 26: 1005–1010.

38. Liu C-C, Baylink DJ. Stimulation of bone formation and bone resorption by fluoride in thyroparathyroidectomized rats. *J Dent Res* 1977; 56: 304–311.
39. Gupta SK, Gambhir S, Mithal A, Das BK. Skeletal scintigraphic findings in endemic skeletal fluorosis. *Nucl Med Commun* 1993; 14: 384–390.
40. Compston JE, Chadha S, Merett AL. Osteomalacia developing during treatment of osteoporosis with sodium fluoride and vitamin D. *Br Med J* 1980; 281: 910–911.
41. Misra UK, Gujral RB, Sharma VP, Bhargava SK. Association of vitamin D deficiency with endemic fluorosis in India. *Fluoride* 1992; 25: 65–70.
42. Faccini JM, Teotia SPS. Histopathological assessment of endemic skeletal fluorosis. *Calcif Tissue Res* 1974; 16: 45–57.
43. Joswey J, Riggs BL, Kelly PJ, Hoffman DL. Effect of combined therapy with sodium fluoride, vitamin D and calcium in osteoporosis. *Am J Med* 1972; 53: 43–49.
44. Srikantia SG, Siddiqui AH. Metabolic studies in skeletal fluorosis. *Clin Sci* 1965; 28: 477–485.
45. Narasingarao BS, Siddiqui AH, Srikantia SG. A study of ^{45}Ca turnover in skeletal fluorosis. *Metabolism* 1968; 17: 366.
46. Rao SR, Murthy KJR, Murthy TVSD. Studies on calcium infusion in endemic fluorosis. *Fluoride* 1978; 11: 166–170.
47. Budden FH, Bayley TA, Harrison TA, *et al.* The effect of fluoride on bone histology depends on adequate fluoride absorption and retention. *J Bone Miner Res* 1988; 3: 127–132.
48. Narasingarao BS, Krishnamachari KAVR, Vijayasarathy C. ^{47}Ca turnover in endemic fluorosis and endemic genu valgum. *Br J Nutr* 1979; 41: 7–14.
49. Dure-Smith BA, Farley SM, Linkhar SG, Farley JR, Baylink DJ. Calcium deficiency in fluoride-treated osteoporotic patients despite calcium supplementation. *J Clin Endocrinol Metab* 1996: 81: 269–275.
50. Ranganathan S. Calcium intake and fluorine poisoning in rats. *Ind J Med Res* 1941; 29: 693–698.
51. Reddy GS, Srikantia SG. Effect of dietary calcium, vitamin C and protein in development of skeletal fluorosis. I. Growth, serum chemistry, and changes in composition, and radiological appearances of bones. *Metabolism* 1971; 20: 642–649.
52. Reddy GS, Narasingarao BS. Effect of dietary calcium, vitamin C and protein in development of experimental skeletal fluorosis. II. Calcium turnover with ^{45}Ca; calcium and phosphorus balances. *Metabolism* 1971; 20: 650–656.
53. Griffiths HJ, Hunt RD, Zimmerman RE, Finberg H, Cuttino J. The role of calcium and fluoride in osteoporosis in Rhesus monkeys. *Invest Radiol* 1975; 10: 263–268.

DISCUSSION

Dr. Gilsanz: Let me see if this scenario explains some of the things you see. We all agree that these children have abnormal bones, that the bone is weak, and weak bone bows. What does a growing child do? The mechanostat tells the body that it needs more bone, even if that bone is not of the best quality. And if you need more bone, you have greater nutrient requirements. If those requirements are unavailable, you will have the primary manifestations of whatever causes the deficiency, which in your case looks like rickets secondary to fluoride plus osteopenia. However, if there is adequate calcium availability, you may have increased bone mass but of poor-quality bone. This is not new. It has been described in children with rickets and renal osteodystrophy and in the very rare cases of primary hyperparathyroidism in childhood; it is also seen in children with fluorosis and in children treated with phosphonates. My concept is that in these children with weak bones and bowing, there is a smaller than normal proportion of calcium. More bone is needed, but you will only get more bone if there is adequate nutrient availability. Curiously, in the areas where the bones are growing fastest—the distal radius and the distal knees—the radiologic osteopenia will be more marked than in the areas that don't grow so fast.

Dr. Mithal: It is clear that there may be factors other than just calcium nutrition. Protein nutrition could also be involved, but the fact remains that if calcium is not available in the right amounts for these bones to mineralize, a lot of abnormal bone will be formed, which is what we see. And the fluoride insult actually increases calcium demand besides producing its own toxicity on the bone. So I think the combination of these is what we see.

Dr. Klish: I was fascinated by the water fluoride levels that you described. You gave a range of 4 to 19 parts per million; 19 ppm is obviously in the toxic range, but 4 ppm is very close to the optimal range with regard to good tooth development, and in the United States there are certain areas that have normal water fluoride content far greater than 4 ppm. Central Texas is one area where we see a lot of dental fluorosis, but I don't think I have ever seen a case of skeletal sclerosis in those children. So my question is related to what you were just discussing. There obviously have to be other factors involved if the children are getting bone defects when they are drinking water in that 4–8 ppm range. This may be as simple as total dose they may be drinking more water; the fluoride may be present in other foods that are grown in that water; or there may be nutrients other than calcium that are involved in this.

Dr. Mithal: This has been a subject of debate for a long time, and as you very rightly pointed out, 4 ppm is perfectly acceptable in some parts of the world. However, in Senegal dental fluorosis occurs with 1 ppm, and they feel that the WHO limit of 1.5 is too high: it should be 0.6. There are problems in China with similar fluoride levels. So I think there are several factors. Some you already enunciated: the fact that there is a major difference in nutrition and that they drink much more water in India, because of sweating in the hot climate. And there may be other factors that we don't know about. But clearly these levels of fluoride are not acceptable in semitropical or tropical scenarios like India and parts of Africa.

Dr. Pettifor: I would like to suggest that a relatively low calcium intake is beneficial to children or adults in endemic fluorosis areas. With a good calcium intake the severe side effects of osteosclerosis are more likely, with intramembranous calcification and all the complications related to excessive bone formation. I wonder whether the low calcium intakes are to a certain extent protective against the severe complications that one sees with the higher calcium intakes.

Dr. Mithal: If you are referring to osteosclerosis on its own, what you are saying is probably right, but when you talk of other manifestations of fluoride toxicity, it is the other way around: an increased calcium intake is desirable. You can't have it both ways. If you increase calcium, you may get more osteosclerosis, but you will get less osteopenia.

Dr. Pettifor: One doesn't want to push calcium intakes up too high, but it certainly should be out of the range that is going to produce rachitic lesions and bone deformities.

Dr. Mithal: Your point is illustrated by the studies from the Punjab, where the dietary calcium intakes are very high because they subsist mainly on dairy products. There you find very severe osteosclerosis with calcification of ligaments, which we certainly don't see to that degree in our population.

Dr. Tsang: How does the amount of fluoride ingested in total compare with therapeutic doses of fluoride advocated for osteoporosis?

Dr. Mithal: If you come from an area where the water contains 35 ppm, you would obviously have a very high fluoride load because you would be consuming at least 3 to 4 l of water per day. In this case the dose that you would get would be significantly higher—maybe three times higher—than you would use in the theraputic treatment of osteoporosis.

Dr. Marini: Can fluoride cross the placenta, and how early can you see these manifestations?

Dr. Mithal: Fluoride does cross the placenta, and the earliest cases that I have seen personally are in children who have just started walking, at 1 year. It is also excreted in breast milk.

Dr. Schofer: Could you explain again the vertebral changes you see in these patients? The deformities look as though there were fractures in the plates of the vertebrae. So is this osteosclerosis from the beginning, or is there osteopenia in the beginning with fractures and then secondary osteosclerosis, maybe of the ligaments mainly?

Dr. Mithal: This is guesswork. I think the child whose spine shows a plate within the vertebral body has been osteopenic from the start and has not developed osteosclerosis. The child with fish-shaped vertebrae has osteosclerosis. We did technetium scintigraphy in 17 of these patients, but we did not find any evidence of stress fractures or microfractures in these cases. Of course, we did find evidence of very high bone turnover, irrespective of other variables.

Dr. Bonjour: What happens to phosphate metabolism in these cases?

Dr. Mithal: I haven't looked at the phosphate metabolism in these cases, but Dr. Pettifor may have.

Dr. Pettifor: We have looked at phosphate excretion in children presenting with clinical rickets associated with endemic fluorosis, and they have high serum phosphate, they have reduced phosphate excretion, and they also have peripheral resistance to parathyroid hormone. I am not sure whether these changes are related to prolonged secondary hyperparathyroidism and renal resistance to parathyroid hormone, or whether it is, as you suggest, an increase in phosphate demand.

Dr. Mithal: I think in your own study when you corrected the calcium you found a reversal of this effect, so you did suggest that the hypocalcemia was probably responsible.

Dr. Pettifor: But to follow on from that, when we correct the calcium we are also correcting the demand for phosphate, because the only way one corrects the calcium is by correcting the osteomalacia, and therefore, the phosphate demands would have decreased, and that may have been one of the factors.

Dr. Arroyo: Could you comment on corrective public health measures that are being implemented and the attempts to eradicate this problem?

Dr. Mithal: The measures being adopted are as follows. Deep wells are being dug and mechanical hand pumps installed to pump up deep water (from 30 m deep or more), which significantly reduces the fluoride concentration, say from 10 ppm to 3 ppm. The concentration may still need to be lower, but in some areas hand pumps have made a significant difference. Then methods are being developed for defluoridation, and there are many teams of engineers working on this, using activated charcoal, etc., but the problem is with logistics. These villages do not have municipal water supplies, and even if you set up a defluoridation plant, you have to set up one in each village, and there are hundreds of villages; and then the plant needs maintenance, it needs replenishment of chemicals, cleaning, and so on, so there are many logistic problems. The government has now formed a National Drinking Water Mission, which is looking at this in a broad public healthcare way.

Dr. Arroyo: Could you also comment on the causes of calcium deficiency and what is being done in this regard?

Dr. Mithal: The cause of calcium deficiency is that there are virtually no milk products, and whatever calcium there is is derived from poor sources such as cereals. This will not improve until the whole system improves.

Dr. Klish: I am curious about fluorosis in terms of what is actually happening from a biochemical point of view. It is my understanding that fluoride is taken up in the hydration shells of the calcium hydroxyapatite crystals and creates a more stable crystalline structure. If that is true, does the sclerosis occur because of a problem of remodeling, that is, do the osteocytes have difficulty in reabsorbing this crystal so that it accumulates in the bone, or is it something more complicated than that?

Dr. Mithal: As of now it has been the hypothesis that the calcium fluorapatite crystal is very stable and does not dissolve easily. Its accumulation is what causes the problem.

Dr. Caverzasio: We have observed that the effects of fluoride on bone-forming cell replication require traces of aluminum, so it is probably a fluoroalumino complex that activates bone-forming cells. This goes along with what we were discussing before, that there are probably other nutrients or factors that are needed for the effect of fluoride on bone forming cells.

Nutrition and Bone Development, edited by
Jean-Philippe Bonjour and Reginald C. Tsang,
Nestlé Nutrition Workshop Series, Vol. 41, Nestec Ltd.,
Vevey/Lippincott–Raven Publishers,
Philadelphia © 1999.

Protein Intake During Childhood and Adolescence and Attainment of Peak Bone Mass

René Rizzoli, Patrick Ammann, Thierry Chevalley, and Jean-Philippe Bonjour

WHO Collaborating Center for Osteoporosis and Bone Diseases, Department of Internal Medicine, Division of Bone Diseases, University Hospital, 1211 Geneva 14, Switzerland

Although a gradual decline in energy intake with age can be considered an adequate adjustment to a progressive reduction in energy expenditure, a commensurate reduction in protein intake may be detrimental to the integrity and function of several organs or systems, including skeletal muscle and bone (1–3). Malnutrition, particularly protein undernutrition, appears to play a key role in the rising incidence of osteoporotic hip fracture observed in elderly people. Protein malnutrition may predispose to hip fracture by increasing the propensity to fall as a result of muscle weakness and impairment of coordination, and by decreasing bone mass.

The amount of bone present at a given age is determined by the mass acquired during growth (the so-called peak bone mass) and by the the subsequent rate of bone loss. The attainment of peak bone mass appears to be highly affected by the state of protein supply and intake during childhood and adolescence, when the need for protein is increased to meet the demands of body growth. It has also been shown that rats treated with growth hormone spontaneously select a high-protein diet (4). During growth, therefore, adaptation to a reduced protein intake should be much more difficult than later in life. Protein undernutrition results in a reduction in height, weight, and overall body protein (5). The recommended daily allowance for protein varies from 2.0 g/kg in children to 1.0 g in adolescents and 0.75 g in adults (6).

DISTURBANCES OF BONE HOMEOSTASIS IN PROTEIN UNDERNUTRITION

Insulin-like growth factor 1 (IGF-1) is an essential factor for longitudinal bone growth (7) as it stimulates proliferation and differentiation of chondrocytes in the epiphyseal plate (8,9). The IGF-1 also plays a role in trabecular and cortical bone formation. This factor can stimulate both proliferation and differentiation of osteoblasts; it increases type 1 collagen synthesis, alkaline phosphatase activity, and osteocalcin production (9). It can also selectively stimulate the transport of inorganic phosphate (Pi) across the plasma membrane in some osteoblastic cell lines (10). This effect could be important in the process of bone formation because Pi is an essential element for cellular growth. Insulin-like growth factor 1 has also been shown to inhibit the degradation of collagen produced by osteoblastic cells (8,9). Plasma levels of IGF-1 are closely related to the growth rate of the organism. It appears to play a key role in calcium-phosphate metabolism during growth by stimulating both the renal transport of Pi and the kidney production of calcitriol (11–13). Because of its renal action on tubular reabsorption of Pi and on the synthesis of calcitriol, IGF-1 can be considered an important controller of the intestinal absorption and extracellular concentration of both calcium and Pi, the main elements of bone mineral (12). This action could well explain the increase in plasma levels of both Pi and calcitriol during the pubertal period of rapid bone accrual (14). Before puberty, a deficiency of IGF-1, as occurs in growth hormone deficiency, or a resistance to its action, results in a diminution of skeletal longitudinal growth (15,16) and of the level of peak bone mass (17,18). Long-term repletion with growth hormone during adolescence can restore peak bone mass to a normal level (18).

Experimental and clinical studies suggest that dietary protein could control bone anabolism by influencing both the production and the action of growth factors, particularly the growth hormone–IGF system (19–21). Decreased levels of IGF-1 have been found in states of undernutrition such as marasmus, anorexia nervosa, celiac disease, or HIV-infected patients (22–26). Refeeding these patients leads to an increase of IGF-1 (27). Furthermore, an increased protein intake can prevent the decrease in IGF-1 usually observed in hypocaloric states (28).

The hepatic production and plasma levels of IGF-1 are under the influence of dietary protein (25,29). Protein restriction has been shown to reduce plasma IGF-1 by inducing a resistance to the action of growth hormone at the hepatic level (25,30,31) and by increasing the metabolic clearance rate of IGF-1 (32). Resistance to growth hormone depends on a decrease in hepatic binding sites for the hormone and on postreceptor defects (33,34). Thus, levels of hepatic IGF-1 mRNA are reduced by protein restriction through an alteration in transcription (35,36), and the hepatic IGF-1 translational process could be affected by protein deprivation (37). The effects of protein restriction on IGF-1 production could also be mediated by a reduction in the hepatic supply of some essential amino acids. Indeed, culture media deprived of tryptophan or lysine caused a selective reduction in the production of IGF-1 by cultured rat hepatocytes without affecting cell viability (38).

On the other hand, protein restriction could also render target systems less sensitive to IGF-1. When IGF-1 was given to rats maintained on a low-protein diet at doses sufficient to normalize its plasma concentration, it failed to restore skeletal longitudinal growth (33). The production of IGF binding proteins (IGFBP) is also influenced by protein energy restriction: IGFBP-1, IGFBP-2, and IGFBP-4, which are possible inhibitors of the action of IGF-1, were found to be increased by protein restriction

(35,39), especially in patients with recent hip fracture, whereas IGFBP-3 levels were lowered (24,40).

Among the hormones that can affect the metabolism and structural integrity of bone, there is no doubt that estrogen plays the most important role in women, at least after pubertal maturation. During the adolescence period, several observations made in pathologic conditions of insufficient estrogen production or inadequate estrogen action have suggested an important role of sex hormones in bone mass acquisition. However, it is not known whether differences in sex hormone secretion or action during pubertal maturation in healthy adolescents contribute to the large biological variability in bone mass gain. In addition to affecting IGF-1 levels, states of energy or protein undernutrition, such as anorexia nervosa, are associated with major hormonal disturbances, and these could also impair the attainment of a normal peak bone mass.

Finally, protein may directly influence osteogenic cells. Indeed, osteoblasts not only are equipped with specific IGF-1 receptors but can also be endowed with IGF-1-producing machinery. Several factors including growth hormone, estradiol, parathyroid hormone, calcitriol, glucocorticoids, and triiodothyronine have the capacity to modulate the expression of IGF-1 mRNA, the accumulation of immunoreactive IGF-1, and its action in bone culture systems (8,9,41,42). The local amino acid environment can also influence IGF-1 production by bone cells. Indeed, the amino acids arginine or lysine increased IGF-1 production in a time- and concentration-dependent manner (43). These results highlight the potential role of locally produced IGF-1 under the influence of extracellular amino acid concentration in the regulation of osteoblast function.

BONE MASS GAIN BEFORE AND DURING PUBERTY

Peak bone mass is defined as the amount of bony tissue present at the end of skeletal maturation (14). This biological variable is an important determinant of osteoporotic fractures later in life (44,45); hence, interest is growing in investigations aimed at understanding how bone mass evolves during development and at identifying the most important genetic and environmental factors, particularly nutritional, that influence its accumulation rate.

Before puberty, no consistent sex difference in bone mass of either the axial or the appendicular skeleton has been reported (14,17). There is no evidence of a gender difference in bone mass at birth. Likewise, the volumetric bone mineral density appears to be similar in both female and male newborns (14,17,46). This absence of sex difference in bone mass is maintained until the onset of the pubertal maturation. During puberty, the gender difference in bone mass becomes expressed. This difference appears to be caused by a more prolonged bone growth period in boys than in girls, with a larger increase in bone size and in cortical thickness (14,17,46–48). Puberty affects bone size much more than volumetric mineral density. There is no significant sex difference in the volumetric trabecular density at the end of pubertal maturation (14). During puberty, the accumulation rate in areal bone mineral density at both lumbar spine and femoral neck levels increases four- to sixfold over a 3- and 4-year period in girls and boys, respectively (47,48). The change in bone mass accumulation rate is less marked in long bone diaphyses. There is an asynchrony between the gain in statural height and bone mass growth (47,48). This phenomenon may be responsible for the occurrence of a transient period of relative increase in bone fragility that may account for the pattern of fracture incidence during adolescence (49,50).

At the beginning of the third decade, there is a large variability in the normal values of areal bone mineral density in both the axial and the appendicular skeleton (14). This large variance, which is observed at sites particularly susceptible to osteoporotic fractures such as the lumbar spine and the femoral neck, is barely reduced after correction for statural height (51) and does not appear to increase much during adult life. The height-independent variance in bone mass thus develops during puberty at sites such as the lumbar spine and the femoral neck, where the accretion rate is markedly increased (47,48,52).

Despite the fact that a majority of studies do not suggest that bone mass continues to accumulate significantly during the third and fourth decades, it is generally accepted that peak bone mass at any skeletal site is attained in both sexes during the mid-30s. However, recent studies indicate that in healthy Caucasian women with apparently adequate intakes of energy, protein, and calcium, bone mass accumulation can be virtually complete before the end of the second decade at both the lumbar spine and the femoral neck (47,48,53).

DETERMINANTS OF PEAK BONE MASS

Many factors, more or less independent of each other, are supposed to influence bone mass accumulation during growth. The list of these determinants classically includes: heredity, sex, dietary components (calcium, protein), endocrine factors (sex steroids, calcitriol, IGF-1), mechanical forces (physical activity, body weight), and exposure to risk factors (54–56). Quantitatively, the most prominent factor appears to be the genetic determinant. However, it is of practical interest that heredity is not the only determinant of peak bone mass. Thus, environmental factors can be modified, and their influence on bone thereby altered. Furthermore, such a modification of environmental factors could also have an impact on the genetic component by affecting the interaction between genes and the environment.

NUTRITIONAL FACTORS

Macronutrient Intakes During Pubertal Maturation

In healthy, apparently well-nourished children and adolescents, the question arises to what extent variations in the intakes of some nutrients (calcium and protein) can affect bone mass accumulation at sites susceptible to osteoporotic fracture. Indeed, as mentioned above, a height-independent broad variability in bone mass develops during puberty, both in the spine and in the proximal femur. Puberty is considered to be a period of major behavioral and life-style change. It is assumed that important modifications in food habits would occur during pubertal maturation, particularly in affluent societies. However, there is still a lack of quantitative and qualitative information on the evolution of macronutrient intakes in relation to pubertal maturation.

In a prospective survey carried out in about 200 female and male adolescents aged 9 to 19 years, food intake was assessed twice, with a 1-year interval, using a 5-day dietary diary method and weighing all consumed foods. Diaries were analyzed for consumption of macronutrients (lipid, carbohydrates, and protein) with nutrition-determining software integrating food composition tables and 103 local food items. The stage of puberty or sexual maturity was rated from stage P1 (prepubertal) to P5 (adult).

With respect to macronutrients, the results indicated that the total energy intake, which remained within the recommended dietary allowances (RDA), was significantly influenced by both pubertal maturation and sex when expressed in absolute terms but only by pubertal stage when adjusted per kilogram of body weight. Compared to the RDA, the macronutrient distribution of the total energy intake showed an excessive quantity of fat (especially saturated fatty acids) and an insufficient intake of carbohydrate-rich fiber. The intake of protein, two-thirds of which was from animal sources, was above the RDA. Overall, these inadequacies in macronutrient intake distribution were remarkably constant throughout pubertal maturation. Thus, our survey did not suggest that adolescence is a period of particular susceptibility to bad food habits (57). However, it did indicate that the affluent type of diet, which has been linked to several chronic diseases in adults from developed countries, is already in place before pubertal maturation, with only mild changes during adolescence.

Protein Intake and Bone Mass Accumulation

Various studies have found a relationship between the level of protein intake and either calcium-phosphate metabolism, bone mass, or the risk of osteoporotic fracture (58). Nevertheless, a long-term influence of dietary protein on bone mineral metabolism and skeletal mass has been difficult to establish. Apparently contradictory information suggests that either a deficient or an excessive protein supply could have a negative effect on calcium balance and on the amount of bony tissue contained in the skeleton (58,59). Therefore, with respect to nutrition, this means that either an increase or a decrease in protein intake could induce an incremental change in the calcium–phosphate balance and decelerate bone mass accrual, according to the prevailing physiological or clinical conditions. There may be several reasons for the present uncertainty about the effect of protein supplementation on calcium balance and bone mass. The outcomes may differ because the protein supplementation was (a) prescribed either to well-nourished people or to subjects showing signs of malnutrition; (b) given in various forms as natural food products (that is, ingested in complex forms) or administered as purified extracts or as mixtures of amino acids; (c) from either animal (for example casein) or vegetable (for example soy) origin; (d) evaluated in either the short or the long term; or (e) assessed in the presence or absence of modifications of other nutritional factors such as energy or calcium. Despite these uncertainties, several studies in both experimental animals and human subjects strongly suggest that a low protein intake *per se* could be particularly detrimental for both the acquisition of bone mass and the conservation of bone integrity with aging. As mentioned above, undernutrition during growth, including an inadequate supply of energy and protein, can severely impair bone development. Studies in experimental animals indicate that isolated protein deficiency leads to reduced bone mass and strength, that is, to osteoporosis, without histomorphometric evidence of osteomalacia (58,60). Thus, an inadequate supply of protein appears to play a central role in the pathogenesis of the delayed skeletal growth and reduced bone mass observed in undernourished children. The possible influences of protein metabolism on calcium phosphate metabolism during puberty are shown in Fig. 1.

In "well-nourished" children and adolescents, the question arises as to whether or not variations in the protein intake within the "normal" range can influence skeletal growth and thereby modulate the genetic potential for peak bone mass attainment (57). In the adolescent cohort described above, we have studied the relationship between bone mass gain at the lumbar and femoral levels and protein intake. Because both increased in the two sexes during adolescence, it was not surprising to find a positive correlation between these two variables. However, the correlation

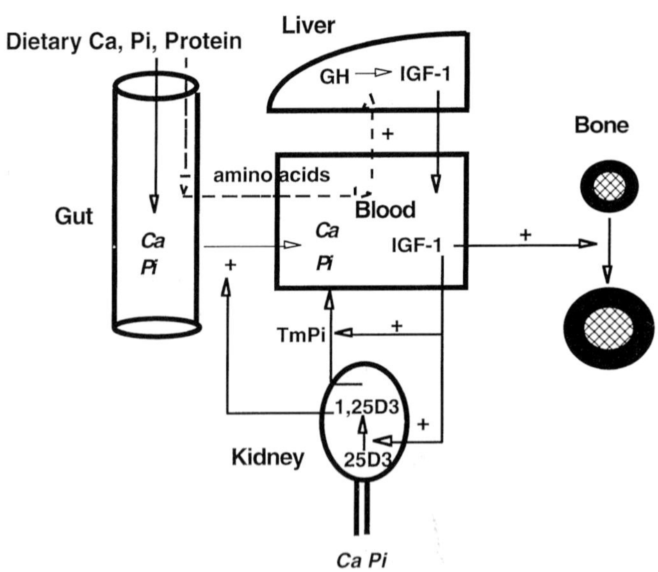

FIG. 1. Changes in calcium phosphate metabolism during puberty and possible influence of dietary protein.

was still statistically significant after correction for the influence of either age or pubertal stage. The association between bone mass gain and protein intake was observed in both sexes at the level of the lumbar spine, the proximal femur, and the midfemoral shaft. The association appeared to be particularly significant from pubertal stage P1 to P4. However, these results should not be interpreted as evidence for a causal relationship between bone mass gain and protein intake. Indeed, it is quite possible that the protein that was related to the overall amount of ingested energy in our cohort was to a large extent determined by growth requirements during childhood and adolescence.

As is the case for other nutrients such as calcium, only prospective interventional studies will ascertain whether variations in protein intake within the range recorded in our Western ''well-nourished'' population can affect bone mass accumulation during growth. Such prospective intervention studies will delineate the crucial years during which modifications in nutrition would be particularly effective for bone mass accumulation in children and adolescents. This kind of information is of importance in order to make credible and well-targeted recommendations in the perspective of setting up osteoporosis prevention programs aimed at maximizing peak bone mass.

CONCLUSIONS

Protein malnutrition appears to play an important role in the underdevelopment of bone and in the eventual bone loss, contributing to the risk of osteoporosis and osteoporotic fracture. Insulin-like growth factor 1 is a key factor in the adjustments of calcium-phosphate metabolism required for normal skeletal development and bone mineralization during growth. Indeed, IGF-1 is considered an essential factor for longitudinal bone growth, as it stimulates proliferation and differentiation of chondrocytes in the epiphyseal plate, and also for bone formation. A deficiency in IGF-1 or a resistance to its action, both of which can occur as a result of an inadequate protein supply, could result in a diminution of skeletal growth and development. In a cohort of 200 adolescents, an association between bone mass gain and protein intake was observed in both sexes at the level of the lumbar spine, the proximal femur, and the midfemoral shaft. This association appeared to be particularly significant from pubertal stages P1 to P4.

REFERENCES

1. Morley JE, Miller DK. Malnutrition in the elderly. *Hosp Pract* 1992; 27: 95–116.
2. Munro H, Schlierf G. *Nutrition of the elderly. Nestlé Nutrition Workshop Series No 29.* New York: Raven Press, 1992.
3. Sullivan DH, Carter WJ. Insulin-like growth factor I as an indicator of protein-energy undernutrition among metabolically stable hospitalized elderly. *J Am Coll Nutr* 1994; 13: 184–191.
4. Roberts TJ, Azain MJ, White DB, Martin RJ. Rats treated with somatotropin select diets higher in protein. *J Nutr* 1995; 125: 2669–2678.
5. Pellett PL. Protein requirements in humans. *Am J Clin Nutr* 1990; 51: 723–737.

6. National Research Council. Recommended Daily Allowances, 10th ed. Washington, DC: National Academy Press, 1989.
7. Froesch ER, Schmid C, Schwander J, Zapf J. Actions of insulin-like growth factors. *Annu Rev Physiol* 1985; 47: 443–467.
8. Canalis E, McCarthy TL, Centrella M. Growth factors and cytokines in bone cell metabolism. *Annu Rev Med* 1991; 42: 17–24.
9. Schmid C, Ernst M. Insulin-like growth factors. In: Gowen M, ed. *Cytokines and Bone Metabolism.* Boca Raton: CRC Press. 1992: 229–265.
10. Caverzasio J, Bonjour J-P. Insulin-like growth factors (IGF-1 and IGF-2) but not insulin selectively stimulate Na-dependent Pi transport activity in osteoblast-like cells (abstract). *J Bone Miner Res* 1990; 5 (Suppl 2): S228.
11. Caverzasio J, Bonjour J-P. Insulin-like growth factor I stimulates Na-dependent Pi transport in cultured kidney cells. *Am J Physiol* 1989; 257: F712–F717.
12. Caverzasio J, Montessuit C, Bonjour J-P. Stimulatory effect of insulin-like growth factor-1 on renal Pi transport and plasma 1,25-dihydroxyvitamin D_3. *Endocrinology* 1990; 127: 453–459.
13. Bonjour J-P, Caverzasio J. IGF-1, a key controlling element in phosphate homeostasis during growth. In: Spencer EM, ed. *Modern Concepts of Insulin-like Growth Factors.* New York: Elsevier Science, 1991: 193–198.
14. Bonjour J-P, Theintz G, Law F, Slosman D, Rizzoli R. Peak bone mass. *Osteoporosis Int* 1994; 4 (Suppl 1): 7–14.
15. Daughaday WH, Trivedi B. Absence of serum growth hormone binding protein in patients with growth hormone receptor deficiency (Laron dwarfism). *Proc Natl Acad Sci USA* 1987; 84: 4636–4640.
16. Merimee TJ, Zapf J, Hewlett B, Cavalli-Sforza LL. Insulin-like growth factors in pygmies. *N Engl J Med* 1987; 316: 906–911.
17. Hyer SL, Rodin DA, Tobias JH, Leiper A, Nussey SS. Growth hormone deficiency during puberty reduces adult bone mineral density. *Arch Dis Child* 1992; 67: 1472–1474.
18. Saggese G, Baroncelli GI, Bertelloni S, Barsanti S. The effect of long-term growth hormone (GH) treatment on bone mineral density in children with GH deficiency. Role of GH in the attainment of peak bone mass. *J Clin Endocrinol Metab* 1996; 81: 3077–3083.
19. Canalis E, Agnusdei D. Insulin-like growth factors and their role in osteoporosis. *Calcif Tissue Int* 1996; 58: 133–134.
20. Rosen CJ, Donahue LR. Insulin-like growth factors: potential therapeutic options for osteoporosis. *Trends Endocrinol Metab* 1995; 6: 235–241.
21. Bonjour J-P, Rizzoli R. Inadequate protein intake and osteoporosis: possible involvement of the IGF system. In: Burckhardt P, Heaney R, eds. *Challenges of Modern Medicine, vol 7.* Rome: Ares-Serono, 1995: 399–406.
22. Pucilowska JB, Davenport ML, Kabir I, *et al.* The effect of dietary protein supplementation on insulin-like growth factors (IGFs) and IGF-binding proteins in children with shigellosis. *J Clin Endocrinol Metab* 1993; 77: 1516–1521.
23. Hill KK, Hill DB, McClain MP, Humphries LL, McClain CJ. Serum insulin-like growth factor-1 concentrations in the recovery of patients with anorexia nervosa. *J Am Coll Nutr* 1993; 4: 475–478.
24. Smith WJ, Underwood LE, Clemmons DR. Effects of caloric or protein restriction on insulin-like growth factor-I (IGF-I) and IGF-binding proteins in children and adults. *J Clin Endocrinol Metab* 1995; 80: 443–449.
25. Thissen JP, Ketelslegers JM, Underwood LE. Nutritional regulation of the insulin-like growth factors. *Endocr Rev* 1994; 15: 80–101.
26. Ketelslegers J-M, Maiter D, Maes M, Underwood LE, Thissen J-P. Nutritional regulation of insulin-like growth factor-I. *Metabolism* 1995; 44: 50–57.
27. Clemmons DR, Underwood LE, Dickerson RN, *et al.* Use of plasma somatomedin-C/insulin-like growth factor-I measurements to monitor the response to nutritional repletion in malnourished patients. *Am J Clin Nutr* 1985; 41: 191–198.
28. Musey VC, Goldstein S, Farmer PK, Moore PB, Phillips LS. Differential regulation of IGF-I and IGF-binding protein-I by dietary composition in humans. *Am J Med Sci* 1993; 305: 131–138.
29. Isley WL, Underwood LE, Clemmons DR. Dietary components that regulate serum somatomedin-C concentrations in humans. *J Clin Invest* 1983; 71: 175–182.
30. Thissen JP, Triest S, Maes M, Underwood LE, Ketelslegers JM. The decreased plasma concentrations

of insulin-like growth factor-I in protein-restricted rats is not due to decreased number of growth hormone receptors on isolated hepatocytes. *J Endocrinol* 1990; 124: 159–165.

31. VandeHaar MJ, MoatsStaats BM, Davenport ML, *et al.* Reduced serum concentrations of insulinlike growth factor I (IGFI) in protein-restricted growing rats are accompanied by reduced IGFI mRNA levels in liver and skeletal muscle. *J Endocrinol* 1991; 130: 30512.
32. Thissen J-P, Davenport ML, Pucilowska J, Miles MV, Underwood LE. Increased serum clearance and degradation of (^{125}I)-labeled IGF-I in protein-restricted rats. *Am J Physiol* 1992; 262: E406–E411.
33. Thissen JP, Underwood LE, Maiter D, Maes M, Clemmons DR, Ketelslegers JM. Failure of insulin-like growth factor-I (IGF-I) infusion to promote growth in protein-restricted rats despite normalization of serum IGF-I concentrations. *Endocrinology* 1991; 128: 885–890.
34. Maiter D, Fliesen T, Underwood LE, *et al.* Dietary protein restriction decreases insulin-like growth factor I independent of insulin and liver growth hormone binding. *Endocrinology* 1989; 124: 2604–2611.
35. Straus DS, Takemoto CD. Effect of dietary protein deprivation on insulin-like growth factor (IGF)-I and (IGF)-II, IGF binding protein-2, and serum albumin gene expression in rat. *Endocrinology* 1990; 127: 1849–1860.
36. Straus DS, Takemoto CD. Effect of fasting on insulin-like growth factor-I (IGF-I) and growth hormone receptor messenger RNA levels and IGF-I gene transcription in rat liver. *Mol Endocrinol* 1990; 4: 91–100.
37. Thissen JP, Triest S, Moats-Staats BM, *et al.* Evidence that pretranslational and translational defects decrease serum insulin-like growth factor-I concentrations during dietary protein restriction. *Endocrinology* 1991; 129: 429–435.
38. Harp JB, Goldstein S, Phillips LS. Molecular regulation of IGF-1 by amino acid availability in cultured hepatocytes. *Diabetes* 1991; 40: 95–101.
39. Straus DS, Burke EJ, Marten NW. Induction of insulin-like growth factor binding protein-1 gene expression in liver of protein-restricted rats and in rat hepatoma cells limited for a single amino acid. *Endocrinology* 1993; 132: 1090–1100.
40. Schürch MA, Rizzoli R, Vadas L, Slosman DO, Bonjour J-P. Protein supplements in elderly with a recent hip fracture increase serum IGF-1, decrease urinary deoxypyridinoline, and prevent proximal femur bone loss (abstract). *J Bone Miner Res* 1996; 11 (Suppl 1): S139.
41. Chen LC, Mallory JB, Hintz RL. Dexamethasone and 1,25$(OH)_2$ vitamin D_3 modulate the synthesis of insulin-like growth factor-I in osteoblast-like cells. *Calcif Tissue Int* 1991; 48: 278–282.
42. Kurose H, Yamaoka K, Okada S, Nakajima S, Seino Y. 1,25-Dihydroxyvitamin-D_3 (1,25-$(OH)_2D_3$) increases insulin-like growth factor-I (IGF-I) receptors in clonal osteoblastic cells. Study on interaction of IGF-I and 1,25-$(OH)_2D_3$. *Endocrinology* 1990; 126: 2088–2094.
43. Chevalley T, Rizzoli R, Manen D, Caverzasio J, Bonjour J-P. Arginine increases IGF-1 production and collagen synthesis in osteoblastic cells (abstract). *J Bone Miner Res* 1996; 11 (Suppl 1): S375.
44. Dempster DW, Lindsay R. Pathogenesis of osteoporosis. *Lancet* 1993; 34: 797–801.
45. Riggs BL, Melton LJ. Drug therapy. The prevention and treatment of osteoporosis. *N Engl J Med* 1992; 327: 620–627.
46. Gilsanz V, Gibbens DT, Roe TF, *et al.* Vertebral bone density in children: effect of puberty. *Radiology* 1988; 166: 847–850.
47. Bonjour J-P, Theintz G, Buchs B, Slosman D, Rizzoli R. Critical years and stages of puberty for spinal and femoral bone mass accumulation during adolescence. *J Clin Endocrinol Metab* 1991; 73: 555–563.
48. Theintz G, Buchs B, Rizzoli R, *et al.* Longitudinal monitoring of bone mass accumulation in healthy adolescents: evidence for a marked reduction after 16 years of age at the levels of lumbar spine and femoral neck in female subjects. *J Clin Endocrinol Metab* 1992; 75: 1060–1065.
49. Bailey DA, Wedge JH, McCullogh RG, Martin AD, Bernhardson SC. Epidemiology of fractures of the distal end of the radius in children as associated with growth. *J Bone Joint Surg [Am]* 1989; 71A: 1225–1230.
50. Fournier PE, Rizzoli R, Slosman DO, Theintz G, Bonjour J-P. Asynchrony between the rates of statureal height gain and bone mass accumulation during puberty. *Osteoporosis Int* 1997; 7: 525–532.
51. Fournier PE, Rizzoli R, Slosman DO, Buchs B, Bonjour J-P. Relative contribution of vertebral body and posterior arch in female and male lumbar spine peak bone mass. *Osteoporosis Int* 1994; 4: 264–272.
52. Glastre C, Braillon P, David L, Cochat P, Meunier PJ, Delmas PD. Measurement of bone mineral

content of the lumbar spine by dual energy x-ray absorptiometry in normal children correlations with growth parameters. *J Clin Endocrinol Metab* 1990; 70: 1330–1333.
53. Slosman DO, Rizzoli R, Pichard C, Donath A, Bonjour J-P. Longitudinal measurement of regional and whole body bone mass in young healthy adults. *Osteoporosis Int* 1994; 4: 185–190.
54. Pocock NA, Eisman JA, Hopper JL, Yeates MG, Sambrook PN, Eberl S. Genetic determinants of bone mass in adults a twin study. *J Clin Invest* 1987; 80: 706–710.
55. Bell NH, Shary J, Stevens J, Garza M, Gordon L, Edwards J. Demonstration that bone mass is greater in black than in white children. *J Bone Miner Res* 1991; 6: 719–723.
56. Dequeker J, Nijs N, Vestraeten A, Geusens P, Gevers G. Genetic determinants of bone mineral content at the spine and radius: a twin study. *Bone* 1987; 8: 207–209.
57. Clavien HH, Theintz G, Rizzoli R, Bonjour J-P. Does puberty alter dietary habits in adolescents living in a Western society? *J Adolesc Health* 1996; 19: 68–75.
58. Orwoll ES. The effects of dietary protein insufficiency and excess on skeletal health. *Bone* 1992; 13: 343–350.
59. Bonjour J-P, Rizzoli R. Bone acquisition in adolescence. In: Marcus R, Feldman D, Kelsey J, eds. *Osteoporosis.* San Diego: Academic Press, 1996: 465–476.
60. Ferretti JL, Tessaro RD, Delgado CJ, Bozzini CE, Alippi RM, Barcelo AC. Biochemical performance of diaphyseal shafts and bone tissue of femur from protein-restricted rats. *Bone Miner* 1988; 4: 329–339.

DISCUSSION

Dr. Tsang: In the P1 study, the increase in protein intake was probably associated with an increase in mineral intake, so was it mineral that was the dominant correlate, or was it protein?

Dr. Rizzoli: In the diary all kinds of foods were recorded, including calcium, phosphate, and other nutrients, and when this was assessed in a multiple regression or stepwise regression, correcting for the intake of calcium and other nutrients, only the protein remained, so it seems that the association was with protein and not anything else.

Dr. Guesry: You showed observational and interventional studies reporting increased growth related to increased protein intake, but you didn't mention the source of the protein. If the source is dairy products, you will increase calcium intake simultaneously, but alternative sources of protein could increase the phosphate intake more, so the type of protein supplement is obviously relevant.

Dr. Rizzoli: I agree. In fact, about two-thirds of the protein were of animal origin, and probably two-thirds of that were dairy products, but even after adjustment for the calcium and phosphate intake, the correlation was still significant in terms of protein and changes in bone mass.

Dr. Haschke: Assuming that IGF-1 is an important factor for growth and bone development, it is worth emphasizing that zinc is very much involved in the regulation of IGF-1 production at the cellular level, and people who work on the relationship between zinc deficiency and impaired growth have always pointed out that marginal zinc supply might be more important than protein or other nutrient supply. In animal experiments it has already been shown that IGF-1 can be efficiently modulated by zinc (1).

Dr. Rizzoli: In our laboratory we have carried out many different manipulations of protein intakes and IGF-1 levels in relation to animal growth, and in all the diets we have used, we have always added trace elements to be certain that the results were not distorted by trace element deficiency. I know that zinc was regularly added to the food in this way.

Dr. Haschke: Of interest is the situation in China, where the prevalence of osteoporotic

TABLE 1. *Age-standardized rates of hip fracture (per 100,000)*

	Men	Women
Beijing	97	88
U.S. Caucasians	207	559

From Xu Ling et al. (2).

hip (Table 1) and vertebral fractures (Table 2) seems to be substantially lower than in the United States.

The data from Xu Ling *et al.* (2) also confirm that calcium intake of Chinese women is lower than that of American women: at ages 50 to 59, 60 to 69, 70 to 79, and beyond 80, mean daily calcium intakes are 328, 347, 325, and 308 mg/day, respectively. The RDA values are between 700 and 1,500 mg/day, and the EU Population Reference intake is 700 mg/day.

Therefore, factors other than calcium intake must be discussed in order to explain the low prevalence of osteoporotic fractures in Chinese women. Indeed, Xu Ling *et al.* (2) show (Table 3) differences in anthropometric parameters between elderly Chinese and American women. The higher level of physical activity in Chinese women is of particular interest. It seems prudent to consider genetic, anthropometric, socioeconomic, and life-style factors as confounders when future studies evaluate the influence of nutritional factors on bone mineral density of the elderly.

Dr. Rizzoli: Regarding the prevalence of osteoporosis in China, this depends on how you define it. In terms of low bone mineral density, normative values for China are only just starting to be published—the first data appeared 2 years ago. So this is a relatively new aspect, and I am not sure that the prevalence of osteoporosis is going to turn out to be especially low, provided you correct for local normative values and age. With an aging population, I suspect that the high incidence of femoral neck fractures will increase.

Dr. Eisman: The decision about whether there is osteoporosis or not depends on the definition you use and on whether people decide that a fracture is normal when related to aging, or whether they decide to apply the term ''osteoporosis.'' I think the primary lack of osteoporosis in China is the lack of the application of the name rather than a lack of fractures or causes of fractures.

Dr. Prentice: I have been working with a colleague at Shenyang Medical College in the Northeast of China. She has been collecting statistics from the hospitals in the city that see orthopedic cases, and they certainly do have a lower rate of femoral neck fractures or hip

TABLE 2. *Age-standardized prevalence of vertebral fractures of women in Beijing and Minnesota*

	Percentage prevalence	
Age (years)	Beijing	Minnesota
50–59	5	11
60–69	16	15
70–79	19	32
80+	37	35

From Xu Ling et al. (2).

TABLE 3. *Some differences between Chinese and U.S. women*

	China	United States
Weight (kg)	55.5	66.6
Height (cm)	152	158
Knee height (cm)	46.5	49.3
Able to squat (%)	93	64
Walking >1 hr/day (%)	94	8

From Xu Ling et al. (2).

fractures in that part of China, and the incidence is greater in men than in women. Fractures also seem to occur earlier than in the West.

Dr. Klish: You alluded to mechanical factors that are involved in the relationship between protein and bone growth. When there is a decrease in these mechanical factors, either with bed rest or with weightlessness during space travel, protein has a negative impact on calcium retention and causes hypercalciuria. My question is, in this extreme situation relating to mechanical factors, could there be a plateau beyond which an increase in protein intake could initiate the same mechanisms that you see in weightlessness?

Dr. Rizzoli: Your question has two parts, the muscle issue and the high-protein issue. I think the muscle issue is very important. In our study in elderly people, where we gave a protein supplement that just corrected, but did not overcorrect the deficiency, we observed not only the effect on bone mass that I showed today but also a small increase in muscle strength at the biceps level. This could be mediated by IGF-1 because we found a higher blood IGF-1 level on protein supplementation. The point you raise is a very important one, that when we look at bone we should look at muscle concomitantly because muscle and bone are two targets for IGF-1. Regarding the protein issue, in a shift from a deficient intake to a relatively normal intake, there is so far no evidence that protein could be detrimental to bone. On the other hand, if you start from a normal intake and increase the intake to supranormal levels, then protein could be detrimental. The pathophysiology of the hypercalciuria is probably related to proton production in urine.

Dr. Rigo: In your group P1 you had a positive correlation with total protein intake, but is the correlation still positive if you adjust for body size or height or if you express protein intake per kilogram body weight per day because total protein intake may also be related to the body size?

Dr. Rizzoli: As I mentioned before, this analysis was done as a multiple regression, in which we included not only the various nutrients but also weight and height. The greatest significance was between bone mass and protein intake, even when we corrected for the size of the individual.

Dr. Marini: You say that the rise in protein intake increases the level of IGF-1. What about binding proteins, because they can neutralize the effect of IGF-1?

Dr. Rizzoli: There is an abundance of data *in vitro,* in animals and in humans, showing that protein depletion is associated with an increase in IGF-BP2 and IGF-BP1 and a decrease in BP3, and the decrease in BP3 could contribute to the higher metabolic rate. When you refeed the animals, you will have the opposite effect—a decrease in IGF-BP1 and BP2 and an increase in BP3. Thus, you are likely to increase the half-life of IGF-1 and have a positive effect. In humans the changes are in the same direction.

Dr. Prentice: Are you suggesting that there is a bell-shaped curve—that a low protein intake is detrimental but a high protein intake is detrimental as well?

Dr. Rizzoli: Yes, that was the point I was making.

Dr. Prentice: And is it the change in protein intake toward the end of childhood that is important rather than the actual level of protein intake during the prepubertal phase? That was what you were implying from your data, I think.

Dr. Rizzoli: Because I don't know the change in the absolute level, I can't answer that.

Dr. Prentice: But if you plotted your graphs against the absolute protein intake of your children in P1, P2, etc., rather than as a change over that year, did you see a relationship?

Dr. Rizzoli: Yes, there is also a relationship.

Dr. Eisman: Much of the focus has been on hip fractures. A comment that was made to me is that in many environments an older woman may just go to bed and not get up, particularly where there is limited access to medical care. This might well be because of a hip fracture. I can't say whether this is true, but it may well be that some of the apparently lower incidences that are recorded in women may not necessarily be accurate.

Dr. Prentice: I have asked that question myself of my colleagues at the medical college in Shenyang, and they say that in the urban areas that is not the case. There is very good access to hospital care, and women with hip fractures would be expected to present to hospital and would probably do so. The situation in rural areas may well be different.

Dr. Seeman: I would like to draw your attention to a paper by Harold Rosen (3). This was an elegant study in rats to which IGF-1 and growth hormone were given. They showed an increase in bone size and in bone mass. However, the bone size increase outstripped the bone mass increase, so the volumetric density went down.

Dr. Rizzoli: I am aware of this paper, and it partly confirmed something we published earlier regarding the effect of IGF-1 in causing increased bone size (4).

Dr. Guesry: In certain parts of the world such as China, the diet is rich in soy protein, which contains very low levels of sulfur amino acids. I think it would be interesting to dissect out the role of different amino acids in relation to IGF-1.

Dr. Rizzoli: This is exactly what we are doing now, but the data are too preliminary to give any results as yet.

Dr. Mithal: In India there are no norms for bone density, and they are just being developed now. There are also no reliable data on osteoporotic fractures. But there were several studies done 20 years or more ago in urban hospitals where people have access to health care, which show exactly what Dr. Prentice has described, that hip fractures seemed to occur more in men than in women and about 10 to 15 years earlier than in the West.

REFERENCES

1. Haschke F, Male C. Trace elements in children and adolescents. In: *Feeding from Toddlers to Adolescence. Nestlé Nutrition Workshop Series, Vol 37.* Nestec Ltd./Vevey/Lippincott–Raven Publishers, Philadelphia, 1996.
2. Xu Ling, Lu Aimin, Zhao Xihe, Chen Xiaoshu, Cummings SR. Very low rates of hip fracture in Beijing, People's Republic of China: The Beijing Osteoporosis Project. *Am J Epidemiol* 1996; 144: 901–907.
3. Rosen HN, Chen V, Greenspan SL, Douglas PS, Moses AC, Beamer WG. Treatment with growth hormone and IGF-1 in growing rats increases bone mineral content but not bone mineral density. *J Bone Miner Res* 1995; 10: 1352–1358.
4. Ammann P, Rizzoli R, Müller K, Slosman D, Bonjour J-P. IGF-I and pamidronate increase bone mineral density in ovariectomized adult rats. *Am J Physiol* 1993; 265: E770–E776.

Nutrition and Bone Development, edited by
Jean-Philippe Bonjour and Reginald C. Tsang,
Nestlé Nutrition Workshop Series, Vol. 41, Nestec Ltd.,
Vevey/Lippincott–Raven Publishers,
Philadelphia © 1999.

Delayed Puberty and Skeletal Growth in Mass, Size, and Density

Ego Seeman

Department of Endocrinology, Austin Hospital, The University of Melbourne, Heidelberg, Melbourne, Victoria 3084, Australia

ROLE OF SKELETAL GROWTH IN THE PATHOGENESIS OF OSTEOPOROSIS

Excessive Bone Loss May Not Be Responsible for the Deficit in Bone Density in Patients with Fractures

Bone mass in adulthood is a function of the amount of bone gained during growth and lost during aging. Because fractures occur late in life, and patients with fractures have low areal bone density relative to age-matched controls, investigators believe that these patients have lost more bone than the rest of the aging population. Although this may be the case in many patients, excessive bone loss may not be the explanation for the lower areal bone density in all patients because: (a) normal or low circulating biochemical measures of bone turnover are often found; (b) bone balance at the basic multicellular unit (BMU) may not be negative; (c) bone balance at the BMU may be negative, but no more negative than in controls (that is, the patients are not losing bone faster than controls) (1).

Bone Mass in the Elderly Is Determined More by the Amount of Bone Gained During Growth Than Lost During Aging

Low volumetric density results when mass is lower (relative to its mean) than size (relative to its mean). Peak bone mass is largely accrued by 18 years. Total body calcium increases from 25 to 30 g at birth to about 1,000 g by 15 to 20 years of age, an increment that is more than twice the loss during adulthood in women and is several times more rapid. Peak total body calcium is 1,200 g in white men and 900 g in white women. Net bone loss from youth to old age is 100 g in men and 250 g in women. The gender difference in bone mass between elderly white men and women is about 400 g, of which about 300 g represents the greater net gain in men during growth and about 150 g results from the greater net loss in women.

Total body calcium is 1,418 g and 1,224 g in pre- and postmenopausal blacks and 1,248 g and 1,018 g in pre- and postmenopausal whites, respectively, giving net losses of 194 g in blacks and 230 g in whites (2). Thus, of the 206 g (1,224 − 1,018 g) greater mass in postmenopausal blacks than whites, 170 g represents the greater net gain in blacks than whites, and 36 g results from the greater net loss in whites than blacks. Similar calculations show that of the 74 g greater upper body bone mass in postmenopausal blacks than whites, 52 g results from greater net gain in blacks, and 22 g from greater net loss in whites. Of the 132 g greater lower body bone mass in postmenopausal blacks, 118 g results from greater net gain in blacks, and 14 g from greater net loss in whites. Thus, the higher bone mass in blacks than whites in the postmenopausal years and the higher bone mass in men than women in old age (when fractures occur) are better accounted for by the greater net gains during growth than by losses during aging.

The Importance of the Large Population Variance in the Volumetric Density

Low volumetric density results when mass is lower (relative to its mean) than size (relative to its mean). Not only are the net increments large during growth, but the variance in peak volumetric bone density is also large; 1 standard deviation (SD) is 10% of the mean (1 SD in height = 4%). Volumetric bone density at the fifth centile is 30% less than that at the 95th centile, a difference greater than found between women with fractures and controls. Thus, the position of peak volumetric density attained during growth is important because it establishes the biological significance of bone loss during aging. This position may vary from region to region. Premenopausal daughters of women with spine fractures have reduced areal bone density at the spine by −0.7 SD compared to controls (3). The premenopausal daughters of women with hip fractures have reduced areal bone density at the femoral neck by −0.5 SD, with slightly higher values at the spine (+0.25 SD, NS) (4). Thus, there may be deficits in peak bone density at the spine, proximal femur, or both that are the result of environmental or genetic factors operating during growth. The site and severity of the deficits may then contribute to the age of onset and types of fractures seen in old age.

These observations imply that the period of growth is important in the development of the pathogenesis of bone fragility in old age. Exposure to illness or risk factors that interrupt either growth or mineral accrual may result in large deficits in bone mass, possibly larger than those resulting from exposure to similar risk factors that may accelerate bone loss in adulthood. Similarly, protective factors may confer a greater benefit when exposure occurs during growth and development. For example, in adults, weight-bearing exercise may increase areal bone density by 1% to 5%, amounts that are unlikely to substantially reduce fracture risk. By contrast, in the prepubertal years, increases in bone mass of 10% to 15% may result, and these may be sustained into adulthood and are large enough to reduce fracture risk (5).

WHAT IS THE QUESTION? PROBLEMS IN THE USE OF DENSITOMETRY TO STUDY GROWTH

An important concern in the study of skeletal growth osteoporosis is the use of the term "density." This is particularly important in the study of skeletal growth, where increasing bone size will be reported and (mis)understood as an increase in density. The densitometric measurement provides an integrated sum of the mineral mass within a projected area or estimated volume of a bony structure, not all of which is bone mineral. Size is not taken into account when bone mass is expressed in grams and is only partly taken into account when it is expressed as an areal apparent density (grams per square centimeter). Failure to adjust for size may result in reporting a reduced bone mass or areal bone density in a bone that has the same amount of bone within its periosteal boundary but is smaller than the reference specimen: both specimens have the same volumetric bone density—the same amount of bone in the bone—they differ only in size.

The structural basis underlying the increase in density during growth is not conveyed by the term "density." Rather than asking about the effects of delayed puberty on bone "density," it may be more instructive to ask about the effects of delayed puberty on trabecular number, thickness, and connectivity; on periosteal apposition, endosteal resorption, and accretion; and on net cortical thickness, bone size, and bone shape (a neglected determinant of bone strength). Are the effects of delayed puberty different at the axial and appendicular skeleton, in boys and girls, or from ethnic group to ethnic group? Are some or all of the effects reversible when puberty begins? Why does puberty occur at the chronological age of 12 to 13 years in girls and 14 to 15 years in boys? Is the pubertal growth response of a trait best at these times and less ideal before or after? If so, what are the physiological events at these ages that make this the most opportune time for puberty to occur? Why are there secular trends in puberty? What effect do they have on bone mass, size, volumetric density at the axial and appendicular skeleton, proximal femoral geometry, and perhaps the epidemiology of fractures? Does puberty occur at different ages in different ethnic groups? If so, why, and what are the effects on the skeleton? We have few answers to these questions.

The failure of densitometric methods to account for size has led to the erroneous view that bone density increases during growth. This view is prevalent because of the conventional graphic display of areal bone density increasing with age as shown in Fig. 1. Cortical bone density does not increase during growth; bone size increases (6,7). When size is taken into account, the amount of bone in the enlarging long bone is constant—volumetric bone density is independent of age because the increase in bone mineral mass and the increase in bone volume are proportional. If this is true, then the factors that determine whether an individual has a higher or a lower volumetric density must do so early in development, perhaps before birth (provided that bone mass tracks, as height does).

The amount of bone mass in the bone does increase out of proportion to the size increase at the spine. Volumetric bone density at the spine increases when measured

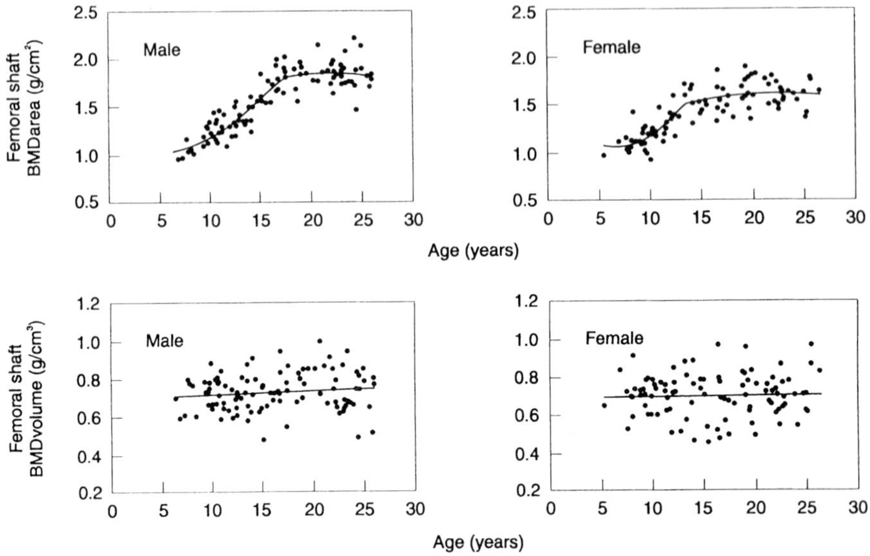

FIG. 1. Areal and volumetric femoral shaft bone mineral density (BMD) plotted against age for male and female subjects. From Lu *et al.* (7).

by quantitative computed tomography in boys and girls to the same degree: volumetric trabecular bone density is the same in both sexes—they have similar numbers of trabeculae of similar thickness. By contrast, the difference in trabecular volumetric density in black and white girls emerges at puberty (8). This may be the result of trabecular thickening or increasing numbers; probably the former, as trabecular numbers are similar in adult black and white women (9). Trabecular number and thickness are the same in men and women (10). (The continued increase in volumetric apparent bone mineral density by the method of Carter *et al.* may be also be the result of a size increase in the posterior processes, which are included in the measurement.)

Whether the variance in volumetric density increases with age and at puberty is uncertain. The variance in height does not appear to increase. If variance in volumetric density increases at puberty, this implies that sex steroids increase trabecular number, thickness, or cortical thickness more in some women than in others. Cortical thickness increases at puberty by increased periosteal apposition, which results in an increase in bone size. In girls, medullary contraction occurs as endosteal bone formation contributes to cortical thickness (11). The increase in medullary contraction occurs earlier at the metacarpal bones than at the midfemur (S. Bass and E. Seeman, *unpublished data*), consistent with the earlier maturation of distal segments than of proximal segments (12). In boys, puberty is associated with an increase in cortical thickness as a result of periosteal expansion, but medullary contraction does not occur, or maybe less than in girls.

Whether the amount of bone in the bone, volumetric density, is lower in patients with delayed puberty than in controls matched either by chronological age or by bone age and bone size is uncertain. The sole study to address this was published in abstract form only. Moore *et al.* report that boys aged 20 years with a history of delayed puberty had normal volumetric bone density (13). These data are seemingly contrary to the data suggesting that delayed puberty results in low areal bone density in males.

Finkelstein *et al.* have suggested that men with constitutionally delayed puberty may have a low peak areal bone density in adulthood (14,15). There were two control groups: 21 men 2 years younger and 39 men 2 years older than the cases. Lumbar spine areal bone density in the cases was 1.03 g/cm^2, 0.10 g/cm^2 less than the younger controls and 0.05 g/cm^2 less than the 60 controls combined. Results for the 39 older controls were not provided but must have been lower than the younger controls to bring the mean from 1.13 g/cm^2 in the younger controls to 1.08 g/cm^2 for all 60 controls; lumbar spine areal bone density should be about 1.03 g/cm^2 in the older controls, no different from the cases. In a follow-up study 2 years later in 18 men, radial and spinal areal bone mineral density were reduced as reported earlier. Femoral neck areal bone mineral density, measured for the first time, was lower than in controls, at 0.88 $\pm$ 0.11 versus 0.98 $\pm$ 0.14 g/cm^2 ($p < 0.02$). The subjects exercised 48 $\pm$ 104 miles/week. Thirty-five percent of the cases ran more than 15 miles per week, and 57% were regular weight lifters. The patients may have had hypogonadotrophic hypogonadism, not constitutionally delayed puberty.

THE VARIANCE IN VOLUMETRIC DENSITY

The Interaction Between Differing Mass and Size as One Possible Mechanism for the Population Variance

What accounts for the variance in volumetric bone density? What factors determine whether the volumetric density is at the fifth or 95th centile? Relative to the fifth centile, persons with volumetric density in the 95th centile have 30% to 40% higher volumetric bone density. This must represent more and/or thicker trabeculae, greater cortical thickness, reduced cortical porosity, or some combination of these. Two individuals with identical volumetric bone density may differ by one having double the number of trabeculae of half the thickness—the same mineral mass with more surface and thinner trabeculae. What factors regulate this heterogeneity? How may deficits in volumetric density develop in a region during growth? How may deficits in volumetric density occur to a greater extent at one site than at another? Could there be mechanisms that result in a reduced volumetric bone density at one site and a high volumetric bone density at another?

The amount of bone calcium (per mass of fat-free tissue) is established in early intrauterine life and is constant from early gestation to old age (16–18). That is, true density, the amount of bone mineral in a volume of bone mineral, is constant. Volumetric density is mistakenly called "true" density. Unstated but implicit in the use of "true" is the notion that this is the best surrogate of strength. There is no evidence to support this view. Density need not be volumetric to be "true." Areal bone density (g/cm^2), bone mineral apparent density (BMAD, g/cm^3), and volumetric density are all *apparent* density measurements—the amount of bone contained within a region, not all of which is bone.

Higher and Lower Volumetric Density: Discordance in Matching of Size and Mass

Volumetric *apparent* density is a function of the amount of bone mineral contained within the periosteal confines of a bone region, not all of which is bone mineral. Thus, volumetric density is determined by the relationship between the numerator—mass and how it is fashioned into cancellous bone or compact bone—and the denominator—bone size or volume as defined by the periosteal membrane. Even if the distinction between cortical and trabecular bone within the periosteum is disregarded for a moment, while bone mass and size are in the same percentile or *z* score (standard deviation, SD) relative to their respective means, volumetric density will be in the midnormal range. If an illness reduces bone size and mineral accrual comparably, then volumetric bone density may be normal. Girls with Turner's syndrome have small bones but normal volumetric bone density (19). High volumetric density results when mass is higher (relative to its mean) than size (relative to its mean). An example of this is in prepubertal gymnasts: they accrue more bone in a smaller bone, and, at least at appendicular sites, a greater percentage of cortical bone as a result of smaller medullary size (20). The data in precocious puberty are scant, but if size is reduced because of sex steroid-dependent epiphyseal closure, and mineral accrual is increased, then volumetric density would be predicted to be high. Low volumetric density results when mass is lower (relative to its mean) than size (relative to its mean). Klinefelter's disease may be an example of the latter. These relationships are illustrated in Fig. 2.

Healthy women aged 20 to 40 years with volumetric density in the lowest tertile have bone mass in the lowest tertile but bone volume in the highest tertile, not the middle tertile as might be expected (Duan Y. and Seeman E., unpublished data). For some reason, some individuals accrue the same mass in a bigger bone by accruing either less cortical thickness, fewer trabeculae, or thinner trabeculae. The genetic and environmental factors regulating bone mass and size are unknown, and the mechanisms responsible for concordance or discordance for the respective trait positions in their respective normal distributions are unknown.

In delayed puberty, volumetric density may be reduced if the epiphyses remain patent and bone size increases as mineral accrual is reduced. If accrual is reduced, this should result in reduced cortical thickness, fewer or thinner trabeculae. That is, compared with either an age-matched or bone-age-matched (but younger) control subjects, trabecular volumetric density should be lower, and cortical thickness should be lower. If delayed puberty results in comparably reduced bone size and reduced accrual, volumetric density may be normal (compared with either control mentioned

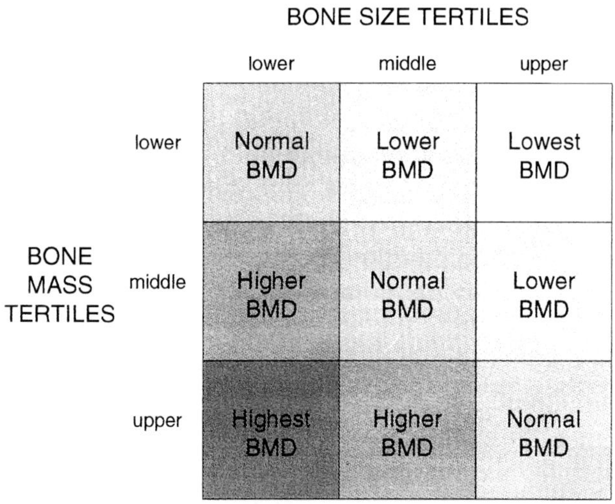

FIG. 2. Volumetric bone density will be in the middle tertile if bone mass and bone size are each in the same tertile of their own trait. High volumetric density results when mass is in a higher tertile than size; lower volumetric density results when mass is in a lower tertile than size.

above); if the reduction in bone size were greater (relative to its mean) than the reduction in accrual (relative to its mean), then volumetric bone density may be high!

When the results are expressed as a bone mineral content (g) and areal density (g/cm^2), as they usually are, the observations are more difficult to interpret as size is not taken into account. Bone mineral content and areal density may be reduced in children with delayed puberty compared with controls matched for chronological age, as the controls must have a skeleton that is more advanced in maturity and nearer its (larger) adult size. If the controls are chosen to be younger, to match for bone size and skeletal age, then chronological age must be less in the controls. Whether areal density or bone mineral content will be lower than these younger controls is not known. There have been no studies done using this approach.

Whatever study is done, it will not be possible to control for both maturational age and chronological age, and there is a case to be made for having two or more control groups. The nature of the control groups will depend on the question being asked and the number of covariates that need to be controlled. It may be possible to use statistical analyses to adjust for covariates, but attention to study design is the preferred approach. Thus, the variance in volumetric density is established, in part, by the relationship between an individual's bone size relative to the population mean and the mineral mass relative to its population mean. If mismatch in size and mass is one means of establishing the variance in volumetric bone density, how can this mismatch occur during growth?

The Differing Rates of Accrual of Cortical and Trabecular Bone Within a Region

In regard to the way bone mass within a volume of bone is fashioned into either cortical or trabecular bone: in adulthood, at the menopause, or during illness, trabecular bone loss is more rapid than cortical bone loss and results in greater deficits at trabecular-rich sites than at cortical sites (Fig. 3, left panel). If the rate of trabecular bone accrual is more rapid than cortical bone accrual during growth, an illness interrupting this growth may result in the opposite pattern of deficits (Fig. 3, right panel)—trabecular bone, being nearer its peak, may have less of a deficit than cortical bone, which accrues more slowly. However, cortical bone accrual occurs by periosteal expansion, which will cease when growth reaches its adult value, and by medullary expansion followed by contraction at puberty in girls but not boys. In this way, at a site with mixed cortical and trabecular bone, the cortical bone may be reduced more than trabecular bone within the same bone.

The Differing Rates of Accrual of the Axial and Appendicular Skeleton and of Proximal and Distal Limb Segments

Longitudinal growth in length of the appendicular skeleton is completed sooner than in the axial skeleton, and distal segments (tibia, radius/ulna) complete their growth before proximal segments (femur, humerus) (12). If the appendicular skeleton completes its growth in size and mass before the axial skeleton, then illnesses may result in greater deficits in size and mass of the axial skeleton because it will be further from its adult peak. If distal segments of a limb complete their growth sooner than proximal segments, deficits in size and mass may be greater in the proximal segments (femur, humerus) than in the distal segments (radius/ulna, tibia). There is evidence

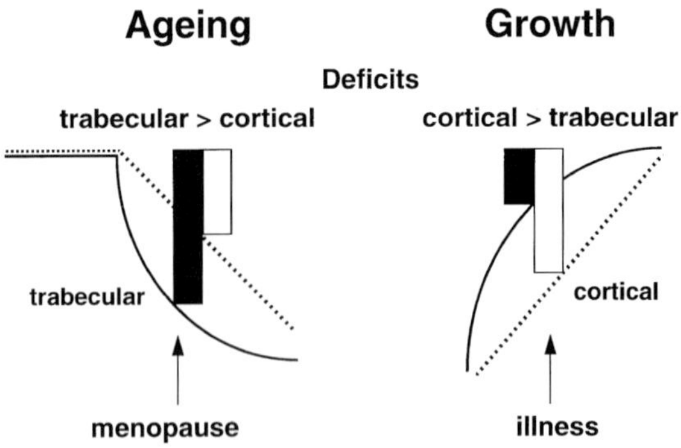

FIG. 3. In adulthood trabecular loss is more rapid than cortical bone loss; greater deficits occur at trabecular than at cortical sites **(left panel).** During growth, if the rate of mineral accrual is more rapid in trabecular than cortical bone, an illness interrupting this growth may result in greater cortical than trabecular deficits **(right panel).**

for more rapid accrual of lumbar spine bone density than of appendicular bone density (21). Data from Fournier *et al.* suggest that the accrual of bone mass at the spine is not more rapid than at the femoral neck (22). Thus, it remains unclear whether the appendicular skeleton has completed its mineral accrual before the axial skeleton.

Unlike in adult life, during growth the effect of a risk factor depends on the maturational stage of a trait or a region, not just the dose and duration of exposure to the risk factor. Deficits occurring when the distal limb segments (tibia) have completed development but not the proximal segments (femur) may again lead to site-specific deficits. This differing tempo of growth in mass and size within a region, of one region compared to another, and of cortical and trabecular bone within a region may have important effects on establishing deficits in volumetric bone density at one region but not at another and within one region at certain times but not in others.

PUBERTAL AND NONPUBERTAL GROWTH IN BOYS AND GIRLS

The differing tempo of growth in size and mass of a region, of the axial and appendicular skeleton, and of cortical and trabecular bone differ because they are regulated differently. Linear growth before puberty probably occurs independently of sex steroids. Most limb length is accrued before puberty, with only a small increase in length resulting from the pubertal component of growth (23–26). Boys have a 2-year longer prepubertal growth period. The pubertal growth spurt is faster and may continue longer than in girls. On average, the prepubertal period contributes 10 cm (5 cm/year for 2 years), and the pubertal growth period contributes 2 to 3 cm to the 12- to 13-cm greater stature of men than women. It is this greater stature that results in a higher bone mass in men than women. Peak bone density is the same in men and women (27).

Of final height, 3.4% (5.5 cm) in women and 5.2% (9.1 cm) in men is attributable to pubertal growth; the rest is nonpubertal. The pubertal contribution to lower limb growth is similar in women and men, accounting for 2.5 cm (3.3% of final limb length) in women and 3.3 cm (3.9% of final limb length) in men. The pubertal contribution to trunk length differs in men and women, accounting for 4.1 cm (4.6% of final trunk length) in women and 6.6 cm (7% of final trunk length) in men. Thus, delayed puberty may result in greater deficits in trunk length in men than in women but in similar deficits in limb length.

As a result of the longer prepubertal growth period in boys than in girls, the proportional contribution of puberty to bone mass differs in boys and girls. Bone size increases during growth, and the rate of growth accelerates at puberty, so that a substantial proportion of peak bone mass, about 40% to 50% at the spine in women, is attained during the pubertal growth spurt. Men are taller than women because they have two more years of prepubertal (or nonpubertal) growth. The nonpubertal/pubertal contributions to total bone mass are 80/20 in males and 50/50 in females

(28). Thus, theoretically, delayed puberty should have a less deleterious effect on peak bone mass in men than in women.

Peak bone mass or volumetric density has a nonpubertal (or prepubertal) and a pubertal component. If puberty is delayed and pre- or nonpubertal growth continues, then these individuals will have a higher proportion of their total peak volumetric bone density as nonpubertal, non-sex-steroid-dependent bone; affected women may be slow bone losers at the menopause. If the extent of pubertal growth in size and mineral accrual depends on the chronological age at which it occurs, then will women and men with delayed puberty have the same final height? Will this height be distributed differently in the upper and lower body? Will the increase in bone mass—trabecular number or thickness, periosteal expansion, and endosteal contraction—be the same in absolute terms? (It will be less in relative terms, as pre- or nonpubertal growth will be greater.) If it is less, then what factors contained in the chronological age at which puberty occurs determine the skeletal response to puberty in size and mass? If total bone mass is lower in delayed puberty, then this must mean that the sex steroid-dependent amount of bone accrued is less than that in women with earlier puberty, and of course a lower proportion of the total bone mass.

ARE THE SEEDS OF OSTEOPOROSIS SOWN 9 MONTHS BEFORE BIRTH, AND ITS PATHOGENESIS ESTABLISHED DURING THE FIRST 20 YEARS?

Attention to the effect of factors influencing mineral accrual before and during puberty may contribute more to the understanding of the pathogenesis of low bone mass late in life than studies in adulthood. The changes during growth are large and occur quickly. The changes during adulthood are smaller and occur slowly. Thus, the changes during growth may have more important biological effects and may be more easily and reliably measured. Changes in adulthood are smaller, more difficult to measure, and may be less biologically important. The effects of risk factors such as delayed puberty need to be defined, by their effect on the structural components that comprise bone density—bone size, mass, cortical thickness, trabecular number and thickness. Evidence suggests that delayed puberty may result in smaller size in some bones, but this may vary from region to region. The reported lower bone mineral content or lower areal bone density may be the result of the size differences. Studies are needed to determine whether delayed puberty may have differing effects on bone size, bone mass, or areal and volumetric bone density at the axial and appendicular skeleton, both within and between sexes and between ethnic groups. Whether the amount of bone in the smaller bone is less remains to be determined; at least in men, this may not be the case.

LOW PEAK BONE MASS AND BONE LOSS: UNIFYING THE PATHOGENESIS OF FRAGILITY FRACTURES

The epidemiology of fractures may be unified by recognizing the central role of reduced peak volumetric bone density in the pathogenesis of the low volumetric density in patients with fractures. Risk and protective factors in the first 20 years of life may have quantitatively larger and qualitatively different effects on the axial and appendicular skeleton than exposure during adulthood. The earlier occurrence of vertebral and forearm fractures and the later occurrence of hip fractures may reflect regional differences in peak volumetric density. As women with reduced peak volumetric density become menopausal, increased bone fragility may appear earlier in the vertebral body than the proximal femur, as accelerated menopausal trabecular bone loss compromises strength in the vertebral body, a structure containing substantial amounts of trabecular bone. Cortical bone loss proceeds more slowly than trabecular bone loss initially, then accelerates as its porosity increases the surface available for resorption, so that increased bone fragility occurs later at the proximal femur (a predominantly cortical structure), at a time when falls occur with increasing frequency, predisposing to hip fractures. Spine fractures may be the result of more severe deficits in peak volumetric bone density, whereas hip fractures—the more serious fracture in terms of morbidity—may be the result of trauma and more moderate degrees of deficit in peak volumetric bone density.

Puberty increases bone size, trabecular thickness, and cortical thickness in women: delayed puberty should reduce bone size, trabecular thickness and cortical thickness. In men, cortical thickness is more a result of periosteal apposition, and there is no contraction of medullary area at puberty in boys. The effect of testosterone is to increase bone size by periosteal growth so that 70% of cortical thickness represents growth in periosteal bone. In boys the effect of delayed puberty will be to result in a smaller bone, but medullary size may be no different, so reduced density is caused by the smaller bone. If trabecular volume in the men depends on conversion to estrogen, then the deficit should be similar to that in women. In women, cortical thickness is caused by periosteal expansion and medullary contraction (65/35); delayed puberty will thus result in a smaller bone with thinner cortices, presumably a worse deficit than in men.

SUMMARY

Bone densitometry does not take size into account. The lower bone mineral content or areal density in children with delayed puberty may reflect their smaller bone size relative to controls of the same chronological age (with larger skeletons of more advanced age). Volumetric bone density takes bone size completely into account. It is uncertain whether children with delayed puberty have lower volumetric bone density compared with controls matched by chronological age or with younger controls of the same skeletal age and bone size. If volumetric density is reduced, whether the deficit results from thinner cortices, fewer trabeculae, or thinner trabeculae is uncertain. Men with a history of delayed puberty have been reported to have reduced areal bone density at the axial and appendicular skeleton, but another study reported normal volumetric spine bone density. The contradictory data may be the result of differences in patient selection and failure to control for differences in bone size, skeletal maturity, and chronological age. It is premature to conclude that delayed puberty results in reduced volumetric bone density or that any purported deficits in bone size, mass, or density are irreversible when puberty eventually occurs.

REFERENCES

1. Seeman E. Relative contributions of low peak bone mass and bone loss to reduced bone density in osteoporosis. *Osteoporosis Int* 1994; 4: 15–25.
2. Perry HM, Horowitz M, Morley JE, *et al.* Aging and bone metabolism in African American and Caucasian women. *J Clin Endocrinol Metab* 1996; 81: 1108–1117.
3. Seeman E, Hopper JL, Bach LA, Parkinson E, Cooper ME, McKay J, Jerums G. Reduced bone mass in daughters of women with osteoporosis. *N Engl J Med* 1989; 320: 554–558.
4. Seeman E, Hopper JL, Tsalamandris C, Formica C. Bone density in daughters of women with hip fractures. *J Bone Miner Res* 1994; 9: 739–743.
5. Kannus P, Haapasalo H, Sankelo M, *et al.* Effect of starting age of physical activity on bone mass in the dominant arm of tennis and squash players. *Ann Intern Med* 1995; 123: 27–31.
6. Dunnill MS, Anderson JA, Whitehead R. Quantitative histological studies on age changes in bone. *J Pathol Bacteriol* 1967; 4: 275–291.
7. Lu PW, Cowell CT, Lloyd-Jones SA, Brody JN, Howman-Giles R. Volumetric bone mineral density in normal subjects aged 5–27 years. *J Clin Endocrinol Metab* 1996; 81: 1586–1590.
8. Gilsanz V, Gibbens DT, Roe TF, *et al.* Vertebral bone density in children: effect of puberty. *Radiology* 1988; 166: 847–850.
9. Han Z-H, Palnitkar S, Rao DS, Nelso D, Parfitt AM. Effect of ethnicity and age or menopause on the structure and geometry of iliac bone. *J Bone Miner Res* 1996; 11: 1967–1975.
10. Aaron JE, Makins NB, Sagreiy K. The microanatomy of trabecular bone loss in normal aging men and women. *Clin Orthop* 1987; 215: 260–271.
11. Garn SM. *The Earlier Gain and Later Loss of Cortical Bone.* Springfield, IL: Charles C Thomas, 1970.
12. Cameron N, Tanner JM, Whitehouse RH. A longitudinal analysis of the growth of limb segments in adolescence. *Ann Human Biol* 1982; 9: 211–220.
13. Moore B, Briody J, Cowell CT, Mobbs E. Does maturational delay affect bone mineral Density? In: *European Society of Paediatric Endocrinology, 5th Joint Meeting.* Stockholm, June 1997.
14. Finkelstein JS, Neer RM, Biller BMK, Crawford JD, Klibanski A. Osteopenia in men with a history of delayed puberty. *N Engl J Med* 1992; 326: 600–664.
15. Finkelstein JS, Klibanski A, Neer RM. A longitudinal evaluation of bone mineral density in adult men with histories of delayed puberty. *J Clin Endocrinol Metab* 1996; 81: 1152–1155.
16. Widdowson EM, Spray CM. Chemical development *in utero. Arch Dis Child* 1951; 28: 205–214.
17. Mitchell HH, Hamilton TS, Steggerda FR, Bean HW. The chemical composition of the adult human body and its bearing on the biochemistry of growth. *J Biochem* 1945; 158: 625–637.
18. Dickerson JWT. Changes in the composition of the human femur during growth. *Biochem J* 1962; 82: 56–61.
19. Neely EK, Marcus R, Rosenfeld RG, Bachrach LK. Turner's syndrome adolescents receiving growth hormone are not osteopenic. *J Clin Endocrinol Metab* 1993; 76: 861–866.
20. Bass S, Pearce G, Young N, Seeman E. Bone mass during growth: effects of exercise. *Acta Univ Carol Med* 1994; 40: 3–5.
21. Slemenda CW, Hui SL, Miller CC, Johnston CC. The effects of physical activity, sexual maturation, and weight gain on bone growth in children. In: Fourteenth Annual Meeting of the ASBMR, Minneapolis, Minnesota (abstract). *J Bone Miner Res* 1992; 7 (Suppl 1): S116.
22. Fournier P-E, Rizzoli R Slosman D-O, Theintz G, Bonjour J-P. Asynchrony between the rates of statural height gain and bone mass accumulation during puberty. *Osteoporosis Int* 1997; 7: 525–532.
23. Preece MA. The development of skeletal sex differences at adolescence. In: Russo P, Gass G, eds. *Human Adaptation.* Sydney: Department of Biological Sciences, Cumberland College of Health Sciences, 1982: 1–13.
24. Preece MA, Pan H, Ratcliffe SG. Auxological aspects of male and female puberty. *Acta Paediatr* 1992; 383: 11–13.
25. Tanner JM, Whitehouse RH, Hughes PCR, Carter BS. Relative importance of growth hormone and sex steroids for the growth at puberty of trunk length, limb length, and muscle width in growth hormone-deficient children. *J Pediatr* 1976; 89: 1000–1008.

26. Tupman GS. A study of bone growth in normal children and its relationship to skeletal maturation. *J Bone Joint Surg [Br]* 1962; 44B: 42–67.
27. Kelly PJ, Twomey L, Sambrook PN, Eisman JA. Sex differences in peak adult bone mineral density. *J Bone Miner Res* 1990; 5: 1169–1175.
28. Gordon CL, Halton JM, Atkinson SA, Webber CE. The contributions of growth and puberty to peak bone mass. *Growth Dev Aging* 1991; 55: 257–262.

DISCUSSION

Dr. Eisman: When you are talking about the delayed puberty, are you implying that these are the findings when you have delayed puberty but before puberty has occurred, so if you then go through normal puberty, would you expect the trunk to develop as normal?

Dr. Seeman: If you have delayed puberty, then once it does begin, do you catch up with size and mass? I don't know; we don't have those data. Patients with Klinefelters' syndrome are generally either taller than normal or have normal height, but it is their segment lengths that are different, this is not controversial.

Dr. Klish: I have had my bone mineral density measured by single-photon absorptiometry across the wrist, and my density by that measurement was so high it was off the scale. However, you have just implied that my bone density should be low. Also, throughout my life I put myself in situations where I could have fractured my bones, though I never have. I have had multiple joint injuries but never bone fractures. So how do I fit into your concept of delayed puberty? I admit I was growing until I was well into college.

Dr. Seeman: One of the most important determinants of the breaking strength of bone is the size of the bone. Many investigators, including Philippe Bonjour, have shown that it is very efficient to put bone on the outside of bone, increasing the bone size. You may have reduced volumetric density, but if you had the measurement done by SPA, your bone density will be off the scale because of your large bone size; that is no surprise whatsoever. Now the amount of bone within your bone may be reduced, or it may be normal. When we look at the higher fracture incidence in women than in men, or at the higher fracture incidence in whites than in blacks, nobody has ever demonstrated that those differences in fracture rates disappear or become less after adjusting in a multivariate analysis for the differences in gender, size, mass, density, or for the ethnic differences in size, mass, and density. We make inferences that the differences in bone mass between men and women and blacks and whites are responsible for the differences in fracture rates, but we have no evidence for that.

Dr. Pettifor: You mentioned that trunk length is decreased in delayed puberty. I would argue with you that if there is a normal delayed puberty, eventually the trunk length will be approximately the same as it would have been if there had been an earlier puberty. What has happened is that leg length has increased, and therefore, the trunk-to-leg length ratio has changed. But if you look at the trunk length *per se,* it is not decreased. Is that not so?

Dr. Seeman: I am not sure if it is so or not. The point is that at puberty trunk length accelerates. If you don't have puberty, that acceleration doesn't occur. So if you compare such individuals to age-matched controls, their trunk length will be shorter. The question that you are asking is very pertinent. If they have their puberty a little later, will they still get that spurt in trunk growth, or will it be less? We don't know. It has not been studied. People with Klinefelters' syndrome are the same height as or taller than age-matched adult 30-year-old controls. Because they are the same height and their legs are longer, their trunks must be shorter. Blacks of the same height as whites will have longer legs. In women and men of the same height, the men will have longer legs and a shorter trunk than the women. Asians of the same height as whites will have shorter legs and a longer trunk with a higher bone mass. So we must take size into consideration when we are comparing genders and across ethnic groups, and until we do that experimentally, we will not know the answer.

Dr. Prentice: I want to thank you for making people aware of the problems of skeletal size. I imagine there are people here who may be worried about what this means in terms of the DXA data or the SPA data that they have already got and how they are now supposed to try to interpret the data. I would like to point out two ways in which you can approach this. First, if you are interested in determinants of bone mineral status—in other words calcium intake, fat mass, and so on—is to make sure that you always incorporate bone area as an independent variable in your multiple regression analysis because most bone mineral density measurements will be correlated with bone area. Once you do that, you will start to find that many seemingly interesting things drop out of your relationships. That, of course, is looking at things in a hard statistical way. For a more pragmatic approach, particularly during growth, I am very impressed with a technique that we have been developing with my colleague Christian Mølgaard, which was published in a recent edition of *Archives of Disease in Childhood* (1). This involves taking whole body bone mineral content measurements and bone area measurements and looking at their *z* scores—a purely pragmatic approach. You ask about a child, is the height appropriate for the age? Is the bone area appropriate for the height? Is the bone mineral content appropriate for the bone area? So you can start to dissect out the relevant aspects of the equation. I would like your comments on that.

Dr. Seeman: The only comment I would make is that if you want to do research in the field, it is absolutely critical that you develop your own normal ranges. Do not use the manufacturers ranges. Then I do not believe there is any reason for concern. You must get your own normal ranges. See the patients and ensure that they don't have major diseases that may influence bone. In fact, let's not use the word ''normal''; let's say a ''reference range,'' and then I think we can work in any country of the world.

Dr. Prentice: But the main point, I think, is to take notice of the bone area results that you get from the DXA and not ignore them. That will help in the interpretation of the data that you have got.

Dr. Guesry: I think the idea that individuals should make their own reference values is a very dangerous one. If you did that, there would be no more obese children in the United States! The same problem is likely to occur with osteoporosis or decreased bone density if people make their own reference values. I don't mean to imply that the reference values provided by the manufacturers of DXA equipment cannot be challenged, but there is danger in people starting to make their own reference ranges.

Dr. Seeman: I disagree with you.

Dr. Bachrach: I have invested heavily for the past 5 years in creating normal standards because I was so frustrated with what was available in the literature. But I don't think everybody can do that. There are many clinicians who are going to turn to a publication for a normal reference standard, perhaps for their own country, although the few comparative studies of adolescents from different countries have come up with remarkably similar results. But my appeal here is for a separate working group of those who do have normative data. For example, we have 5-year longitudinal data in a mixed population with Asians, Hispanics, and blacks as well as Caucasians. We need to get together and amalgamate our data as far as possible, given the limitations of the different software used. And then we need to bring in everybody who has a slant on the best correction to use, whether it is your correction by area of the bone or our correction that involves area as well, or other people who wish to correct for weight, because that gets around the difficulties of measuring the margins of the error in calculating areas. But I think that those of us who really are concerned about this issue need to sit down together and come up with a composite that can become a gold standard.

Dr. Seeman: I disagree with that too.

Dr. Eisman: In relation to errors, I am concerned that bone area measurement, and particularly head measurements in children where the head forms a relatively large part of the total, is very dependent on the orientation of the head. If the child turns his head to the side, you will see a very big change in the projected area. This is true for many measurements of bone area, for example, the hip in terms of its rotation: if it is internally rotated, you will get a different projected area. So although I agree these are important measurements, I think one should be a little bit cautious about using them.

Dr. Bonjour: You stated that the difference between boys and girls at the end of puberty arose because boys have 2 extra years before entering the period of accelerated growth, but I think you forgot that boys also have an additional year of accelerated bone growth. This also is important at the end of the day.

Dr. Seeman: Yes, absolutely. Girls switch off more rapidly, and boys continue longer; that is quite true.

Dr. Bonjour: I think the difference between boys and girls during puberty is not so much the velocity of bone mass accrual, it is caused more by the duration over which it occurs. This is certainly true for the femoral neck and femoral diaphysis, where you don't see a difference in velocity.

Dr. Specker: Girls are not necessarily concordant as far as breast development and pubic hair development are concerned. How does this affect bone development?

Dr. Seeman: That is an excellent question. It raises the broader issue of how we define our reference ranges, and I certainly believe that for a start we must define the puberty stage as well as possible. I also believe we should measure bone age, but I am unsure what ossification centers we should be using. Should we, for example, be using the iliac crest as a marker of skeletal maturity for spinal growth? Should we even be developing atlases where each bone's ossification center is defined, the mineral mass is defined, and the size is defined? So your point is very well taken, that girls of the same breast stage could be at a different skeletal age, and I think this is a problem.

Dr. Specker: My question really is that sometimes you have breast development without pubic hair development, and the estrogen and androgen profiles in such girls are very different. Are you aware of any information on how this affects skeletal growth?

Dr. Seeman: Nobody has done that work yet.

Dr. Bachrach: I think it is very important to try to dissect the part of puberty that is breast tissue, which is presumably estrogen-mediated, from the part of puberty that is axillary and pubic hair, which represents adrenal androgens. In general, children with idiopathic premature adrenarche, where you get androgen production before true puberty, have some degree of skeletal advancement in bone age, of the order of 1 year, whereas children with true precocious puberty, who have high levels of estrogens and breast development, tend to have a greater acceleration of bone age. Those are generalities only. I think it would tell us a lot about the relative impact of the sex steroids on bone mineralization to do a study of children with premature adrenarche versus those with precocious puberty.

REFERENCE

1. Mølgaard C, Thomsen BL, Prentice A, Cole TJ, Michaelsen KF. Whole body bone mineral content in healthy children and adolescents. *Arch Dis Chld* 1997; 76: 9–15.

Nutrition and Bone Development, edited by
Jean-Philippe Bonjour and Reginald C. Tsang,
Nestlé Nutrition Workshop Series, Vol. 41, Nestec Ltd.,
Vevey/Lippincott–Raven Publishers,
Philadelphia © 1999.

Malnutrition, Endocrinopathies, and Deficits in Bone Mass Acquisition

Laura K. Bachrach

Department of Pediatrics, Division of Endocrinology, Stanford University School of Medicine, Stanford 94305, California, USA

Childhood and adolescence are normally dynamic periods for skeletal growth and acquisition of bone mineral. In healthy young people, the tempo of bone mineral acquisition parallels the pace of linear growth. Gains in bone mineral are most rapid between 11 and 14 years in girls and 14 and 17 years in boys, following peak height velocity by a year (1). Half of the peak bone mass, the bone bank for adulthood, is acquired during the teenage years, making this a critical period for establishing bone health. The magnitude of peak bone mass is strongly influenced by heritable factors (2), but 20% to 40% of the variability between individuals reflects nutrition, physical activity, body mass, and hormonal factors. The genetic potential for peak bone mass is reached only when the modifiable factors that contribute to bone acquisition are favorable.

Several disorders of childhood may disrupt the process of bone mineral acquisition and result in low bone mass. In some disorders, such as Turner's syndrome, glucocorticoid excess, or growth hormone deficiency, the osteopenia has been attributed to abnormalities in a single hormone. In illnesses such as anorexia nervosa, exercise-associated amenorrhea, and cystic fibrosis, malnutrition, sex steroid deficiency, and other factors combine to increase the risk of osteopenia.

Several noninvasive techniques are available for evaluating bone mass, with considerably more sensitivity than standard radiographs. Dual-energy x-ray absorptiometry (DXA) is available widely and offers the advantages of speed, precision, and a low radiation exposure. The limitations of this method are discussed in detail in the chapter by Gilsanz on assessment of bone mass development. The greatest challenge in the interpretation of densitometry in children relates to the dramatic changes in bone size that occur during normal growth. The DXA quantifies bone mass in terms of bone mineral content (BMC) and density (BMD), both of which are influenced by bone size. True bone density may be underestimated in smaller bones and overestimated in larger ones. To address this problem, estimates of volumetric bone density have been applied to examine whether the apparent deficits in bone mineral can be attributed to small bone size (3). Only quantitative computed tomography (QCT) provides a direct measure of volumetric bone density, but this technique is generally less available than DXA and requires a greater radiation dose.

The interpretation of bone densitometry in children is also challenging because pediatric norms for all skeletal sites are generally not included in the DXA software. Densitometry data must be compared with data from locally derived control subjects or with published gender- and age-specific norms measured on similar densitometry equipment. Interpretation of the bone mineral data should also take into account slow growth, delayed puberty, and retarded skeletal maturation, often present in patients with the disorders listed above. Despite these challenges, densitometry serves to identify young patients with deficits in bone mineral and to provide a means to monitor response to therapy. A moderate deficit in bone mineral is termed osteopenia, meaning low bone mass for age. Osteoporosis is used to describe a greater reduction in bone mineral and disruption of normal bone architecture sufficient to permit atraumatic fractures.

In this chapter I briefly examine the disorders of malnutrition and endocrine function associated with osteopenia in childhood and adolescence. The bone mineral deficits, pathogenesis, therapy, and outlook for recovery are discussed.

ANOREXIA NERVOSA

Osteopenia and osteoporotic fractures are well described complications of anorexia nervosa (4,5). In studies of young adult women with chronic anorexia nervosa, significant deficits in both trabecular and cortical bone have been observed, which may result in pathologic fractures (4). Mean bone density for anorexics has been reported to be 1 SD below normal (4), but spine densities more than 2 SD below normal have been observed in as many as 50% of patients in some studies. Osteopenia also occurs frequently in younger patients and may be apparent early in the course of the illness. In a study of adolescents with anorexia nervosa (mean age 16 years), Bachrach *et al.* found that the mean lumbar spine and whole bone densities were more than 20% and 25% below that of healthy controls, respectively (5). Twelve of the 18 patients studied had BMD measurements more than 2 SD below expected. Half of these osteopenic women had been diagnosed with anorexia nervosa within the previous 1.5 years.

Multiple risk factors are likely to contribute to the low bone mass frequently seen in this disorder (4), which begins typically in mid- to late adolescence. A morbid fear of weight gain results in malnutrition and low body mass, known risk factors for osteopenia. Low body weight may have a direct effect on bone mass because of the reduced mechanical stress on bone or may be associated with osteopenia as a manifestation of malnutrition. Intake of protein and calcium is inadequate, and the deficit may be compounded by increased urinary calcium loss (4). Estrogen deficiency and glucocorticoid excess interrupt normal acquisition of bone mineral and may contribute to increased bone loss.

The treatment of osteopenia in anorexia nervosa must address the multiple risk factors associated with this disorder. Gains in bone density have been observed in anorexic patients who gain weight in most (4,6) but not all (7) studies. The changes in BMD observed using DXA must be interpreted with caution because the increased body fat that accompanies weight gain will influence BMD measurements using this technique (8). However, gains in volumetric bone density have also been demonstrated in recovering anorexic patients using QCT, a technique that is unaffected by body composition (9). Calcium supplementation has not been proven to increase bone mineral, although it is prudent to ensure adequate intake, especially because women with anorexia nervosa have increased urinary calcium loss (4). Weight-bearing physical activity has been found to preserve bone mineral at weight-bearing sites in some studies (4,10) but not in others (5). The potential benefits of exercise must be weighed against the risk of fracture, slowed weight gain, and prolonged amenorrhea.

Most controversial of all is the value of estrogen replacement in anorexia nervosa. In a retrospective study, Seeman *et al.* found that women with anorexia nervosa who had taken oral contraceptives had greater spine BMD than those without a history of estrogen use (10). No differences were found at the femoral neck between contraceptive users and nonusers, and all patients had low bone mass for age. Other retrospective studies have failed to show an effect of sex hormone therapy on bone mass in anorexia nervosa (4). The only controlled, prospective trial reported to date compared gains in spine BMD in 19 young women given estrogen and progestin with gains in 25 untreated controls (9). The changes in BMD for the two groups were not significantly different after 1.5 years. However, sex hormone therapy prevented the bone loss seen in patients who were less than 70% of ideal weight. Thus, estrogen replacement is not a substitute for weight rehabilitation, although this treatment may be of benefit in severely malnourished patients. Estrogen should be avoided in patients with open epiphyses because this treatment accelerates skeletal maturation and may compromise final adult height.

Even with treatment, the recovery from osteopenia in anorexia nervosa may be incomplete (4,6,7,11). In adolescent girls with anorexia nervosa, mean BMD increased after 15 months in therapy (Fig. 1); however, eight of 15 patients still had BMD measurements more than 2 SD below the expected value for age (6). Persistent deficits in bone mineral in spine (6,11) and radius (7,11) have been observed in several follow-up studies of adults with a history of anorexia nervosa. In one study, gains in radius bone mass were not significantly different in patients without or with weight gain, resumption of menses, sex steroid or calcium use, or exercise (7). Patients who continued to have signs of their eating disorder were found to have more severe osteopenia at both lumbar spine and radius. However, even women who had recovered from anorexia nervosa had mean bone densities at lumbar spine and radius of −0.26 and −0.68 SD below normal, respectively (11). These data indicate that recovery of cortical bone is slower than recovery of trabecular bone,

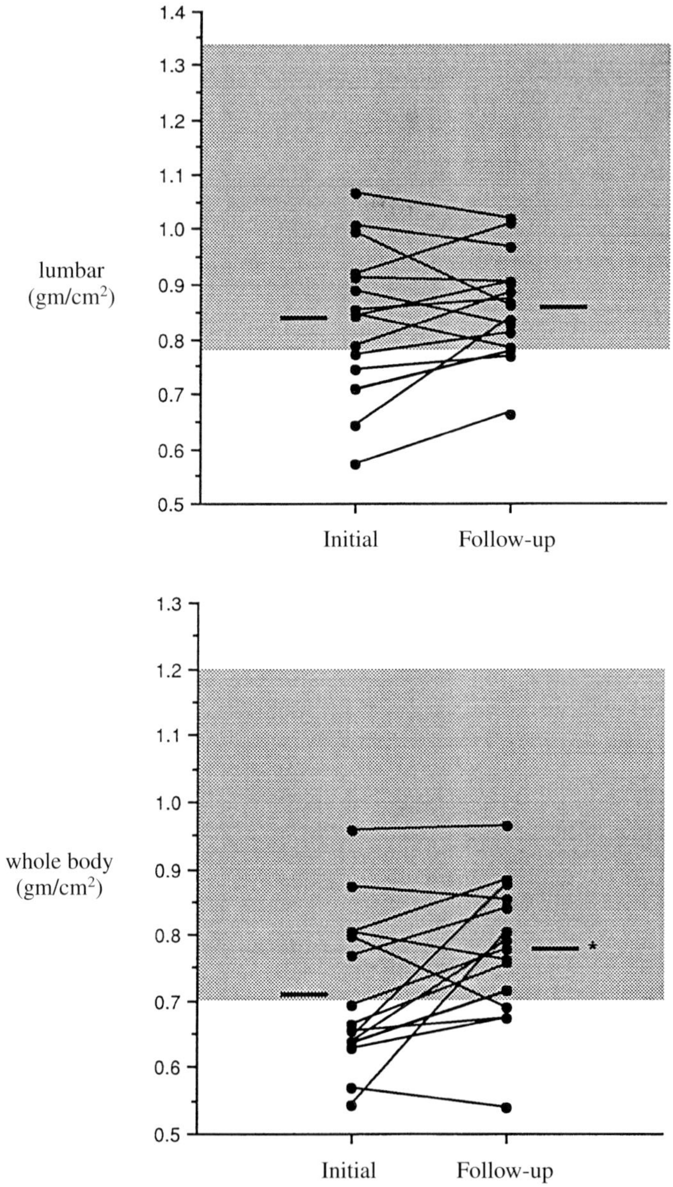

FIG. 1. Initial and follow-up lumbar spine and whole body bone mineral densities in adolescents with anorexia nervosa. The *asterisk* indicates a significant change ($p < 0.05$), and the *shaded region* indicates the 95% confidence interval for normal bone density. Reprinted with permission from Bachrach *et al.* (6).

and recovery of bone mass may be incomplete even in patients with a good outcome following anorexia nervosa.

EXERCISE-ASSOCIATED AMENORRHEA

Exercise has variable effects on skeletal health depending on its intensity. In moderation, weight-bearing activity appears to enhance bone mineral acquisition in children and young adults (1). However, osteopenia occurs commonly when hypogonadism and low body mass accompany intensive physical activity (12–14). Increased fracture risk accompanies the osteopenia (12).

The likelihood that osteopenia will develop and the skeletal site(s) affected have been shown to vary by the type of sport. For distance runners, deficits have been observed at all skeletal sites including spine, hip, proximal femur, radius, and tibia (12,13). By contrast, bone mass may be preserved at weight-bearing sites in ballet dancers (15) and in gymnasts (16) despite low body mass and hypogonadism. The authors theorized that hypogonadism contributed to trabecular bone loss while the mechanical loading from dance was sufficient to stimulate cortical bone acquisition at weight-bearing sites in young, growing athletes (15).

As in anorexia nervosa, both nutritional and hormonal factors are proposed as risk factors for osteopenia (14). Intake of energy, protein, and calcium may be inadequate as athletes go on diets to maintain the idealized physique for their sport. Intensive training during childhood may contribute to the later onset and completion of puberty. For women who begin training intensively after menarche, an estimated 5% to 50% will develop oligomenorrhea or amenorrhea. Increased endogenous glucocorticoid levels have also been implicated.

Evaluation and treatment of athletes with osteopenia should address all risk factors for the condition (14). A clinical and laboratory evaluation is indicated to exclude pregnancy, thyroid disorders, hyperprolactinemia, or ovarian failure as causes of amenorrhea. Bone densitometry is appropriate to determine if osteopenia is present. Nutritional support should be directed at ensuring adequate intake of calcium and energy. Weight gain or reduced activity may be needed before regular menses will resume. As in anorexia nervosa, the efficacy of estrogen replacement to preserve or increase bone mass has not been established. In a retrospective study, Myburgh *et al.* observed that athletic women with a history of stress fractures were less likely to have used oral contraceptives than athletes without fractures (12). However, there are no prospective, randomized studies published to date which have examined the efficacy of sex steroids for preserving bone mass in amenorrheic athletes. Until such studies are available, calcium or estrogen supplementation should not be viewed as a substitute for adequate nutrition and reduced exercise intensity.

The reversibility of exercise-associated osteopenia in adolescence is unknown. Adult women regain bone mineral with the return of menses, although deficits may not be fully restored (17). The long-term effects may also vary by the type of activity, as noted above. Indeed, intensive exercise in younger children may foster gains that are not achieved at a later age. Further studies are needed to define the risks and benefits of weight-bearing activity in younger athletes.

CYSTIC FIBROSIS

Bone mineral deficits in cystic fibrosis are common and often a significant cause of morbidity as more patients survive to adulthood. Decreased bone mineral has been observed in cystic fibrosis patients of all ages, suggesting that inadequate gains in bone mass begin early in life. Gibbens *et al.* observed the mean lumbar spine BMD to be 10% lower than expected in children and adolescents with cystic fibrosis, and 19% of the patients had significant osteopenia (18). In a study of 8- to 48-year-old patients (Fig. 2), Bhudhikanok *et al.* reported mean BMD z scores (standard deviations) of -1.7 at lumbar spine, -1.9 at femoral neck, and -1.2 for whole body (19). Estimates of hip and spine volumetric bone densities (bone mineral apparent density, BMAD) were also significantly lower than those of controls, indicating that the low bone mass could not be explained as an artifact of the small bones of cystic fibrosis patients. More than half of the subjects (38% of those under the age of 18) were osteopenic with BMD z scores less than -2.0, and 12% of the subjects had sustained atraumatic or minimally traumatic bone fractures.

Several nutritional and endocrine factors combine to set the stage for osteopenia in cystic fibrosis (19). Fat malabsorption and chronic illness commonly lead to low body mass, vitamin D deficiency, and slow growth. However, serum 25-hydroxyvitamin D concentrations and calcium intake did not correlate with bone mineral at any site in one study (19). Delayed puberty and early gonadal dysfunction are common in cystic fibrosis, and bone mineral has been shown to be significantly lower in patients with reproductive dysfunction (19). Patients receiving chronic glucocorticoid therapy for pulmonary symptoms had significantly lower bone mass than those not on steroids (19). Finally, physical activity may be restricted by chronic illness, although the contribution of inactivity to osteopenia in cystic fibrosis has not been established.

Treatment to prevent or reverse the osteopenia in cystic fibrosis should include appropriate nutritional and hormonal support. Diet should be optimized to foster weight gain and to ensure adequate intake of protein, calcium, and phosphorus. Vitamin D supplementation in excess of 800 IU daily may be required to achieve normal levels of 25-hydroxyvitamin D. The dose of glucocorticoids should be reduced to the minimum that controls pulmonary symptoms; inhaled steroids may have a greater bone-sparing effect than those taken orally. Sex hormone replacement should be provided for adults with hypogonadism and for adolescents with significantly delayed puberty. Osteopenia may develop despite these general supportive measures, particularly in patients with more severe disease and those requiring glucocorticoid therapy (19). Controlled treatment trials with antiresorptive or anabolic agents have not been published; these studies are urgently needed to determine the safety and efficacy of such agents in cystic fibrosis. As with all forms of osteoporosis, strategies to prevent osteopenia are likely to prove more effective than efforts to

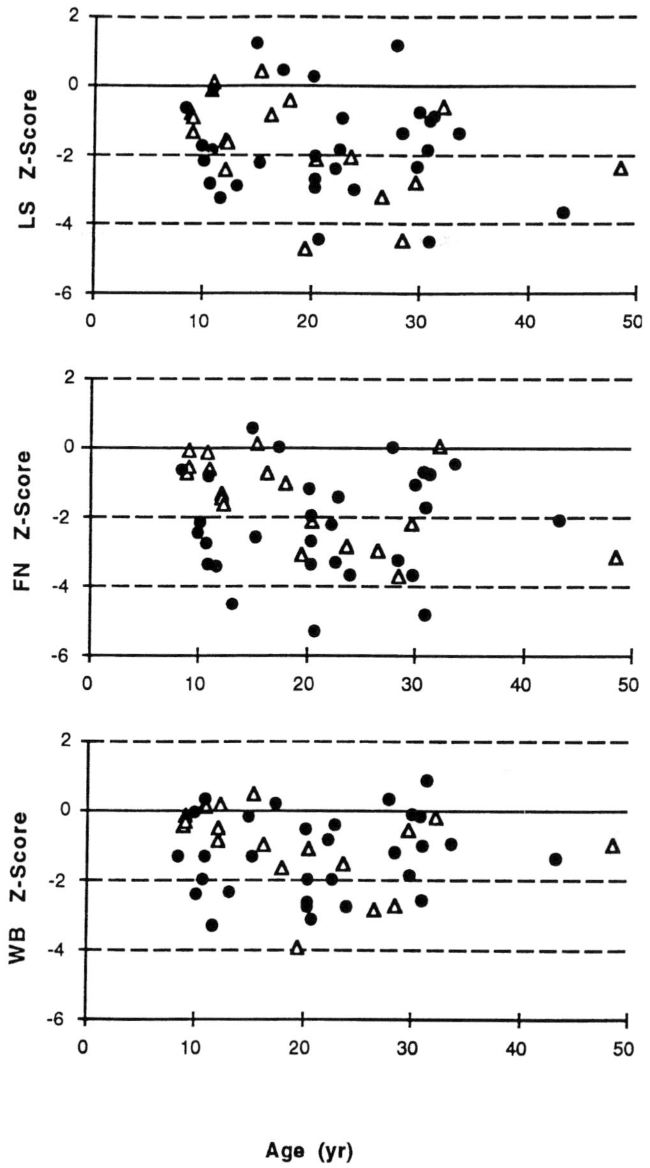

FIG. 2. Lumbar spine (LS), femoral neck (FN), and whole body (WB) age-adjusted bone mineral densities for males *(triangles)* and females *(circles)* with cystic fibrosis. Reprinted with permission from Bhudhikanok *et al.* (19).

reverse established deficits. Attention to skeletal health should be considered an essential component of the health care program for cystic fibrosis patients from childhood.

ISOLATED HYPOGONADISM

Adolescent gains in bone mass are most rapid during puberty, reflecting the contribution of sex steroids to skeletal health. Sex hormones appear to foster gains in bone mineral in addition to preventing the bone loss seen in postmenopausal women. Not surprisingly, osteopenia has been observed in teenagers who have hypogonadism without other identifiable risk factors for osteopenia.

Osteopenia develops commonly in adolescents and young adults with hypogonadotropic hypogonadism. In one study of 23 men, mean radial and spine bone densities were 19% and 40% lower than controls, respectively; more than half of the subjects had BMD measurements 2 SD or more below expected (20). Bone histomorphometry indicated low turnover, supporting the hypothesis that the deficits in bone mass reflected inadequate gains in bone mineral rather than accelerated loss.

Studies in women with hypothalamic amenorrhea have been more difficult to interpret because they include subjects with anorexia nervosa or exercise-associated menstrual disorders. In these patients, it is not possible to determine the relative contributions of hypogonadism, low body mass, and malnutrition to the observed osteopenia. Bone studies in women with primary ovarian failure offer the opportunity to evaluate the effects of sex steroid deficiency without confounding risk factors. In several studies to date, a high prevalence of osteopenia has been observed in adolescents with Turner's syndrome, a chromosomal disorder associated with ovarian dysgenesis. However, many of these failed to adjust for the short stature, delayed skeletal maturation, and delayed puberty characteristic of this syndrome. As a result, the magnitude of bone mineral deficits may have been overestimated. Neely *et al.* addressed these issues in a study comparing bone mineral in 19 adolescents with Turner's syndrome (mean age 14 years) with that in controls (21). All but two of the Turner's girls had been treated for short stature with recombinant human growth hormone (hGH), but none had begun estrogen replacement. The bone mineral content of lumbar spine and whole body in Turner's subjects was significantly lower than that in controls, reflecting in part the smaller bone size. However, BMD was not significantly reduced, and estimates of volumetric bone density (BMAD) were identical in the two groups. In fact, when Turner's subjects were compared with normal girls matched by bone age and pubertal stage, BMD and BMAD were equal to or greater than control values.

Osteopenia has also been noted in rare disorders of estrogen resistance (22) or aromatase deficiency, in which estrogen synthesis is impaired (23). Men and women with these disorders have delayed epiphyseal closure and low bone mass, suggesting that estrogen is essential for normal skeletal maturation and mineral acquisition in both sexes.

The obvious treatment for osteopenia in sex steroid deficiency is hormone replacement. However, controversy surrounds the optimal time to start this treatment and how effectively deficits in bone mineral can be prevented or reversed. Adult men with hypogonadism have been shown to gain bone mass with testosterone therapy; increases are greater in patients with open epiphyses at the start of treatment than in older men (24). Despite sex steroid replacement, peak bone mass was below expected adult norms. Similarly, several studies have observed that estrogen replacement in hypogonadal females reduces, but does not eliminate, deficits in peak bone mass (25). Unfortunately, none of these studies followed the subjects from the time sex steroids were initiated until peak bone mass was reached, and no standardized replacement protocol or monitoring of compliance was employed. Nevertheless, these data suggest that treatment may need to be initiated earlier to optimize peak bone mass. Alternatively, there may be other factors contributing to the osteopenia in hypogonadal patients, and these must be identified and addressed. Further longitudinal studies are needed to define the most effective sex steroid replacement to optimize adolescent gains in bone mineral in hypogonadal patients.

GROWTH HORMONE DEFICIENCY

Relative osteopenia has been observed in growth-hormone-deficient children before treatment. Saggese *et al.* reported a mean z score of -2.9 for radius bone mineral content in classical growth hormone deficiency (26). However, when radius bone mass was corrected for height, age, or bone age, mean z score was only -1.4. Thus, much of the apparent deficit in bone mineral reflects the smaller bone size and delayed skeletal maturation characteristic of this disorder. No increased fracture incidence has been reported in this disorder.

The presumed mechanism for osteopenia in growth hormone deficiency is inadequate stimulation of bone mineral acquisition. The pivotal role of growth hormone and the insulin-like growth factors (IGF) for bone growth is well accepted. The contribution of these peptides to accrual of bone mineral remains more controversial. Studies carried out *in vitro* and *in vivo* indicate that growth hormone and the IGFs act directly to stimulate osteoblast proliferation and production of bone matrix factors. Growth hormone also appears to work indirectly by increasing the conversion of 25-hydroxyvitamin D to its more active metabolite, 1,25-dihydroxyvitamin D and by increasing the sensitivity of intestinal cells to parathyroid hormone (PTH). These actions result in greater calcium absorption, which may enhance bone mineral accretion.

Growth hormone replacement is the treatment of choice to address this deficit. When given in adequate doses, growth hormone has been shown to reduce or to eliminate the deficit in bone mass in children (26). However, peak bone mass is reduced in many adults who received treatment for growth hormone deficiency in childhood (27). De Boer *et al.* found a mean BMD z score of -1.5 at the lumbar spine and -1.2 at the femoral neck in 70 adult male patients; 33% of the adults had spine areal bone densities more than 2 SD below expected (27). Even when estimates of volumetric bone density were used to adjust for small bone size, bone mineral remained significantly below that of controls (z scores of -0.90 and -0.74

for spine and hip, respectively); 14% of the patients had spine volumetric bone densities more than 2 SD below normal. Several explanations have been proposed to account for the persistent deficits in bone mass seen after childhood growth hormone deficiency. Patients may have been treated with suboptimal doses of growth hormone because of the limited supply of the hormone in earlier decades. Alternatively, they may have lacked other pituitary factors required for optimal gains in bone mineral. This explanation appears unlikely because the bone mass of patients with isolated growth hormone deficiency did not differ significantly from that of patients with multiple pituitary hormone deficits. Finally, it may be that growth hormone treatment must be sustained after linear growth is completed to maintain bone mineral. Again, this hypothesis seems less likely because longitudinal studies in untreated patients have failed to show increased bone loss. Rather, the low bone mineral in this condition appears to reflect inadequate acquisition of bone during childhood and adolescence. Further studies are needed to determine if normal peak bone mass can be achieved with optimal growth hormone replacement and if low-dose growth hormone must be continued in deficient adults to maintain bone mineral.

DIABETES MELLITUS

Mild osteopenia has been observed in diabetic patients for more than 50 years. However, the prevalence, severity, and pathogenesis of low bone mineral are still unresolved. As summarized in a recent review (28), reduced bone mass at the radius in children and adolescents with type I diabetes has been observed in several studies. Osteopenia has commonly been found, with 18% to 54% of subjects showing significant reductions in bone mineral at the radius for age. When present, the osteopenia in insulin-dependent diabetes appears to be mild, with deficits of 6% to 14% (0.7 to 1.2 SD) below expected (28). By contrast, studies in diabetic children found spine BMD to be similar to that of controls matched for race, sex, and age (29). Cortical bone is more affected than trabecular bone. No increased fracture incidence has been reported in younger patients. Osteopenia has been detected at the time of diagnosis in some diabetic children, with continued bone loss over the first 2 to 5 years of insulin therapy (28). Several studies have found no relationship between diabetic control and the magnitude of deficit in bone mass or the rate of change in bone mass over time.

The pathogenesis of osteopenia remains unsettled (28). Some histomorphometry data and the finding of hypercalciuria have suggested increased bone loss. However, alterations in insulin, insulin-like growth factors, and their binding proteins may result in reduced bone formation. In some but not all cases, poor diabetic control (as assessed by hemoglobin A_{1C}) has been linked to osteopenia. Because the etiology of diabetic bone disease remains elusive, it is difficult to target therapy. As noted above, osteopenia may or may not progress over time and may not be prevented by improved metabolic control. Larger studies are needed to determine the magnitude of the problem and the best approach to treatment in the young patient with type I diabetes.

HYPERTHYROIDISM

Variable degrees of osteopenia have been reported in children and adults with endogenous or iatrogenic hyperthyroidism. Profound osteopenia and vertebral fractures have developed in children with Graves' disease; bone mineral deficits were reversed with treatment of thyrotoxicosis (30). Osteopenia has also been found in patients given high-dose L-thyroxine treatment for thyroid cancer or goiter (31). In general, the bone mineral deficit increases with the severity and duration of hyperthyroidism and the presence of other risk factors.

Thyroid hormone excess stimulates bone resorption, which increases serum calcium levels. This leads to suppression of PTH and 1,25-dihydroxyvitamin D production, reduced calcium absorption, increased urinary calcium excretion, and a negative calcium balance. Management of osteopenia in this setting includes prompt medical or surgical treatment of spontaneous hyperthyroidism. For patients on L-thyroxine, the dose should be adjusted to avoid suppression of thyroid-stimulating hormone except in cases of thyroid cancer.

GLUCOCORTICOID EXCESS

The skeletal complications of glucocorticoid excess are often the most profound and challenging to treat of all the endocrine disorders (32). Although these problems develop commonly in Cushing's disease, this disorder is rare in childhood. Most steroid-induced bone disease is seen in young patients who require glucocorticoid therapy for asthma, rheumatoid arthritis, inflammatory bowel disease, or following organ transplantation (33). The typical skeletal manifestations of glucocorticoid excess are osteopenia and osteoporosis; avascular necrosis of the femoral head occurs far less commonly (32). The greatest deficits occur in the trabecular bone of the spine and femoral neck, with relative sparing of cortical bone in the peripheral skeleton. In severe cases, pathologic bone fractures occur, typically at the spine and proximal hip. Bone loss begins within 6 months of initiating chronic steroids, and osteopenia develops in as many as 50% of adult patients (32). There are fewer data on the childhood incidence of steroid-induced osteopenia. However, deficits in bone mineral may be even more profound because bone loss is compounded by impaired bone growth and mineral acquisition. Growth failure and delayed puberty occur commonly with chronic steroid administration. Deficits in bone mass persist even when appropriate adjustments are made for small bone size and delayed skeletal maturation (33).

The mechanisms involved in steroid-induced bone disease are complex (32). In supraphysiological concentrations, glucocorticoids act directly to inhibit osteoblast differentiation and production of osteocalcin, a key bone matrix protein. Indirectly, steroids interfere with calcium absorption from the gut and reduce renal tubular calcium resorption. This negative calcium balance leads to secondary hyperparathyroidism, which results in increased bone resorption. Steroids also inhibit local production of bone growth factors such as insulin-like growth factor 1 (IGF-1) and prostaglandin E_2 and reduce the response of bone cells to transforming growth factor. β Glucocorticoid excess also alters hypothalamic–pituitary function, resulting in reduced production of both growth hormone and gonadotropins. The net effect of these local and systemic actions is a state of increased bone loss and reduced bone formation. For many patients on glucocorticoid therapy, factors related to the underlying disease add to the risks from the steroids. Chronic inflammation and reduced physical activity exacerbate bone loss in patients with arthritis and asthma; marginal nutrition complicates the course in inflammatory bowel disease; in organ transplant patients, previous renal or hepatic disease and bone-destructive drugs such as cyclosporine add to the risk of osteopenia.

Treatment for steroid-induced osteopenia is generally only partially effective if glucocorticoid excess continues. Rare cases of Cushing's disease should be treated promptly; once treated, these patients have rapid catch-up gains in bone mineral, although full recovery may not occur. For patients who require chronic glucocorticoid therapy, steroids should be limited to the minimum dose that controls the underlying disorder. Although the risk of osteopenia is dose-related, there is no established threshold below which bone loss will not occur. Alternate-day steroid dosing may result in less bone loss than daily administration, and inhaled steroids may offer advantages over oral medication. Preliminary data indicate that newer steroid derivatives, such as deflazacort, may effectively control inflammation with fewer adverse effects on bone (34)

Other general supportive measures should be instituted in young patients on glucocorticoids. Adequate vitamin D should be given to maintain 25-hydroxyvitamin D in the high normal range, and calcium intake of 1,500 mg/day should be encouraged to offset increased urinary calcium excretion. If hypercalciuria develops, this may be treated with thiazide diuretics. Serum calcium should be monitored to avoid hypercalcemia. Gentle weight-bearing physical activity should be encouraged on a daily basis. Sex steroid treatment may be appropriate in teenagers with significantly delayed puberty. Growth hormone has been shown to be marginally effective in increasing growth velocity in some studies; its benefits for counteracting steroid-induced osteopenia remain uncertain. When these general measures fail, other therapeutic agents may be appropriate. Calcitonin has been shown to improve bone mineral status in small numbers of glucocorticoid-treated children (35). Sodium fluoride increases markers of bone formation in steroid-dependent adults. Controlled randomized trials of these agents in children are needed.

CONCLUSION

The management of osteopenia in childhood poses many challenges. Assessment of bone mineral is complicated by delayed growth, puberty, and skeletal maturation that commonly accompany endocrine and nutritional disorders. Once recognized, osteopenia may be difficult to treat. Often, several factors are present that interrupt the normal acquisition of bone mineral. In general, treatment is most effective only when all risk factors are addressed simultaneously. For example, calcium supplementation is unlikely to increase bone mass in patients who remain hypogonadal or underweight. Many therapeutic agents that have proven useful and safe in adults have not been tested adequately in children. Furthermore, antiresorptive agents may not be the drugs of choice in younger patients whose deficits reflect failure to gain bone rather than accelerated loss. Anabolic agents such as parathyroid hormone or sodium fluoride may prove more effective but must be tested in controlled trials. There is an urgent need to explore these treatment options and to increase awareness of the risk factors for childhood osteopenia. Early recognition and intervention are the keys to fostering the skeletal health of these youth.

REFERENCES

1. Bonjour JP. Bone mineral acquisition in adolescence. In: Marcus R, Feldman D, Kelsey J, eds. *Osteoporosis*. San Diego: Academic Press, 1996: 465–476.
2. Kelly PJ, Eisman JA, Sambrook PN. Interaction of genetic and environmental influences on peak bone density. *Osteoporosis Int* 1990; 1: 56–60.
3. Carter DR, Bouxsein ML, Marcus R. New approaches for interpreting projected bone densitometry data. *J Bone Miner Res* 1992; 7: 137–145.
4. Carmichael KA, Carmichael DH. Bone metabolism and osteopenia in eating disorders. *Medicine* 1995; 74: 254–267.
5. Bachrach LK, Guido D, Katzman D, Litt IF, Marcus R. Decreased bone density in adolescent girls with anorexia nervosa. *Pediatrics* 1990; 86: 440–447.
6. Bachrach LK, Katzman DK, Litt IF, Guido D, Marcus R. Recovery from osteopenia in adolescent girls with anorexia nervosa. *J Clin Endocrinol Metab* 1991; 72: 602–606.
7. Rigotti NA, Neer RM, Skates SJ, Herzog DB, Nussbaum SR. The clinical course of osteoporosis in anorexia nervosa. A longitudinal study of cortical bone mass. *JAMA* 1991; 265: 1133–1138.
8. Hamgarttner T. Influence of fat on bone measurements with dual-energy x-ray absorptiometry. *Bone Miner* 1990; 9: 71–78.
9. Klibanski A, Biller BK, Schoenfeld DA, Herzog DB, Saxe VC. The effects of estrogen administration on trabecular bone loss in young women with anorexia nervosa. *J Clin Endocrinol Metab* 1995; 80: 898–904.
10. Seeman E, Szmukler GI, Formica C, Tsalamandris C, Mestrovic R. Osteoporosis in anorexia nervosa: the influence of peak bone density, bone loss, oral contraceptive use and exercise. *J Bone Miner Res* 1992; 7: 1467–1474.
11. Herzog W, Minne H, Deter C, *et al.* Outcome of bone mineral density in anorexia nervosa patients 11.7 years after first admission. *J Bone Miner Res* 1993; 8: 597–605.
12. Myburgh KH, Hutchins J, Fataar AB, Hough SF, Noakes TD. Low bone density is an etiologic factor for stress fractures in athletes. *Ann Intern Med* 1990; 113: 754–759.
13. Rencken ML, Chesnut CH, Drinkwater BL. Bone density at multiple skeletal sites in amenorrheic runners. *JAMA* 1996; 276: 238–240.
14. Snow-Harter CM. Bone health and prevention of osteoporosis in active and athletic women. *Clin Sports Med* 1994; 13: 389–404.
15. Young N, Formica C, Szmukler G, Seeman E. Bone density at weight-bearing and nonweight-bearing sites in ballet dancers: the effects of exercise, hypogonadism, and body weight. *J Clin Endocrinol Metab* 1994; 78: 449–454.
16. Robinson TL, Snow-Harter C, Taaffe DR, Gillis D, Shaw J, Marcus R. Gymnasts exhibit higher bone mass than runners despite similar prevalence of amenorrhea and oligomenorrhea. *J Bone Miner Res* 1995; 10: 26–35.
17. Drinkwater BL, Nilson K, Ott S, Chestnut CH III. Bone mineral density after resumption of menses in amenorrheic athletes. *JAMA* 1986; 256: 380–382.
18. Gibbens DT, Gilsanz V, Boechat MI, Dufer D, Carlson ME, Wang C-I. Osteoporosis in cystic fibrosis. *J Pediatr* 1988; 113: 295–300.
19. Bhudhikanok GS, Lim J, Marcus R, Harkins A, Moss RB, Bachrach LK. Correlates of osteopenia in patients with cystic fibrosis. *Pediatrics* 1996; 97: 103–111.

20. Finkelstein JS, Klibanski A, Neer RM, Greenspan SL, Rosenthal DI, Crowley WF. Osteoporosis in men with idiopathic hypogonadotropic hypogonadism. *Ann Intern Med* 1987; 106: 354–361.
21. Neely EK, Marcus R, Rosenfeld RG, Bachrach LK. Turner syndrome adolescents receiving growth hormone are not osteopenic. *J Clin Endocrinol Metab* 1993; 76: 861–866.
22. Smith EP, Boyd J, Frank GR, *et al.* Estrogen resistance caused by a mutation in the estrogen-receptor gene in a man. *N Engl J Med* 1994; 331: 1056–1061.
23. Morishima A, Grumbach MM, Simpson ER, Fisher C, Qin K. Aromatase deficiency in male and female siblings caused by a novel mutation and the physiologic role of estrogens. *J Clin Endocrinol Metab* 1995; 80: 3689–3698.
24. Finkelstein JS, Klibanski A, Neer RM, *et al.* Increases in bone density during treatment of men with idiopathic hypogonadotropic hypogonadism. *J Clin Endocrinol Metab* 1989; 69: 776–783.
25. Davies MC, Guleki B, Jacobs HS. Osteoporosis in Turner syndrome and other forms of primary amenorrhea. *Clin Endocrinol* 1995; 43: 741–746.
26. Saggese G, Baroncelli BI, Bertelloni S, Cinquanta L, Di Nero G. Effects of long-term treatment with growth hormone on bone and mineral metabolism in children with growth hormone deficiency. *J Pediatr* 1993; 122: 37–45.
27. De Boer H, Block GJ, Van Lingen A, Teule GJJ, Lips P, Van Der Veen EA. Consequences of childhood-onset growth hormone deficiency for adult bone mass. *J Bone Miner Res* 1994; 9: 1319–1326.
28. Selby PL. Osteopenia and diabetes. *Diabetes Med* 1988; 5: 423–428.
29. Roe TF, Mora S, Costin G, Kaufman F, Carlson ME, Gilsanz V. Vertebral bone density in insulin-dependent diabetic children. *Metabolism* 1991; 40: 967–971.
30. Saggese G, Bertelloni S, Baroncelli GI. Bone mineralization and calciotropic hormones in children with hyperthyroidism. Effects of methimazole therapy. *J Endocrinol Invest* 1990; 13: 587–592.
31. Radetti G , Castellan C, Tato L, Platter K, Gentili L, Adami S. Bone mineral density in children and adolescent females treated with high doses of L-thyroxine. *Horm Res* 1993; 3: 127–131.
32. Luckert B. Glucocorticoid-induced osteoporosis. In: Marcus R, Feldman D, Kelsey J, eds. *Osteoporosis.* San Diego: Academic Press, 1996: 801–820.
33. Kotaniemi A, Savolainen A, Kautiainen H, Kroger H. Estimation of central osteopenia in children with chronic polyarthritis treated with glucocorticoids. *Pediatrics* 1993; 91: 1127–1130.
34. Loftus J, Allen R, Hesp R, *et al.* Randomized, double-blind trial of deflazacort versus prednisone in juvenile chronic (or rheumatoid) arthritis: a relatively bone-sparing effect of deflazacort. *Pediatrics* 1991; 88: 428–436.
35. Nishioka T, Kurayama H, Yasuda T, Udagawa J, Matsumura C, Niimi H. Nasal administration of salmon calcitonin for prevention of glucocorticoid-induced osteoporosis in children with nephrosis. *J Pediatr* 1991; 118: 703–707.

DISCUSSION

Dr. Klish: I agree with you that anorexia nervosa is probably the most common form of severe malnutrition we see in the United States. However, it is not a very good model of malnutrition, as you well know, because these girls do so many things to abuse their bodies. Some of the things done by anorexics affect factors that influence bone growth. For example, they tend to avoid foods that are high in calcium, and as a result their calcium intake is very low; they are frequently on laxatives and diuretics; and they exercise obsessively, which changes the mechanical forces on bone. Are any of these other factors predictive for the risk of developing the osteopenia, at least in the severe forms that we occasionally see in the anorexic?

Dr. Bachrach: I will address the specific issue of exercise, which is still controversial. There are those who believe that exercise provides some degree of protection at the femoral neck, and there are others who believe there is no protection; certainly there is no protection at sites such as the radius. The bottom line is that in both anorexia nervosa and underweight athletes, the benefits of exercising an underweight skeleton with other nutritional deficits are not as obvious as in a nutritionally replete individual. Exercising without adequate nutrient intake may not be sufficiently protective.

Dr. Seeman: We compared about 70 girls with anorexia with age-matched controls, and we also had another control group of ballet dancers of equivalent weight. It is very difficult to control for all of the variables, but we found that bone density at the proximal femur was normal in all these girls, though it was reduced in the spine in the anorexics (1).

Dr. Eisman: In relation to glucocorticoid osteoporosis I agree there need to be properly done randomized controlled studies of potential treatments. I am surprised, however, that you don't mention the one treatment that has actually been shown to be of prophylactic benefit, at least in adults, and that is calcitriol. This certainly stops the loss at the spine, though maybe it is less effective at the hip. I have a question. You mentioned that some of the anorexics were given oral contraceptives. That would imply that they had a return of menses or that the decision about their use may not have been related to what the child wanted but what the family wanted. I am concerned about compliance with treatments of this kind, and just as anorexic girls don't necessarily comply with diet, they also tend not to comply with hormone replacement. I think that is also true in athletes who develop amenorrhea because they believe that it is protective. So my question is, do you believe that those girls were really having adequate hormone replacement?

Dr. Bachrach: Again, because I did not do the study, I can only go by what is written, and the article states that the three women who elected to take oral contraceptives wished them as a means of birth control. They did not state that they were menstruating. Obviously they should not have been included in the study if they were menstruating spontaneously. But there is a fact that women with anorexia nervosa can get pregnant because if they are in the midst of their nutritional rehabilitation, they never know when they may ovulate. So it is potentially possible that the women who elected to get the oral contraceptives were not menstruating but were just sexually active, which of course in itself is unusual for anorexics. The other point was the compliance issue. As to compliance, I could not agree with you more. Even if we knew that sex steroid therapy was 100% effective, we would have a horrendous time trying to sell it either to athletes or to anorexics. Acceptance and compliance are both important issues, and I can only report what is in the study.

Dr. Eisman: In relation to the gymnasts, you made the comment that you could make an adjustment in these sorts of studies for volumetric density, and you said that not only was the bone density high but when you did the adjustment for volumetric density it was even higher, though that was presumably because their bones were smaller. It is fine to know precisely what the bone size is and precisely what the bone density is or even, if such a thing exists, what the true bone density is. But the strength of a bone depends not only on its density and its structural integrity but also on its actual size in relation to the individual, so I wonder, particularly in relation to the gymnasts, whether there was a suggestion that their total bone was better, or was it worse but not seeming to be so bad, because their bones were smaller?

Dr. Bachrach: Even if we decided that the volumetric density was normal or increased in gymnasts, we would still have the issue that gymnasts end up with smaller bones because of stunting of pubertal growth. So then we need to look at ultimate lifetime fracture risk in terms of both bone quality and bone size.

Dr. Seeman: In the gymnasts we studied, the vertebral size was normal, and the size of the tibia was reduced. When we did metacarpal morphometry, the difference that we found was not in the external diameter of the bone, but the medullary cavity of the femur was reduced, so that the higher bone mass within the bone resulted from the smaller medulla. Not everybody has found that, and I suspect that exercise may have differing effects on those surfaces depending on the rate of growth and the length of time that exercise is undertaken.

Dr. Gilsanz: You found a 20% decrease in BMD in lumbar spine in anorexics and no reduction in the radius. To what degree is the reduction in BMD values in the lumbar spine caused by changes in body size? How much do you think that the difference of 20% loss in the lumbar spine and no loss in the radius reflected errors in measurements of body size?

Dr. Bachrach: It is not that there was no deficit at the radius; it didn't reach statistical significance. I think there are two possibilities. One is the issue of what we are truly measuring. What I reported was BMD and not some estimate to correct for the smaller size. The other potential explanation is that there is a greater contribution of trabecular bone at that site, and we are seeing a greater deficit at that site because the girls were at puberty, if we agree with Dr. Seeman's theory about the timing of the impact. That argument is diluted a little because our whole body measurements were also reduced. The best correction might be whole body BMC divided by height or divided by total area, as suggested by others.

Dr. Pettifor: Do you have any evidence that those with mainly a formation problem respond better to treatment than those who have increased resorption? I would suspect that those who have lost trabeculae are not going to reform them, but those who have just got a decrease in bone formation on the trabeculae and whose trabecular number remains relatively normal may well recover their bone mass adequately during treatment.

Dr. Bachrach: This question is clearly confounded by age of intervention. If one intervenes in an age where you believe you are dealing with interrupted acquisition, I think potential gains may be much greater. Theoretically I would have to agree with you.

Dr. Gilsanz: Obese children who lose weight through puberty will have marked changes in BMC or BMD, and you will not know what those changes are caused by. We have very useful precise tools, and it is very important to ask what we are measuring. But to measure children with eating disorders by these techniques is very difficult because we don't know which of the variables is the one that influences the results. My question is to what degree do you think that 20% decrease in BMD reflects body size?

Dr. Bachrach: I don't believe we will explain it all away by correcting for bone size. I don't believe it because of our experience with cystic fibrosis, where we used our own techniques to obtain a correction for the bone size; I don't believe it also because when individuals go on to develop fractures, that tells us something about their bones. My best guess is that bone size explains between 40% and 60% at most and that you will have real deficits that remain, and they are deficits of acquisition, potentially compounded by some loss if the hypogonadal state continues.

Dr. Prentice: I was interested in your comments about new antiresorptive agents, where you said you had reservations about that approach for the growing child. I wonder if you can give me some information about something that has been puzzling me for a long time, which is about our understanding of remodeling in the growing child and how it is effected. High intakes of calcium are used as antiresorptive agents for postmenopausal bone loss, and in calcium supplementation studies in peripubertal children at least some of the effect seems to be an effect on remodeling. I have asked various people what they would expect that to mean for the growing child in terms of peak bone mass. Will it be of benefit? Will it be detrimental? I wonder if you have any information on that.

Dr. Bachrach: I don't have any information. My opinion is that the adult model, where increasing calcium acts by interfering with resorption, does not fully explain what goes on in children. There are convincing data that the potential anabolic effects of calcium are independent of blocking the increased resorption. I think that the model of what calcium does in children is different. My concern about using antiresorptive drugs in children is that, although we think the effect of these drugs is heavily weighted toward greater inhibition of resorption than formation, there are nevertheless potential direct effects on formation, and we also know that all markers of bone turnover increase dramatically during adolescence, which I presume reflects the coupling of resorption that precedes acquisition at some sites, so I worry about blocking resorption in a child who is growing.

REFERENCE

1. Young N, Formica C, Szmukler G, Seeman E. Bone density at weight-bearing and nonweight-bearing sites in ballet dancers: the effects of exercise, hypogonadism, and body weight. *J Clin Endocrinol Metab* 1994; 78: 449–454.

Nutrition and Bone Development, edited by
Jean-Philippe Bonjour and Reginald C. Tsang,
Nestlé Nutrition Workshop Series, Vol. 41, Nestec Ltd.,
Vevey/Lippincott–Raven Publishers,
Philadelphia © 1999.

Conclusion of the Workshop

Dr. Tsang: I want to thank all the attendees—speakers from ten countries and participants from 20 countries—for their participation. The comments have been interesting, and the discussions raised many issues that we need to attend to. Several participants asked that we produce a short summary. We clearly can't repeat everything, but we want to highlight a few of the issues, and I will share this task with my co-chairman, Dr. Bonjour.

We are all very interested in early bone development, and many comments have been made about the fact that there is a crucial period before the age of 15 to 17 years when most of the bone mass is accreted, and the traditional focus on this part of the curve needs to be reexamined.

We talked about genes—master genes, *Hox* genes, PDR genes—and we are beginning to understand that there are many major influences on bone development very early in life, beginning at conception. The placenta is obviously a major transfer organ that transports calcium and phosphorus at phenomenal rates to the fetus. The influences on placental transfer in the clinical setting are very poorly understood, but we do understand that there are many maternal disturbances that conceivably affect transport, including vitamin D nutrition and season.

In the premature infant who is deprived of placental transport of minerals, we have traditionally approached the problem by replacement or restoration of what we think is needed in terms of calcium and phosphorus, both enterally and parenterally. This has been effective in restoring bone mass near to what it would have been *in utero* except in very small or very sick premature babies. The issue of human milk feeding for preterm infants has been highlighted, and the need for phosphate supplementation in particular. An important area of current study is how much mineral to provide for premature babies when they are sent home. Do we need to replenish their mineral status to the level of the term infant? Is imprinting important? These are issues that are currently being studied and debated.

In the term infant, it is also clear that one can manipulate the dietary intake of calcium and phosphorus and produce changes in bone mass. However, these changes may not be permanent, and follow-up studies beyond the period of supplementation appear to show that they are restored to their original track. The issue of excess phosphate and the secondary hyperparathyroidism has been discussed and needs further study.

The effect of exercise and its interactions with diet are extremely interesting in my view, reminding us that what may seem to be apparent is not necessarily so when one studies it, in particular that with a normal dietary intake of minerals, exercise appears if anything to have an adverse effect on bone. The issue of standing and walking in infants and its effects on bone loading seem to be important, but the cause-and-effect equation and the influence of genetics and muscle mass are still being debated.

The issue of prepuberty has been discussed intensively at this meeting. Mineral supplementation may be effective in improving bone mineral content in prepubertal children, and the type of calcium salts used may be important. Previous discussion focused on a milk-extracted calcium and phosphate supplement, which is somewhat different from what has been used in other studies. In prepuberty, exercise seems to have a bearing on the risk of later osteoporosis and fractures, and this is an exciting goal for study. The genetic interactions with the vitamin D receptor (VDR) and the response to dietary calcium intake are also interesting and deserve future study.

Puberty has been discussed in detail. Delayed puberty especially, and its effects on trunk–limb dimensions and bone mass measurements, are of particular relevance.

Pregnancy has really not been much talked about at this meeting, but as you may know there have been rather large trials of calcium supplementation during pregnancy, particularly in Central and South America, that seem to provide evidence for a reduction in pregnancy-induced hypertension and its associated conditions–low birth weight, etc. Those studies are really impressive, but multicenter trials of calcium supplementation during pregnancy in the United States have recently been reported and show no effect under conditions of higher basal calcium intake.

Lactation was covered very nicely, especially in regard to the natural development of bone, with its significant drop of 4% of bone mass during the lactation period, which is generally restored at weaning. If anything, there might even be an overshoot phenomenon. The finding that women from different parts of the world have quite varying amounts of calcium in their breast milk is something that deserves future study. Whether the amounts are appropriate to that population, what adaptive mechanisms may be present, and any genetic components are obvious questions to be explored. Calcium supplementation during lactation does not seem to confer any particular advantage in terms of either reducing the fall in bone mass or affecting its restoration at weaning.

Other areas that have been covered during this conference are the hormonal relationships with bone mass, other nutrients such as protein and fluoride, and diseases that appear to have an effect on bone mass. These are all new areas of study and are very exciting for the future. We need to be reminded that the common comment that "you need more calcium" is not as simple as that because there are many interactions that we have covered and many caveats that need to be taken into account.

Dr. Bonjour: I would like to thank Nestlé and of course the speakers, who in my view have done a beautiful job. After Dr. Tsang's very full summary I shall confine myself to some brief comments.

We have heard about several elements that can influence bone growth, and it is clear that we have to start to understand the molecular mechanism by which calcium, phosphate, and protein can stimulate bone growth. I think the key issue is the interaction between genetics and the environment, which includes the necessary nutrients and physical activity. Candidate genes for osteoporosis include those controlling hormones, cytokines, receptors, transporters, transduction factors, and transcription factors, and all these genes are regulated by the *Hox* gene, as was beautifully described by Dr. Potter. It is clear that much remains to be done with respect to the relationship between these different factors and bone mass accrual. It is also clear that we can interfere with plant genetics to alter the calcium yield of cereal grains, and this will give firms like Nestlé ideas for developing products for preventing osteoporosis in the future.

Subject Index

R